Handbook of Experimental Pharmacology

Volume 282

The *Handbook of Experimental Pharmacology* is one of the most authoritative and influential book series in pharmacology. It provides critical and comprehensive discussions of the most significant areas of pharmacological research, written by leading international authorities. Each volume in the series represents the most informative and contemporary account of its subject available, making it an unrivalled reference source.

HEP is indexed in PubMed and Scopus.

Stella E. Tsirka • Maricedes Acosta-Martinez
Editors

Sex and Gender Effects in Pharmacology

Springer

Editors
Stella E. Tsirka
Department of Pharmacological Sciences
Renaissance School of Medicine/Stony Brook University
Stony Brook, NY, USA

Maricedes Acosta-Martinez
Department of Physiology and Biophysics
Renaissance School of Medicine/Stony Brook University
Stony Brook, NY, USA

ISSN 0171-2004 ISSN 1865-0325 (electronic)
Handbook of Experimental Pharmacology
ISBN 978-3-031-42647-6 ISBN 978-3-031-42648-3 (eBook)
https://doi.org/10.1007/978-3-031-42648-3

This Springer imprint is published by the registered company Springer Nature Switzerland AG
The registered company address is: Gewerbestrasse 11, 6330 Cham, Switzerland

Paper in this product is recyclable.

Preface

The field of pharmacology has long been dominated by a "one-size-fits-all" approach, with little consideration given to the potential impact of sex and gender on drug efficacy and safety. However, a growing body of evidence suggests that sex and gender can significantly influence pharmacokinetics, pharmacodynamics, and pharmacotherapy. This volume on "*Sex and Gender Effects in Pharmacology*" aims to highlight some of these critical differences and their implications for clinical practice. In the chapters, we proceed from a more basic principles approach to effects of sex and gender on individual organ systems.

The first chapter, "*The impact of sex and gender in medicine and pharmacology*," provides a comprehensive overview of the biological and physiological differences related to sex and gender. It delves into the role of hormones, reproduction, and menopause, and how these factors can influence drug metabolism and response.

In "*Sex differences in pharmacokinetics*," the authors explore how sex can affect the absorption, distribution, metabolism, and excretion of drugs. This chapter underscores the importance of considering sex in drug dosing and administration, as well as in the design of clinical trials.

The chapter on "*Clinical pharmacological considerations in transgender medicine*" is particularly timely, given the unique and increasing recognition of transgender health needs. It discusses how sex and gender transitions can affect drug response over time and the need for personalized pharmacotherapy in transgender individuals.

"*Sex and gender differences in the pharmacology of the overactive urinary bladder*" further elaborates on the need for sex and gender-based analyses in clinical trials. Focusing on pharmacological treatments for overactive urinary bladder, it highlights this is one of the few indications in which women are overrepresented in these trials despite similar prevalence of the condition in both genders.

As we move to specific diseases and pharmacological treatments, the book first delves into CNS pathologies. "*Sex differences in the evaluation and treatment of stroke*" and "*Sex differences in pain and its treatment*" highlight the disparities in disease prevalence, presentation, and response to treatment between sexes. Similarly, "*Therapeutics for substance-using women: The need to elucidate sex-specific targets for better-tailored treatments*" and "*Intersection of sex and depression: Pathogenesis, presentation and treatments*" underscore the need for sex-specific approaches in psychiatry and neurology.

In "*Biological and clinical implications of sex-specific differences in Alzheimer's disease,*" the intriguing link between sex and neuroimmunity is investigated. This chapter provides insights into how sex can influence the pathogenesis and progression of neurodegenerative diseases, like Alzheimer's, and how this knowledge can inform treatment strategies.

The final chapters of the book focus on metabolic diseases, a field where sex and gender differences are particularly pronounced. "*Gender differences in cardiovascular health: Hormonal effects on cardiovascular risk and management,*" "*Sex differences in glucose homeostasis,*" "*Sex-gender-based differences in metabolic diseases,*" and "*Hypothalamic pituitary gonadal axis disorders impacting fertility in both sexes and the potential of kisspeptin-based therapies to treat them*" delve into the role of sex in conditions like diabetes, cardiovascular disease, osteoporosis, and infertility.

The Handbook of Experimental Pharmacology on "*Sex and gender effects in pharmacology*" is a comprehensive exploration of the intersection between sex, gender, and pharmacology. It underscores the need for a more nuanced, personalized approach to pharmacotherapy, one that takes into account the unique biological and physiological characteristics of each individual. Whether a clinician, researcher, or student, the book will provide valuable insights into the role of sex and gender in drug response and the potential implications for clinical practice.

Stony Brook, NY, USA Stella E. Tsirka

Contents

Part I

Pharmacological Basic Principles

The Impact of Sex and Gender in Medicine and Pharmacology

Eva Becher and Sabine Oertelt-Prigione

Contents

Abstract

Sex and gender play a pivotal role in health and disease. Differences can be identified in symptoms, biomarkers, lifetime experiences of diseases, incidence, prevalence, therapeutic options, health-related behavior, and resiliency. However, awareness of sex and gender differences in medicine is still limited. Systematic

E. Becher
Sex- and Gender-Sensitive Medicine Unit, Medical Faculty OWL, Bielefeld University, Bielefeld, Germany

S. Oertelt-Prigione (✉)
Sex- and Gender-Sensitive Medicine Unit, Medical Faculty OWL, Bielefeld University, Bielefeld, Germany

Gender Unit, Departement of Primary and Community Care, Radboud University Medical Center, Nijmegen, The Netherlands
e-mail: sabine.oertelt-prigione@radboudumc.nl

S. E. Tsirka, M. Acosta-Martinez (eds.), *Sex and Gender Effects in Pharmacology*, Handbook of Experimental Pharmacology 282,
https://doi.org/10.1007/164_2023_688

implementation of sex and gender-sensitive research is not yet the norm, resulting in gaps in evidence especially in the diagnosis and treatment of diseases in women. For decades research has predominantly included male persons and animals, leading to a lack of information about symptoms in female individuals or the classification of their symptoms as "atypical". Currently, the inclusion of female participants in clinical marketing access trials is mandatory. However, this does not automatically translate into sex-disaggregated analyses potentially limiting the discovery of sex-specific targeted therapeutic schemes. Consistent consideration of sex and gender in planning, conducting, analyzing, and dissemination of pharmacological research projects is an important prerequisite for closing the gender data gap. Targeted implementation strategies might help to include sex and gender aspects in different parts of the health system and thereby support the improvement of health care for all patients. Health economic aspects could be a further drive for the implementation of sex- and gender-sensitive medicine.

The current chapter focuses on the role of sex and gender in biomedical research and, consequently, their potential role in pharmacology. We will explore the commonly used terminology in the field, the historical development of sex and gender-sensitive medicine (SGSM), the relevance of sex and gender to research and clinical practice and conclude with an outlook on future developments in the field.

Keywords

Sex · Gender · Gender medicine · Sex and gender-sensitive medicine · Pharmacology · Awareness · Implementation · Sex and gender-sensitive research · Gender-data gap · Personalized medicine

The present chapter focuses on the role of sex and gender in biomedical research and their impact on pharmacology. We will explore the commonly used terminology in the field, the historical development of sex and gender-sensitive medicine (SGSM), the relevance of sex and gender to research and clinical practice and conclude with an outlook on future developments in the field.

The role of sex and gender as modulators of health and disease has been widely acknowledged (Mauvais-Jarvis et al. 2020), especially the impact of sex as a biological variable (SABV) on disease development and as modulator of pharmacological interventions. Regardless of this progress, the "sex/gender" terminology is still often used interchangeably (Nieuwenhoven and Klinge 2010) contributing to methodological challenges, such as potential limited reproducibility. In biomedicine, *sex* is defined by biological and physiological characteristics, including chromosomes, sex organs, and endogenous hormonal profiles. These characteristics are often addressed with the acronym "3G," encompassing genes, gonads (hormones), and genitalia to define biological sex (Joel 2012). According to the Canadian Institute of Health Research (CIHR) sex is operationalized as female,

Table 1 Gender dimensions

Gender dimension	Description
Gender identity	Subjective perception of one's gender (e.g., being a woman or a non-binary person). If binary definitions are used (female/male; woman/man), people can be classified as cis or trans-gender. E.g., if one's gender identity matches sex assigned at birth (female/woman or male/man), the person is described as *cis*-gender, if not the person is considered *trans*-gender. Non-binary individuals do not identify as woman or man, agender individuals do not identify with any gender
Gender expression	Describes how an individual manifests their gender identity to the world. This can be through behavior, clothing, hairstyle, etc.
Gender roles and norms	Gender roles and norms encompass the perception of femininity and masculinity in a society at a given time and place and the impact that these perceptions can exert on individuals living within that society. Nonconformity with these norms and roles can lead to potential challenge, exclusion, and rejection by others in a given society
Gender relations	Represent the dynamics of human interaction, the power structures that characterize them and the influence that gender has on the negotiation ability of individuals in the context of a personal or professional relationship
Institutionalized gender	Defines the (oftentimes) informal gendered assumptions and practices that shape laws, institutions, and organizations. Although not explicitly mentioned in these practices and contexts, many structures have been designed with specific gendered ideas and concepts in mind

male, and intersex. It is, however, important to always consider that there is a degree of variation in the biological attributes that define sex in an organism or individual, and in how those attributes are expressed (Government of Canada, What is Gender? What is Sex? 2018). In fact, the karyotype of circulating blood cells might vary over time, with sex chromosome monosomy increasing with age (Guttenbach et al. 1995; Machiela et al. 2016). Hormone levels change during the day, the month, and the course of our lives (Bailey and Silver 2014) and anatomy is not always unequivocal or binary, but characterized by differences and variations in a variable number of individuals in the general population (Fausto-Sterling 2000). State-of-the-art sex-specific analysis will have to take these variations into account and provide specific details about the operationalization of sex to achieve optimal reproducibility and rigor.

Gender is a complex multidimensional construct that encompasses characteristics established in social interactions. The National Institutes of Health (NIH) describe gender as socially constructed and enacted roles and behaviors, which occur in a historical and cultural context and vary across societies and over time (National Institute of Health, Sex and Gender 2018). In current quantitative biomedical research gender is commonly analyzed as one of the following dimensions: gender identity, gender expression, gender roles and norms, gender relations, institutionalized gender (Table 1). Each dimension addresses a different facet of the overall construct of gender and disentanglement of the different influences is essential for application in clinical practice (Oertelt-Prigione 2023). Briefly, gender identity describes the subjective perception of one's gender, e.g. being a woman or a non-binary person. Gender roles and norms address the perception of femininity and masculinity in society at a given time and the impact that these perceptions can exert on the individual. Gender expression denotes how an individual manifests their gender identity to the world. Gender relations denote the dynamics of human interaction, power structures that characterize them and the influence that gender has on the negotiation ability of individuals in a personal or professional relationship. Institutionalized gender represents the oftentimes informal gendered assumptions and practices that shape laws, institutions, and organizations (Heise et al. 2019; Tannenbaum et al. 2016a). Different instruments are available to capture different gender dimensions and analyze their impact on health outcomes (Horstmann et al. 2022; Oertelt-Prigione 2023).

In our practice, we employ the term sex- and gender-sensitive medicine (SGSM), as it reflects the different contributing perspectives. SGSM includes both a focus on biological differences between male and female phenotypes (hormones, gene expression, enzyme activity, X-chromosome-linked genes) and a consideration of gender aspects, such as gendered norms, roles, and relationships (Oertelt-Prigione 2020).

1 Historical Development

Sex- and gender-sensitive medicine has evolved from the women's health movement of the 1960 and 1970 in the USA and Europe. In the USA, in 1969, a group of politically-active college-educated women professionals met at a Women's Liberation Conference at Emmanuel College in Boston. Although not trained healthcare workers themselves, they recognized the striking lack of knowledge about women's bodies and health and started the Women's Health Book Collective. "Women and their Bodies – a Course," a comprehensive description of relevant women's health issues, such as sexuality and abortion, emerged as the product of their labor. Over time the initiative has been renamed "Our Bodies Ourselves," but is still active as a collaboration with the Center for Women's Health and Human Rights at Suffolk University and features trustworthy, up-to-date, curated information on the health and sexuality of women, girls, and gender-expansive people (https://www.ourbodiesourselves.org,). This collaboration was one of the first events spearheading a broad societal discussion about women's health.

In the following decades institutionalization progressed. The National Institutes of Health (NIH) played a major role in fostering equal opportunities in science and promoting knowledge and research on women's health. In 1990, the Women's Health Equity Act was passed by the U.S. Congress. Subsequently, the NIH established the Office of Research on Women's Health (ORWH), the first national agency focusing on women's health issues. Since the 1990s the IOM (Institute of Medicine) recommended the inclusion of women in Clinical Trials, after a lengthy period of exclusion (Wizemann and Pardue 2001). The NIH Health Revitalization Act 1993 acknowledged sex differences in the physiology of male and female individuals at the molecular level and acknowledged that sex differences were not limited to gynecology. In Canada, Health Canada started requesting the inclusion of women in clinical trials in 1997 and in 2002 the Sixth Research Framework Program (FP6) of the European Commission addressed the topic of gender for the first time in the European research area. Furthermore, in 2004 the International Conference on Harmonization of Technical Requirements for Registration of Pharmaceuticals for Human Use (ICH) published the first regulation calling for the inclusion of women and men in clinical trials. ICH, however, argued against the need for a separate ICH guideline on women as special population in clinical trials (Singh 2015). A number of ICH Guidelines, in particular M4E (CTD- efficacy) and E3 (structure and content of clinical study reports), call for a demographic characterization of the patient population, which should include demographic variables such as age and sex (ICH 2009). The ICH guideline E8 (R1) on "General considerations for clinical trials" published in 2022, mentions sex and gender aspects exclusively in the context of pregnancy and breast feeding. Women are listed as "special populations" along with geriatric patients and children. Subpopulations with potentially different metabolism are mentioned in the context of pharmacokinetics. Special attention should be paid for patients with renal or hepatic impairment, geriatric patients, children, and ethnic subgroups. Consideration of possible differences in the pharmacokinetics between the sexes is not explicitly mentioned (ICH 2022).

These structural developments have fostered awareness and change, but a systematic implementation of sex and gender-sensitive research is not yet the norm. The systemic blocks and the needed change were summarized in a series of articles in the scientific journal *Nature* in 2010 (Baylis 2010; Kim et al. 2010; Zucker and Beery 2010). The editorial "Putting Gender on the agenda," argues for the implementation of sex- and gender-sensitive research because "medicine, as it is currently applied to women, is less evidence-based than that being applied to men" ("Putting gender on the agenda," 2010). This statement was followed by three more articles describing sex and gender inequalities in biomedical research as a persistent problem. The authors appealed to journals, funding agencies, and researchers to give women parity with men in studies and the clinic (Kim et al. 2010). It was pointed out that pregnant women are routinely excluded from clinical trials, which is unethical and unscientific and regulators were urged to mandate change (Baylis 2010). Last, female animals are lacking in the vast majority of studies in animals and more stringent measures are needed to correct this imbalance (Zucker and Beery 2010).

In the following sections we will report on the growing body of evidence supporting sex- and gender-sensitive analysis and highlight why this approach should become standard practice.

2 Basic Research

Basic research primarily serves to gain knowledge and develop theories. In the medical field, this motivation is furthered by the prospect of the development of novel therapeutic and preventive options. Cell cultures or model organisms, e.g. mice, rats, or flies, are often used to elucidate pathomechanisms of human diseases. However, different animal models are differentially suited for the study of certain organ systems and diseases. Pragmatic reasons often play a decisive role in the choice of model, such as breeding speed, costs, size, etc. No matter which animals or cells are used, the results of these studies cannot be directly transferred to humans. They can, however, support the development of hypotheses, clinically applicable therapies and support initial testing of compounds. Age and sex are important factors impacting disease development, pharmacokinetics and pharmacodynamics, as described in the field of cardiovascular disease (Oertelt-Prigione and Regitz-Zagrosek 2009). Contributing factors such as the hormonal regulation of gene expression, the role of genes on the X chromosome, or sex differences in biomarkers should be taken into account throughout the research process (Regitz-Zagrosek 2006). In the following sections, we will provide more detail to substantiate the need for a thorough consideration of sex and gender in the research process.

2.1 Immune Response

Many pathological conditions are caused or exacerbated by a dysregulation of the immune response, which makes the immune system an ideal target for pharmacological interventions, such as immunosuppressive drugs, immunomodulators, or preventative agents such as vaccines. Oftentimes, however, therapeutic approaches do not take potential sex differences in pharmacokinetics and pharmacodynamics into account (Farkouh et al. 2020). The immune response and the intensity of inflammatory processes differ clearly between male and female bodies (Klein and Flanagan 2016), impacting disease progression, severity, incidence, and therapy (Sirufo et al. 2022). The identified differences can be found at the genetic, hormonal, and environmental level.

At the genetic level, the differential expression of sex chromosome-linked genes is one possible mechanism for the mediation of sex differences. Several genes with immune functions are located on the X chromosome such as Toll-like receptors 7 and 8, cytokine receptors IL2RG and IL13 RA2, and transcriptional factors like FOXP3 (fish). Toll-like receptors are a family of key regulators of the innate and the adaptive immune system, which have a proven role in various human diseases (Cook et al. 2004). Cytokines are important key mediators of the immune response. FOXP3 (a transcription factor of the forkhead family) is critically important for the development and function of regulatory T-cells (Ziegler 2006).

Historically, the inactivation of the X chromosome affecting one of the two copies of the X chromosome was assumed to balance the levels of male and female X-related gene expression (Lyon 1961). However, in the last decades we learned that some regions on the X chromosome can escape inactivation, leading to a proportionally elevated expression of these genes in female animals and humans compared to males (Carrel and Willard 2005). Furthermore, the fact that females generally carry two X chromosomes, harboring two potentially different allelic options, entails a potentially broader range of physiological response options compared to males, who usually only carry one X chromosome (Libert et al. 2010).

Sex differences are influenced not only by sex chromosomes but also by gonadal hormone effects (Arnold 2020). Steroid hormones like estrogen, progesterone, and androgens contribute to the differential regulation of immune responses between the sexes (Bhatia et al. 2014). For example, the activity of Toll-like receptors, which play an important role as mediators of innate immunity, fluctuates throughout the menstrual cycle demonstrating the effect of hormonal variations (Dennison et al. 2012). Receptors for estrogen (17ß-estradiol), ER-α and ER-β, are expressed in various lymphoid tissue cells, lymphocytes, macrophages, and dendritic cells and exhibit differential expression patterns among immune cell subsets. ERs are also able to show non-classical ER signaling via protein–protein interaction with transcription factors like NF-κB, SP1, and AP1 in immune cells (Kovats 2015). Specifically, inflammatory stimuli suppress ER-α expression via the activation and subsequent binding of NF-κB to the ERα promoter, and 17β-estradiol/ER- may antagonize the inhibitory effect of NF-κB (Mahmoodzadeh et al. 2009), further suggesting an interplay between estrogen/estrogen receptors and the immune response. Sex differences in immune response change throughout life and are influenced by age and reproductive status of an individual. However, regardless of age, females tend to show greater antibody response than males, higher basal immunoglobulin levels, and higher B cell numbers (Abdullah et al. 2012; Furman et al. 2014; Teixeira et al. 2011).

Environmental factors, including nutrition status and the composition of the microbiome, also alter the development and functioning of the immune system differently in male and female organisms (Klein and Flanagan 2016). Sex differences can be found in autoimmune diseases, inflammatory disorders, and allergies (Spoletini et al. 2012), yet the role of the gut microbiome as a contributor and modulator of systemic chronic inflammation is still under investigation. Recent studies indicate that the gut microbiota is shaping sex differences in immunity by influencing the hormonal milieu that governs differences between the sexes. A bi-directional cross-talk between microbiota and the endocrine system is emerging with bacteria being able to produce hormones (e.g., serotonin, dopamine, and somatostatin), respond to host hormones (e.g., estrogens), and regulate host hormones' homeostasis (e.g., by inhibiting gene prolactin transcription or converting glucocorticoids to androgens) (Rizzetto et al. 2018). Therefore, it is of utmost importance to research this innovative and future-oriented field of immunological research, which could lead to promising new therapeutically approaches, in a sex- and gender-sensitive way.

2.2 Animals and Cells

The first steps to disentangle the pathophysiology of diseases are studies in cell cultures and experimental animals. These models are essential for our understanding of the pathogenesis of disease and to identify possible therapeutic target molecules. However, cells and animals also have a biological sex, which can impact experimental results, and which is often overlooked as highlighted by a study in 2010 in

10 biological fields. Male bias was present overall and most prominent in neuroscience and studies of both sexes frequently failed to disaggregate results by sex (Beery and Zucker 2011).

One reason for hesitation to include female animals in preclinical research has been the expected higher variability of the results due to the female estrus cycle. However, a meta-analysis of 293 articles could demonstrate that the variability was not significantly greater in females compared to males for different behavioral, morphological, physiological, and molecular neurological endpoints (Prendergast et al. 2014). The assumption that non-human female mammals are intrinsically more variable than males, and too troublesome for routine inclusion in research protocols, is considered to be without foundation (Beery and Zucker 2011). Most likely, the lack of cycle-related differences in experimental animals compared to humans can be attributed to the different duration of the various cycle phases. While the average estrus cycle in humans lasts 28 days, exposing cells to several days of elevated hormone concentration that can impact transcriptional profiles, the average cycle in rodents is 4 days, which probably does not suffice to trigger transcriptional changes in the different phases.

Cells and cell cultures, which serve as a model for many physiological processes, have a sex. Mammalian cells, which are diploid in their chromosome set, harbor either an XX or XY chromosome set, or variations thereof. Sex differences in gene expression proliferation and/or behavior have been reported for primary cell cultures, organoids, embryonic and induced pluripotent stem cells (Miguel-Aliaga 2022). Gonadal hormones and sex chromosomes both play a role in sex-specific cell differentiation. The role of sex chromosome effects compared to hormonal effects, i.e. which one is more prominent in driving potential sex-related differences, is still debated. Traditional methods, which have uncovered the largest sex differences in the context of reproductive cells and areas of the brain controlling reproduction, might have overestimated the role of gonadal hormones relative to sex chromosomes (Arnold 2020).

In 2015, the National Institutes of Health (NIH) released a policy on sex as a biological variable (SABV) to address the overreliance on men and male animals in biomedical research and the lack of attention to sex-based responses to medical treatments (NIH Policy on Sex as a Biological Variable 2015). An analysis in the year 2020 described that over the past decade the proportion of biological studies that included both females and males increased, but the proportion in which sex was treated as a variable has not (Woitowich et al. 2020). In fact, the analysis of 151 articles in biological science that included both males and females and reported data by sex (Woitowich et al. 2020) revealed misreporting and misinterpretation of sex differences. The frequency of reporting of sex differences depended on the medical discipline: sexes were most commonly compared in the field of Endocrinology (93%) and least often in the field of Neuroscience (33%). Interestingly, when sex differences were identified, the majority of the analyzed articles defined them as a major finding, and half of them even mentioned the identified sex difference in the title. However, not all of these differences were supported by statistical evidence. Some articles claimed sex differences without having conducted the appropriate statistical analysis, other articles claimed the absence of sex differences without having tested for them. Results from male and female samples were pooled very often, at least for some of the analysis. As described before, the term "gender" was used for non-human animals, sometimes exclusively, sometimes in combination with the term "sex" (Garcia-Sifuentes and Maney 2021).

Overall, these findings highlight how the inclusion of male and female samples and/or participants into studies does not necessarily lead to sex- and gender-sensitive research. Inclusion is the first step, but sex-disaggregated reporting and proper statistical analysis need to follow to guarantee rigorous and reproducible results.

3 Clinical Trials

Currently, it is becoming a standard practice to include female and male subjects into clinical trials, yet this does not always occur in appropriate numbers and has not always been the case. In 1977, the FDA ruled that female participants of childbearing potential should be excluded from clinical trials in the aftermath of the thalidomide tragedy in the 1960 and 1970 (Mercurio et al. 2017). The exclusion of female participants led to a substantial lack of evidence about efficacy and safety of newly developed pharmaceutical products for this group. Given the absence of information during clinical trials, pharmacovigilance became the first source of sex-specific information about unwanted pharmacological side effects. Ten drugs had to be removed from the US market between 1997 and 2000, of which 80% bore a greater health risk in female users (Caplan and Friesen 2017). Revision of the guidance to exclude women from clinical trials followed in 1993 with the Revitalization Act, which for the first time mandated the inclusion of women and minorities in research funded by the NIH. Inclusion of racial and ethnic minorities remains another important aspect to consider for future clinical trials. In fact, 20 years after the Revitalization Act, the proportion of minority ethnic patients enrolled in cancer clinical trials remained persistently low (Chen et al. 2014). In 2016, the Twenty-First Century Cures Act mandated the NIH to make information regarding the study population of NIH-funded clinical research publicly available, to update guidelines on the inclusion of women and minorities in clinical research, and to develop guidelines on reporting analysis by sex/gender, race, and ethnicity in Phase III clinical trials (Twenty-First Century Cures Act, pub L No. 114–255, 130 stat 1065–1068 (2016). 2016. Available at: https://www.congress.gov/114/plaws/publ255/PLAW-114publ255.pdf)).

In 2022 a study analyzing 1,442 manuscripts published in the years 2015 to 2019 in three highly reputable international journals [Journal of the American Medical Association (JAMA), The Lancet, and The New England Journal of Medicine] found that significantly more male than female participants were included in clinical trials (56% vs. 44%, $p < 0.0001$). The authors concluded that, despite recognizing the importance of sex inclusiveness in clinical research and the recommendations and requirements that have been enacted, sex bias remains prevalent in biomedical research (Barlek et al. 2022). A recent study evaluating FDA's publicly available drug registration dossiers of commonly prescribed drugs, however, rejected any systematic underrepresentation of women in clinical trials and suggested that some form of sex-specific analysis has been performed in most cases. Nevertheless, the authors found that sub-analysis of sex is not fully reported in the publicly available data, with the majority (79%) of reports lacking either sex-disaggregated safety or efficacy analysis. In the selected sample of 38 drugs, the majority of them were equally effective in males and females. However, a higher proportion of side effects was identified in females compared to males, but these differences were relatively small and appeared to be of limited clinical relevance. The authors emphasize that many other factors, including weight, age, genotype, phenotype, ethnicity, hormonal status, fasting conditions, polymorphisms of metabolizing enzymes, receptor expression and sensitivity, co-medication interactions, co-morbidities, pregnancy status, and gut microbiome status cause variability in drug response for efficacy and/or safety in a target population (Labots et al. 2018).

A recent study of marketing authorization application dossiers (MAAs), submitted to the European Medicines Agency (EMA), demonstrated that female participants were included in all phases of drug development, but their number in the phase III clinical trials was not always similar to disease prevalence rates in the general population. Female participants were underrepresented in pharmacokinetic studies and in phase III trials, and the representation of female participants in clinical studies differed across investigated diseases (hepatitis C, HIV, schizophrenia, heart failure and hypercholesterolemia). In studies on depression, epilepsy, thrombosis, and diabetes no underrepresentation was identified (Dekker et al. 2021). A previous exploratory study about the underrepresentation of women in trials of cardiovascular drugs suggested that inclusion and exclusion criteria might have had only a minor effect and that the underrepresentation may have already occurred before screening (Scott et al. 2018). In another study, female and male participants appeared equally willing to participate in clinical trials and attitudes toward trials were generally more favorable among women than among men (Gruca et al. 2018). Interestingly, this study described more women with adverse events not only in treatment group, but also in some of the placebo groups (Dekker et al. 2021) suggesting potential sex differences in nocebo effects as previously reported (Vambheim and Flaten 2017).

A 2016 study published in the Cochrane Database of Systematic Reviews evaluated the frequency, validity, and relevance of statistically significant ($p < 0.05$) sex-treatment interactions in randomized controlled trials. The study demonstrated that statistically significant sex–treatment interactions are only slightly more frequent than expected by chance and that there is little evidence of subsequent corroboration or clinical relevance of sex-treatment interactions. Furthermore, the review concluded that meta-analyses rarely corroborate sex-based subgroup findings from individual randomized trials and that they are rarely included in clinical guidelines or recommendations. The authors recommend to carefully scrutinize the credibility of subgroup analysis and rank isolated sex-based subgroup analyses as simply hypothesis generating (Wallach et al. 2016). Unfortunately, the authors did not point out a fundamental issue of their study sample. In fact, only 41 out of 1,141 eligible articles actually provided sufficient data for the subsequent analysis, leading to a substantially biased sample which highlights the gross lack of sex-disaggregated data for analysis (Tannenbaum et al. 2016b).

Notwithstanding its limitations, the Wallach review (Wallach et al. 2016) does, however, highlight another major issue in the analysis of clinical trial data. Data on sex differences are often obtained by post hoc analysis, which might not allow for sufficiently powered analyses. A better understanding of the basic mechanisms of sex differences needs large-scale prospective studies with a primary focus on this topic (Soldin et al. 2011). Although sex and gender differences are increasingly emerging in every area of medicine, specific sex-targeted studies are still too infrequent (Oi Yan Chan et al. 2022; Sirufo et al. 2022). The potential influence of sex on the exposure-response relationship has not been fully explored for many drugs used in clinical practice, though population-based pharmacokinetic/pharmacodynamic modeling is well-suited to explore this effect (Oi Yan Chan et al. 2022).

Despite increased enrolment of female participants in recent clinical studies, knowledge gaps about sex differences in pharmacokinetics and pharmacodynamics for many compounds remain, particularly for anticancer drugs. Female participants very often exhibit higher exposure than males (characterized by higher AUC, Cmax, and lower CL). Higher exposure in females often translated to sex-related differences in pharmacodynamics, efficacy, or adverse drug reactions (Oi Yan Chan et al. 2022). These aspects will be discussed in further detail in the following section.

4 Pharmacology

Sex differences in pharmacology can be mediated by sex-specific and sex-hormone-related regulation of gene expression. Body composition, drug-metabolizing enzyme activity, and kidney function are relevant factors for sex-related differences in pharmacology. Pharmacodynamics and pharmacokinetics play a key role in drug efficacy and safety profiles. Sex and gender can influence several aspects of both. Sex-related differences have been reported for pharmacokinetics and pharmacodynamics, revealing differences in therapeutic efficacy and side effects (Spoletini et al. 2012).

Certain pharmacological side effects are reported more often in women compared to men. Sex-biased *pharmacokinetics* can predict adverse drug reactions (ADRs) in female users for certain drugs. A systematic analysis searching the ISI Web of Science and PubMed for sex- or gender-related differences in pharmacokinetics, pharmacodynamics, and adverse drug reactions identified 86 drugs where ADRs were described for males and females together with the pharmacokinetic values (PK). Seventy-six displayed higher pharmacokinetic values in female users. For 59 drugs with clinically identifiable ADRs, sex-biased PKs predicted the direction of sex-biased ADRs in 88% of cases (Zucker and Prendergast 2020). Several metabolic steps in the processing of pharmaceuticals can display sex-related differences, as illustrated by the examples below.

Absorption: Females have slower gastrointestinal transit time and lower gastric acidity than males (Freire et al. 2011). Two frequent examples for these differences are ethanol and salicylate formulations (i.e., aspirin). Ethanol bioavailability is higher in females than males. Gastric enzyme activity (e.g., alcohol dehydrogenase), which is generally lower in females, contributes to these findings (Anderson 2005). Age diminishes the strength of this association (Freire et al. 2011).

Distribution: Females typically have a higher percentage of total body fat than males, increasing the volume of distribution of lipophilic drugs (e.g., benzodiazepines) (Hanley et al. 2010). Conversely, lean body mass is on average higher in males, increasing the volume of distribution of hydrophilic medications like the beta-adrenergic blocking agents atenolol or sotalol (Schwartz 2003).

Metabolism: There are remarkable differences between the sexes regarding activity of drug metabolism, both in drug modification and conjugation. Sex hormones or sex hormone regulators affect the pharmacokinetics of drugs via the regulation of different members of the cytochrome P450 family (Zou et al. 2022). Conjugating enzymes, e.g. enzymes of the Phase II drug metabolism, display a sex-dependent activity (Farkouh et al. 2020).

Clearance: Data support sex-related differences in the three renal processes of glomerular filtration, tubular secretion, and tubular reabsorption (Schwartz 2003). The measured glomerular filtration rate (GFR), an index of overall kidney function, is slightly lower in females after adjusting for body surface area compared to males (10%) (Meibohm et al. 2002).

Sex-related differences in *pharmacodynamics* are well described for frequently prescribed drugs, such as analgesics, tranquillizers, statins, or beta-blockers. Some drugs are more effective in males than females (e.g., ibuprofen) or vice versa (e.g., opioids, benzodiazepine) due to pharmacodynamic processes (Farkouh et al. 2020). Furthermore, drug transporter expression or levels of sex hormones can all contribute to different responses to medications (Oi Yan Chan et al. 2022).

4.1 Sex Differences

The impact of the gut microbiota on drug metabolism has been extensively described. Microbiota can exert its influence via different mechanisms: drugs can be directly activated or inactivated, the availability and uptake of drugs might be influenced by the microbiota or by co-administration of probiotics, toxicity of drugs can be influenced by microbial β-glucuronidase activity and can be selectively inhibited by antibiotics or specific microbial β-glucuronidase inhibitors (Enright et al. 2016). Sex-specific differences in the gastrointestinal microbiota in humans have been described and might contribute to sex differences in digestion, absorption, distribution, and elimination (Mauvais-Jarvis et al. 2021). It is important to remember that the interaction between microbiota and the host is a two-way process. For example, microbiota can metabolize estrogen-like compounds, which in turn may induce proliferation and growth of certain types of bacteria (Campesi et al. 2018). The microbiome of postmenopausal women is more similar to that of men in comparison to that of premenopausal women demonstrating a potential impact of circulating estrogen levels. This does not only apply to endogenous, but likely also to exogenous sex steroids. In fact, oral contraceptives appear to alter both microbial species abundance and functional pathways. The microbiota itself might act as an important regulator of circulating estrogens and estrogenic molecules (Kim et al. 2020).

4.2 Gender Differences

Although biological differences play an important role in the efficacy and safety of pharmacological therapies, gender accounts for the choice and administration of therapy, and, thus influences the potential incidence of side effects. Gender can also play a role in health-related behavior like caloric intake, choice of food, alcohol consumption and consumption of other drugs, and smoking. Thereby, gender indirectly influences these habits and the efficacy and safety of pharmacological drugs (Oertelt-Prigione and Regitz-Zagrosek 2009).

An example of the consequences of gender-related bias in pharmacotherapy can be found analyzing statin therapies in the USA. Women have historically received less aggressive lipid management than men. In a nationwide registry study (the PALM registry about cholesterol management) the access to statin therapy, the compliance of statin dosing regimens with guidelines and potential reasons for undertreatment were analyzed. Even after adjusting for sociodemographic characteristics such as age, insurance status, education, numeracy, and income, women remained significantly less likely to access statin treatment and obtain it according to ACC/AHA guideline-recommendations if they had access to it. Contrary to the expectations, the study identified important sources of bias in the participants beliefs and perceptions surrounding statins and cardiovascular disease. Women were less likely to believe that high cholesterol levels correlated with a higher risk of having a heart attack. Furthermore, they were less likely to believe that statins were safe and were more likely to report believing that statins can cause diabetes, muscle symptoms, and liver damage. As a result, women were more frequently declining and discontinuing treatment although they would have qualified for it and were offered access to it (Nanna et al. 2019). Overall, a combination of gendered stereotypes, misinformation, and systemic barriers prevented these patients from obtaining the best care.

5 Epidemiology, Health Care Research, and Prevention Research

The consideration of sex and gender as causal factors or modulators in the exposure-outcome relation should be integrated in state-of-the-art experimental design. Lack of sex- and gender-sensitive analyses can inhibit the detection of meaningful and reproducible effects (Miguel-Aliaga 2022). Several points need to be considered during research design to achieve appropriate integration of these aspects, yet they are still frequently disregarded.

One problematic approach is the pooling of data from both sexes, which can lead to wrong conclusions due to masking. Pooling data not only assumes that there are no differences between the sexes; it takes for granted that the statistical distributions of the outcome values before treatment are similar in male and female participants ignoring potential differences in the baseline values, e.g. a higher baseline in females and a lower baseline in males. If data is not disaggregated, both baseline differences and differences in outcomes will be overlooked (Tannenbaum et al. 2019).

Another important aspect is subgroup analysis. Many analytical claims based on subgroup analysis from randomized clinical trials or meta-analysis are questionable (Wallach et al. 2016). Oftentimes it is not evident whether the subgroup characteristic was measured at baseline or after randomization, if the suggested effect was a comparison between or within studies. A number of criteria should be considered in design, analysis, and context. For example, subgroups should be defined on baseline characteristics, independence of the subgroup effect, a priori specification of the direction of the subgroup effect. Furthermore, consistency across related outcomes is needed to differentiate between spurious and real subgroup effects (Sun et al. 2010).

The analysis of gender in quantitative health studies is a specific challenge. A recent scoping review based on systematic literature analysis had identified 72 instruments, which were designed to measure dimensions of sex and/or gender. The instruments defined gender through external assignment, self-assignment, and agreement with statements/stereotypes about gender. Most of the instruments operationalize sex and/or gender in a binary way and only a very limited number of instruments considered societal context (Horstmann et al. 2022).

Gender may lead to differences in health outcomes due to differences in health-related exposures, in health behaviors and in access to health care (Heise et al. 2019). These aspects arise from differences in gender roles, gender identities, and gender relations. The socially ascribed gender roles and responsibilities cause different exposures to health risks and hazards. Women are more likely to care for family members, especially ones with chronic medical condition and often experience negative effects on their own health. They tend to have higher level of stress and mental health issues and are more likely to experience symptoms of depression (Heise et al. 2019). The links between a broad range of masculine behaviors and negative health outcomes have been established across settings and age groups, in areas such as help-seeking behavior for medical care, reckless driving, substance use, aggression, and poor body image (Ragonese and Barker 2019). In low-income settings, men, mothers-in-law, or older family members take decisions for younger women's access to health care. When women lack financial autonomy, they are dependent on men to meet their transport and treatment costs (Heise et al. 2019). But, also in high-income countries, women are more likely to work in lower paid jobs and therefore might be under- or uninsured.

Evident gender differences have been reported in preventive behavior. Although men have more socioeconomic resources on average, they die earlier nonetheless (Austad and Fischer 2016). This might partially be explained by differences in willingness to participate in preventive health programs. A population-based assessment of masculinity beliefs showed that men with strong masculinity beliefs are less likely than men with more moderate masculinity beliefs to receive preventive care. Preemptive use of health care can be related to perceived concern about one's health, whereas treating an acute problem can be rationalized as a stereotypically masculine framework of "fixing a problem" (Springer and Mouzon 2011). As masculinity ideals are always part of a specific cultural and timely context, this cannot be generalized (Gottgens and Oertelt-Prigione 2023). One could, however, speculate that refuting an ideal of hegemonic masculinity might have a positive effect on the demand of preventive care offers.

6 Sex and Gender and Personalized Medicine

Human beings differ in their biology and due to the different social and physical environments they are exposed to. Both are sources of variability between the individuals and both are intertwined and confounded with each other (Arnold 2020). The consideration of sex and gender as modulators of health and disease represents the first step toward individualized or precision medicine. The FDA defines precision medicine as treatments that are tailored to specific characteristics of individuals, such as a person's genetic makeup, or the genetic profile of an individual's tumor (FDA 2022) mostly ignoring social and cultural influences. Next generation sequencing identifies or sequences large sections of a person's genome and can contribute to advances in the clinical applications of precision medicine; yet, interpersonal differences related to their social gender and other environmental factors are not part of the analysis. Many models in the context of precision medicine operationalize precision along the P1-P4 model, where the Ps stand for prediction, prevention, personalization, and participation (Hood and Friend 2011). We recently proposed an expansion of the P4 model to include gender-related and community-based factors with the intent to offer a more holistic approach to precision medicine. The proposed $P3^2$ model incorporates the dimensions of P4-P6 (participatory, psychosocial, and percipient) and P7-P9 (population-informed, partnered with community and public-engaging) (Sapir-Pichhadze and Oertelt-Prigione 2023) proposing a more holistic model of personalized medicine.

7 Implementation of Sex and Gender Sensitive Medicine

The implementation of sex- and gender-sensitive approaches in pharmacology will need a concerted multi-stakeholder effort (Fig. 1). Generation of knowledge about sex- and gender specific differences in health, disease, and pharmacological therapeutic options is necessary, but not sufficient. Translation needs knowledge, awareness, and action. Many stakeholders will need to be included in the process. Patients could play a crucial role in the implementation process, if they are informed about the potential implications of sex and gender on diagnostics and treatment options and

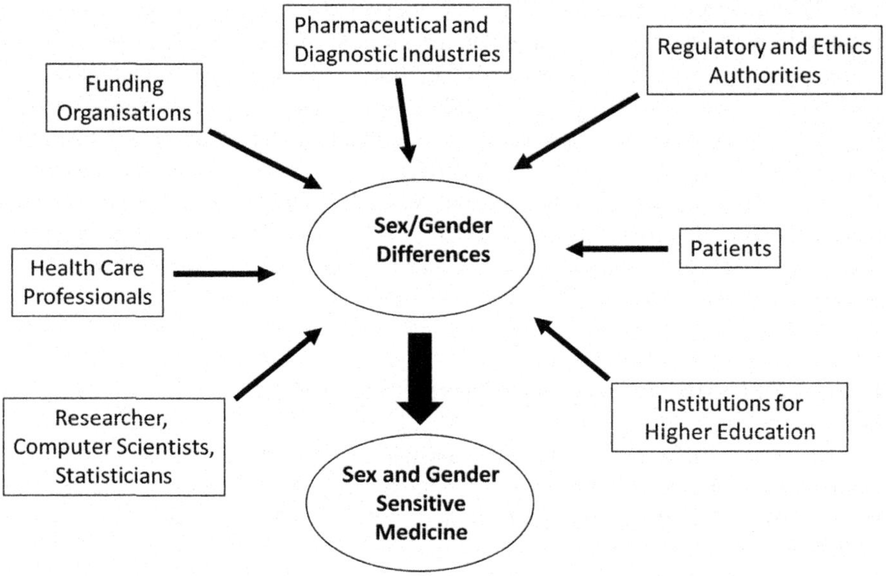

Fig. 1 Important players for successful implementation of sex/gender-sensitive medicine in education, research and health care. Awareness for sex and gender differences and active consideration is necessary in different fields simultaneously. Political and cultural frameworks can strongly support the structural incorporation of sex and gender aspects

if they feel empowered to ask their doctors for a shared decision-making process. Doctors and all medical professionals, including pharmacists, must be educated during their training and post-gradually. To reach that goal, teachers at universities and higher education institutions must be aware and educated themselves. Furthermore, the medical and pharmacological curricula and examinations need to incude sex- and gender-specific content. Awareness is also needed in funding organizations, which can have an impact by defining their priorities and funding conditions. Public sponsors can contribute to raising awareness for sex- and gender-sensitive biomedical research by designing specific funding measures. The quality of medical care depends on robust scientific evidence as foundation for the development of health care interventions. Evidence-based care is unattainable without the consideration of possible sex- and gender-related effects. Importantly, not every therapeutic intervention will have to differ based on sex. However, a lack of differences can only be ascertained after investigation.

Progress has been made in sex- and gender-sensitive requirements by regulatory and ethics authorities. Compliance with these is necessary to change research and development in pharmaceutical and diagnostic industries. Pharmaceutical and diagnostic industries are still reluctant to acknowledge the need to investigate and develop sex-specific drug interventions or dosing schemes. However, sex-specific investigation could increase safety and efficacy for a large proportion of the population. Higher treatment efficacy and reduction of adverse drug reactions would also contribute to the economic success of the proposed pharmaceutical for the company and an overall decrease of societal and health care costs due to the avoidance of trickle-down costs of ADRs. Overall, the implementation of sex and gender in the field of health needs to focus on raising awareness, defining intervention targets and priority issues, producing and integrating high-quality data, and developing of translational implementation strategies and political support (Oertelt-Prigione et al. 2017).

8 Conclusion

Sex and Gender are important modulators of health and diseases. Pharmacological therapies are the result of long and costly research processes. After the investigation of amendable pathways and processes in basic research, pharmacological compounds are selected and tested in clinical trials. Marketing and pharmacovigilance will then follow to confirm the success of the therapy in a real-world setting. Lack of attention to possible sex and gender differences during the whole process of research and development may lead to the development of therapeutic options that are not fitting for all patients.

The exclusion of women from clinical trials in the past century still leads to knowledge gaps for a number of widely-used medications approved in those years. Currently, the inclusion of women in clinical marketing access trials is mandatory. However, sex-disaggregated data analysis, systematic publication of these analysis, and proposal of targeted therapeutic schemes (if applicable) are still not standard practice. Consistent consideration of sex and gender in planning, conducting, analyzing, and dissemination of pharmacological research projects is an important prerequisite for closing the sex and gender-data gap and provision of the best possible care for all patients.

References

Abdullah M, Chai PS, Chong MY, Tohit ER, Ramasamy R, Pei CP, Vidyadaran S (2012) Gender effect on in vitro lymphocyte subset levels of healthy individuals. Cell Immunol 272(2): 214–219. https://doi.org/10.1016/j.cellimm.2011.10.009

Anderson GD (2005) Sex and racial differences in pharmacological response: where is the evidence? Pharmacogenetics, pharmacokinetics, and pharmacodynamics. J Womens Health (Larchmt) 14(1):19–29. https://doi.org/10.1089/jwh.2005.14.19

Arnold AP (2020) Sexual differentiation of brain and other tissues: five questions for the next 50 years. Horm Behav 120:104691. https://doi.org/10.1016/j.yhbeh.2020.104691

Austad SN, Fischer KE (2016) Sex differences in lifespan. Cell Metab 23(6):1022–1033. https://doi.org/10.1016/j.cmet.2016.05.019

Bailey M, Silver R (2014) Sex differences in circadian timing systems: implications for disease. Front Neuroendocrinol 35(1):111–139. https://doi.org/10.1016/j.yfrne.2013.11.003

Barlek MH, Rouan JR, Wyatt TG, Helenowski I, Kibbe MR (2022) The persistence of sex bias in high-impact clinical research. J Surg Res 278:364–374. https://doi.org/10.1016/j.jss.2022.04.077

Baylis F (2010) Pregnant women deserve better. Nature 465(7299):689–690. https://doi.org/10.1038/465689a

Beery AK, Zucker I (2011) Sex bias in neuroscience and biomedical research. Neurosci Biobehav Rev 35(3):565–572. https://doi.org/10.1016/j.neubiorev.2010.07.002

Bhatia A, Sekhon HK, Kaur G (2014) Sex hormones and immune dimorphism. ScientificWorldJournal 2014:159150. https://doi.org/10.1155/2014/159150

Campesi I, Marino M, Cipolletti M, Romani A, Franconi F (2018) Put "gender glasses" on the effects of phenolic compounds on cardiovascular function and diseases. Eur J Nutr 57(8): 2677–2691. https://doi.org/10.1007/s00394-018-1695-0

Caplan A, Friesen P (2017) Health disparities and clinical trial recruitment: is there a duty to tweet? PLoS Biol 15(3):e2002040. https://doi.org/10.1371/journal.pbio.2002040

Carrel L, Willard HF (2005) X-inactivation profile reveals extensive variability in X-linked gene expression in females. Nature 434(7031):400–404. https://doi.org/10.1038/nature03479

Chen MS Jr, Lara PN, Dang JH, Paterniti DA, Kelly K (2014) Twenty years post-NIH Revitalization Act: enhancing minority participation in clinical trials (EMPaCT): laying the groundwork for improving minority clinical trial accrual: renewing the case for enhancing minority participation in cancer clinical trials. Cancer 120(Suppl 7):1091–1096. https://doi.org/10.1002/cncr.28575

Cook DN, Pisetsky DS, Schwartz DA (2004) Toll-like receptors in the pathogenesis of human disease. Nat Immunol 5(10):975–979. https://doi.org/10.1038/ni1116

Dekker M, de Vries ST, Versantvoort CHM, Drost-van Velze EGE, Bhatt M, van Meer PJK, Havinga IK, Gispen-de Wied CC, Mol PGM (2021) Sex proportionality in pre-clinical and clinical trials: an evaluation of 22 marketing authorization application dossiers submitted to the European Medicines Agency. Front Med (Lausanne) 8:643028. https://doi.org/10.3389/fmed.2021.643028

Dennison U, McKernan DP, Scully P, Clarke G, Cryan J, Dinan T (2012) Menstrual cycle influences toll-like receptor responses. Neuroimmunomodulation 19(3):171–179. https://doi.org/10.1159/000331424

Enright EF, Gahan CG, Joyce SA, Griffin BT (2016) The impact of the gut microbiota on drug metabolism and clinical outcome. Yale J Biol Med 89(3):375–382. https://www.ncbi.nlm.nih.gov/pubmed/27698621

Farkouh A, Riedl T, Gottardi R, Czejka M, Kautzky-Willer A (2020) Sex-related differences in pharmacokinetics and pharmacodynamics of frequently prescribed drugs: a review of the literature. Adv Ther 37(2):644–655. https://doi.org/10.1007/s12325-019-01201-3

Fausto-Sterling A (2000) The five sexes, revisited. Sciences 40(4):18–23. https://doi.org/10.1002/j.2326-1951.2000.tb03504.x

FDA (2022) Personalized medicine at FDA: the scope & significance of progress in 2022. https://www.personalizedmedicinecoalition.org/Userfiles/PMC-Corporate/file/report.pdf

Freire AC, Basit AW, Choudhary R, Piong CW, Merchant HA (2011) Does sex matter? The influence of gender on gastrointestinal physiology and drug delivery. Int J Pharm 415(1–2): 15–28. https://doi.org/10.1016/j.ijpharm.2011.04.069

Furman D, Hejblum BP, Simon N, Jojic V, Dekker CL, Thiebaut R, Tibshirani RJ, Davis MM (2014) Systems analysis of sex differences reveals an immunosuppressive role for testosterone in the response to influenza vaccination. Proc Natl Acad Sci U S A 111(2):869–874. https://doi.org/10.1073/pnas.1321060111

Garcia-Sifuentes Y, Maney DL (2021) Reporting and misreporting of sex differences in the biological sciences. Elife 10. https://doi.org/10.7554/eLife.70817

Gottgens I, Oertelt-Prigione S (2023) Moving beyond gender identity: the need for contextualization in gender-sensitive medical research. Lancet Reg Health Eur 24:100548. https://doi.org/10.1016/j.lanepe.2022.100548

Government of Canada, What is Gender? What is Sex? (2018) Retrieved 17 Aug 2022 from https://cihr-irsc.gc.ca/e/48642.html

Gruca TS, Hottel WJ, Comstock J, Olson A, Rosenthal GE (2018) Sex and cardiovascular disease status differences in attitudes and willingness to participate in clinical research studies/clinical trials. Trials 19(1):300. https://doi.org/10.1186/s13063-018-2667-7

Guttenbach M, Koschorz B, Bernthaler U, Grimm T, Schmid M (1995) Sex chromosome loss and aging: in situ hybridization studies on human interphase nuclei. Am J Hum Genet 57(5): 1143–1150. https://www.ncbi.nlm.nih.gov/pubmed/7485166

Hanley MJ, Abernethy DR, Greenblatt DJ (2010) Effect of obesity on the pharmacokinetics of drugs in humans. Clin Pharmacokinet 49(2):71–87. https://doi.org/10.2165/11318100-000000000-00000

Heise L, Greene ME, Opper N, Stavropoulou M, Harper C, Nascimento M, Zewdie D, Gender Equality N, Health Steering C (2019) Gender inequality and restrictive gender norms: framing the challenges to health. Lancet 393(10189):2440–2454. https://doi.org/10.1016/S0140-6736(19)30652-X

Hood L, Friend SH (2011) Predictive, personalized, preventive, participatory (P4) cancer medicine. Nat Rev Clin Oncol 8(3):184–187. https://doi.org/10.1038/nrclinonc.2010.227

Horstmann S, Schmechel C, Palm K, Oertelt-Prigione S, Bolte G (2022) The operationalisation of sex and gender in quantitative health-related research: a scoping review. Int J Environ Res Public Health 19(12). https://doi.org/10.3390/ijerph19127493

ICH (2009) International conference on harmonisation of technical requirements for registration of pharmaceuticals for human use. Sex-related considerations in the conduct of clinical trials. https://admin.ich.org/sites/default/files/2019-04/ICH_Women_Revised_2009.pdf

ICH (2022) General considerations for clinical studies E3(R1). Retrieved from https://database.ich.org/sites/default/files/ICH_E8-R1_Guideline_Step4_2021_1006.pdf

Joel D (2012) Genetic-gonadal-genitals sex (3G-sex) and the misconception of brain and gender, or, why 3G-males and 3G-females have intersex brain and intersex gender. Biol Sex Differ 3(1):27. https://doi.org/10.1186/2042-6410-3-27

Kim AM, Tingen CM, Woodruff TK (2010) Sex bias in trials and treatment must end. Nature 465(7299):688–689. https://doi.org/10.1038/465688a

Kim YS, Unno T, Kim BY, Park MS (2020) Sex differences in gut microbiota. World J Mens Health 38(1):48–60. https://doi.org/10.5534/wjmh.190009

Klein SL, Flanagan KL (2016) Sex differences in immune responses. Nat Rev Immunol 16(10): 626–638. https://doi.org/10.1038/nri.2016.90

Kovats S (2015) Estrogen receptors regulate innate immune cells and signaling pathways. Cell Immunol 294(2):63–69. https://doi.org/10.1016/j.cellimm.2015.01.018

Labots G, Jones A, de Visser SJ, Rissmann R, Burggraaf J (2018) Gender differences in clinical registration trials: is there a real problem? Br J Clin Pharmacol 84(4):700–707. https://doi.org/10.1111/bcp.13497

Libert C, Dejager L, Pinheiro I (2010) The X chromosome in immune functions: when a chromosome makes the difference. Nat Rev Immunol 10(8):594–604. https://doi.org/10.1038/nri2815

Lyon MF (1961) Gene action in the X-chromosome of the mouse (Mus musculus L.). Nature 190: 372–373. https://doi.org/10.1038/190372a0

Machiela MJ, Zhou W, Karlins E, Sampson JN, Freedman ND, Yang Q et al (2016) Female chromosome X mosaicism is age-related and preferentially affects the inactivated X chromosome. Nat Commun 7:11843. https://doi.org/10.1038/ncomms11843

Mahmoodzadeh S, Fritschka S, Dworatzek E, Pham TH, Becher E, Kuehne A, Davidson MM, Regitz-Zagrosek V (2009) Nuclear factor-kappaB regulates estrogen receptor-alpha transcription in the human heart. J Biol Chem 284(37):24705–24714. https://doi.org/10.1074/jbc.M109.000463

Mauvais-Jarvis F, Bairey Merz N, Barnes PJ, Brinton RD, Carrero JJ, DeMeo DL, De Vries GJ, Epperson CN, Govindan R, Klein SL, Lonardo A, Maki PM, McCullough LD, Regitz-Zagrosek V, Regensteiner JG, Rubin JB, Sandberg K, Suzuki A (2020) Sex and gender:

modifiers of health, disease, and medicine. Lancet 396(10250):565–582. https://doi.org/10.1016/S0140-6736(20)31561-0
Mauvais-Jarvis F, Berthold HK, Campesi I, Carrero JJ, Dakal S, Franconi F, Gouni-Berthold I, Heiman ML, Kautzky-Willer A, Klein SL, Murphy A, Regitz-Zagrosek V, Reue K, Rubin JB (2021) Sex- and gender-based pharmacological response to drugs. Pharmacol Rev 73(2): 730–762. https://doi.org/10.1124/pharmrev.120.000206
Meibohm B, Beierle I, Derendorf H (2002) How important are gender differences in pharmacokinetics? Clin Pharmacokinet 41(5):329–342. https://doi.org/10.2165/00003088-200241050-00002
Mercurio A, Adriani G, Catalano A, Carocci A, Rao L, Lentini G, Cavalluzzi MM, Franchini C, Vacca A, Corbo F (2017) A mini-review on thalidomide: chemistry, mechanisms of action, therapeutic potential and anti-angiogenic properties in multiple myeloma. Curr Med Chem 24(25):2736–2744. https://doi.org/10.2174/0929867324666170601074646
Miguel-Aliaga I (2022) Let's talk about (biological) sex. Nat Rev Mol Cell Biol 23(4):227–228. https://doi.org/10.1038/s41580-022-00467-w
Nanna MG, Wang TY, Xiang Q, Goldberg AC, Robinson JG, Roger VL, Virani SS, Wilson PWF, Louie MJ, Koren A, Li Z, Peterson ED, Navar AM (2019) Sex differences in the use of statins in community practice. Circ Cardiovasc Qual Outcomes 12(8):e005562. https://doi.org/10.1161/CIRCOUTCOMES.118.005562
National Institute of Health, Sex and Gender (2018) Retrieved 17 Aug 2022 from https://orwh.od.nih.gov/sex-gender
Nieuwenhoven L, Klinge I (2010) Scientific excellence in applying sex- and gender-sensitive methods in biomedical and health research. J Womens Health (Larchmt) 19(2):313–321. https://doi.org/10.1089/jwh.2008.1156
NIH Policy on Sex as a Biological Variable (2015) National Institute of Health. https://orwh.od.nih.gov/sex-gender/nih-policy-sex-biological-variable
Oertelt-Prigione S (2020) Putting gender into sex- and gender-sensitive medicine. EClinicalMedicine 20:100305. https://doi.org/10.1016/j.eclinm.2020.100305
Oertelt-Prigione S (2023) The operationalization of gender in medicine. In: Legato MJ (ed) Principles of gender-specific medicine sex and gender-specific biology in the postgenomic era, 4th edn. Elsevier, pp 503–512
Oertelt-Prigione S, Regitz-Zagrosek V (2009) Gender aspects in cardiovascular pharmacology. J Cardiovasc Transl Res 2(3):258–266. https://doi.org/10.1007/s12265-009-9114-9
Oertelt-Prigione S, Dalibert L, Verdonk P, Stutz EZ, Klinge I (2017) Implementation strategies for gender-sensitive public health practice: a European workshop. J Womens Health (Larchmt) 26(11):1255–1261. https://doi.org/10.1089/jwh.2017.6592
Oi Yan Chan J, Moullet M, Williamson B, Arends RH, Pilla Reddy V (2022) Harnessing clinical trial and real-world data towards an understanding of sex effects on drug pharmacokinetics, pharmacodynamics and efficacy. Front Pharmacol 13:874606. https://doi.org/10.3389/fphar.2022.874606
Prendergast BJ, Onishi KG, Zucker I (2014) Female mice liberated for inclusion in neuroscience and biomedical research. Neurosci Biobehav Rev 40:1–5. https://doi.org/10.1016/j.neubiorev.2014.01.001
Putting gender on the agenda (2010) Nature 465(7299):665. https://doi.org/10.1038/465665a
Ragonese C, Barker G (2019) Understanding masculinities to improve men's health. Lancet 394(10194):198–199. https://doi.org/10.1016/S0140-6736(19)31609-5
Regitz-Zagrosek V (2006) Therapeutic implications of the gender-specific aspects of cardiovascular disease. Nat Rev Drug Discov 5(5):425–438. https://doi.org/10.1038/nrd2032
Rizzetto L, Fava F, Tuohy KM, Selmi C (2018) Connecting the immune system, systemic chronic inflammation and the gut microbiome: the role of sex. J Autoimmun 92:12–34. https://doi.org/10.1016/j.jaut.2018.05.008
Sapir-Pichhadze R, Oertelt-Prigione S (2023) P3(2): a sex- and gender-sensitive model for evidence-based precision medicine: from knowledge generation to implementation in the field

of kidney transplantation. Kidney Int 103(4):674–685. https://doi.org/10.1016/j.kint.2022.12.026
Schwartz JB (2003) The influence of sex on pharmacokinetics. Clin Pharmacokinet 42(2):107–121. https://doi.org/10.2165/00003088-200342020-00001
Scott PE, Unger EF, Jenkins MR, Southworth MR, McDowell TY, Geller RJ, Elahi M, Temple RJ, Woodcock J (2018) Participation of women in clinical trials supporting FDA approval of cardiovascular drugs. J Am Coll Cardiol 71(18):1960–1969. https://doi.org/10.1016/j.jacc.2018.02.070
Singh J (2015) International conference on harmonization of technical requirements for registration of pharmaceuticals for human use. J Pharmacol Pharmacother 6(3):185–187. https://doi.org/10.4103/0976-500X.162004
Sirufo MM, De Pietro F, Ginaldi L, De Martinis M (2022) Sex, allergic diseases and omalizumab. Biomedicine *10*(2). https://doi.org/10.3390/biomedicines10020328
Soldin OP, Chung SH, Mattison DR (2011) Sex differences in drug disposition. J Biomed Biotechnol 2011(5):187103. https://doi.org/10.1155/2011/187103
Spoletini I, Vitale C, Malorni W, Rosano GM (2012) Sex differences in drug effects: interaction with sex hormones in adult life. Handb Exp Pharmacol 214:91–105. https://doi.org/10.1007/978-3-642-30726-3_5
Springer KW, Mouzon DM (2011) "Macho men" and preventive health care: implications for older men in different social classes. J Health Soc Behav 52(2):212–227. https://doi.org/10.1177/0022146510393972
Sun X, Briel M, Walter SD, Guyatt GH (2010) Is a subgroup effect believable? Updating criteria to evaluate the credibility of subgroup analyses. BMJ 340:c117. https://doi.org/10.1136/bmj.c117
Tannenbaum C, Greaves L, Graham ID (2016a) Why sex and gender matter in implementation research. BMC Med Res Methodol 16(1):145. https://doi.org/10.1186/s12874-016-0247-7
Tannenbaum C, Regitz-Zagrosek V, Miller VM (2016b) Rapid response to: sex based subgroup differences in randomized controlled trials: empirical evidence from Cochrane meta-analyses. BMJ:355
Tannenbaum C, Ellis RP, Eyssel F, Zou J, Schiebinger L (2019) Sex and gender analysis improves science and engineering. Nature 575(7781):137–146. https://doi.org/10.1038/s41586-019-1657-6
Teixeira D, Longo-Maugeri IM, Santos JL, Duarte YA, Lebrao ML, Bueno V (2011) Evaluation of lymphocyte levels in a random sample of 218 elderly individuals from Sao Paulo city. Rev Bras Hematol Hemoter 33(5):367–371. https://doi.org/10.5581/1516-8484.20110100
Vambheim SM, Flaten MA (2017) A systematic review of sex differences in the placebo and the nocebo effect. J Pain Res 10:1831–1839. https://doi.org/10.2147/JPR.S134745
Wallach JD, Sullivan PG, Trepanowski JF, Steyerberg EW, Ioannidis JP (2016) Sex based subgroup differences in randomized controlled trials: empirical evidence from Cochrane meta-analyses. BMJ 355:i5826. https://doi.org/10.1136/bmj.i5826
Wizemann TM, Pardue ML (2001) Exploring the biological contributions to human health: does sex matter? J Womens Health Gend Based Med 10(5):433–439. https://doi.org/10.1089/152460901300233902
Woitowich NC, Beery A, Woodruff T (2020) A 10-year follow-up study of sex inclusion in the biological sciences. Elife *9*. https://doi.org/10.7554/eLife.56344
Ziegler SF (2006) FOXP3: of mice and men. Annu Rev Immunol 24:209–226. https://doi.org/10.1146/annurev.immunol.24.021605.090547
Zou P, Heath A, Sewell C, Lu Y, Tran D, Seo SK (2022) EXOGENOUS sex hormones and sex hormone receptor modulators in COVID-19: rationale and clinical pharmacology considerations. Clin Pharmacol Ther 111(3):559–571. https://doi.org/10.1002/cpt.2508
Zucker I, Beery AK (2010) Males still dominate animal studies. Nature 465(7299):690. https://doi.org/10.1038/465690a
Zucker I, Prendergast BJ (2020) Sex differences in pharmacokinetics predict adverse drug reactions in women. Biol Sex Differ 11(1):32. https://doi.org/10.1186/s13293-020-00308-5

Sex Differences in Pharmacokinetics

Irving Zucker and Brian J. Prendergast

Contents

Abstract

Because women have been excluded from most clinical trials, assessment of sex differences in pharmacokinetics is available for a minority of currently prescribed drugs. In a 2020 analysis, substantial pharmacokinetic (PK) sex differences were established for 86 drugs: women given the same drug dose as men routinely generated higher blood concentrations and longer drug elimination times than men. 96% of drugs with higher PK values in women were associated with a higher incidence of adverse drug reactions (ADRs) in women than men; in the small number of instances when PKs of men exceeded those of women, this sex difference positively predicted male-biased ADRs in only 29% of cases. The absence of sex-stratified PK information for many medications raises the concern

I. Zucker (✉)
Departments of Psychology and Integrative Biology, University of California, Berkeley, CA, USA
e-mail: irvzuck@berkeley.edu

B. J. Prendergast
Department of Psychology Institute for Mind and Biology and Committee on Neurobiology, The University of Chicago, Chicago, IL, USA

S. E. Tsirka, M. Acosta-Martinez (eds.), *Sex and Gender Effects in Pharmacology*, Handbook of Experimental Pharmacology 282,
https://doi.org/10.1007/164_2023_669

that sex differences in pharmacokinetics may be widespread and of clinical significance, contributing to sex-specific patterns of ADRs. Administering equal drug doses to women and men neglects sex differences in pharmacokinetics and body weight, risks overmedication of women, and contributes to female-biased ADRs. Evidence-based dosing adjustments are recommended to counteract this sex bias.

Keywords

Adverse drug reactions · Drugs · Pharmacokinetics · Sex differences

Abbreviations

ADR	Adverse drug reaction
AUC	Area under the curve
ClT	Clearance time, exposure, or plasma concentration after a fixed time interval
Cmax	Maximum circulating concentration
PD	Pharmacodynamics
PK	Pharmacokinetics
SysExp	Systemic exposure
$t_{1/2}$	Elimination half-life
Tmax	Time required to reach Cmax value

1 Introduction

This review chapter draws on narratives in Zucker and Prendergast (2020) and Zucker et al. (2022), with updates since 2020.

In the past decade inclusion of women in clinical trials and post-marketing clinical research has increased (Bierer and Meloney 2022; Rechlin et al. 2022), but key steps such as sex-based analysis and sex-specific drug dosing remain to be implemented (Rechlin et al. 2022; Zucker et al. 2022). Until recently researchers labored under the assumption that information garnered from studies of males could be generalized without modification to females. Since then, sex differences in mechanisms underlying basic biological processes, including drug metabolism, have been detailed, with important consequences for women's health (Heinrich 2011; Klein et al. 2015; Zucker et al. 2022; Zucker and Prendergast 2020). Sex-inclusive research practices have increased since 2009, although male bias remains in several biological disciplines (Woitowich et al. 2020) and has increased in some fields (e.g., cardiovascular research; Ramirez et al. (2017)). A recent review of NIH-funded randomized control trials enrolling men and women found that just 26% of studies reported even a single outcome by sex or included both sexes as a covariate (Geller et al. 2018); in 72% of studies, the analyses excluded sex altogether. There has been no concomitant increase in the percentage of studies that assess sex or gender as a factor in pharmacokinetics: fewer than half of sex-inclusive studies refer to such types of analyses (Mamlouk et al. 2020; Rechlin et al. 2022; Woitowich et al. 2020; Zucker et al. 2022).

Many currently prescribed drugs were approved by the US Food and Drug Administration (FDA) without adequate enrollment of women in clinical trials. The sedative-hypnotic drug zolpidem (Ambien), for example, was first approved in 1992 with just 19 women and 49 men as the sole subjects. A marked elevation of zolpidem concentrations in women and longer elimination times was evident in this study, but no recommendation for dose reductions in women was forthcoming. It was only after years of post-marketing reports of cognitive deficits in women treated with zolpidem that sex-based dose adjustments were recommended, and women were advised to receive half the dose given to men. Physicians in several European countries still tend to prescribe zolpidem without considering the FDA recommendations of a maximum dose of 5 mg for women (Greil et al. 2022). Many other drugs also require re-evaluation for sex-specific dose adjustments, but the relevant data are lacking for almost all currently prescribed pharmaceuticals. A survey of clinical pharmacology data for 300 new drug applications (NDAs) evaluated by the FDA from 1994 to 2000 found that 31% of NDAs identified a possible sex effect, based on pharmacokinetic (PK) differences >20% between the sexes (Fadiran and Zhang 2015). The existing knowledge base for sex-aware drug prescribing lacks information on sex differences in PKs for one-third of all medications (Fadiran and Zhang 2015; Lind et al. 2017). Most drugs are not administered on a mg/kg body mass basis (Pai 2012); women are given the same dose as men, despite on average lower body weights in women and numerous sex differences in drug absorption, distribution, bioavailability, metabolism, and excretion. Consequently, women may be overmedicated.

Across all drug categories, adverse drug reactions (ADRs) are substantially more common in women than in men (Brabete et al. 2022; de Vries et al. 2019; Park et al. 2021) and across all regions of the world, ADRs are reported in greater numbers by females than males (Watson et al. 2019). Women are also more likely to be hospitalized due to an ADR (Damien et al. 2016; Nakagawa and Kajiwara 2015; Tharpe 2011). Developmentally, ADRs peak two decades earlier in women (30–39 years of age) than men (50–59 years of age; (Martin et al. 1998)). For many drugs, PKs differ in men and women (Chen et al. 2000; Franconi and Campesi 2014, 2017; Gandhi et al. 2004; Harris et al. 1995; Meibohm et al. 2002; Schwartz 2003; Soldin and Mattison 2009) which impacts drug efficacy and also toxicity, but PK information is included in only a small minority of approved drug labels (Fadiran and Zhang 2015).

Here, we review a recent examination of relations between sex differences in drug PKs and ADRs, in which we critically evaluated the hypothesis that drug exposure (PKs) and clinically unintended, harmful effects of drugs (ADRs) should be considered together in the development of rational, sex-based dosing adjustments. Such considerations are currently uncommon. We recommend that sex-based dosing adjustments be developed, disseminated into clinical practice, and appear on drug labels.

2 Methods

To examine whether sex differences in PKs are associated with sex differences in ADRs, we reviewed empirical studies that examined PKs in females and males treated with FDA-approved drugs and quantitative reports of ADRs in both sexes. ADRs were identified from relevant reports and recorded as either female-biased, male-biased, or not-biased. Multiple searches of the ISI Web of Science database were conducted throughout 2018 and 2019 and again in December 2022 with the terms: drugs and sex differences, pharmacokinetics drugs and gender, pharmacokinetics drugs and sex differences, pharmacodynamics drug safety and dose, drug safety and dose, gender and adverse drug reactions, sex and adverse drug reactions, and gender and adverse drug reactions, which yielded over 5,600 articles, with substantial overlap among searches. Only publications that contained data on sex differences in pharmacokinetics and/or ADRs were included in the final analyses reported here. For additional details of the first iteration of this literature review, see methods and results reported in our original analysis (Zucker and Prendergast 2020).

3 Results and Discussion

Table 1 lists the specific PK measures for each drug, the direction of sex bias in the measure, whether any reported ADRs were female- or male-biased, and whether PK findings and ADR data were sex-concordant (i.e., the PK bias is in the same direction as the ADR bias) or sex-discordant. In addition to drugs listed by Zucker and Prendergast (2020), 5 additional drugs that were identified in a 2022 analysis are included in Table 1. Many drugs with striking sex differences in ADRs did not make it onto this list because there were no available PK data, almost always because drugs were approved prior to the year 2000, and the relevant information is not available in the online FDA database. These data and their implications for gender-informed approaches to pharmacology are considered below.

3.1 Sex Differences in PKs Correlate with Sex Differences in ADRs

Sex differences in PKs corresponded strikingly with sex differences in ADRs. In 89% of instances, a sex difference in PKs (in either direction) was associated with a similar sex difference in ADRs (i.e., 58 of 65 drugs were concordant; Table 1). This incidence is notably higher than the 46% sex difference in ADRs across all drugs, when assessed without regard to PK sex differences (Yu et al. 2016). This outcome suggests that when PK data are included in the consideration of ADRs and the analyses are stratified both by the presence and by the direction of PK differences,

Table 1 Summary of sex-biased PK measures and concordance with clinical ADRs. Modified from Zucker and Prendergast (2020), with additional drugs from 2019-2022

WHO ATC category	Drug[a]	PK measure[b]	Female-biased ADRs	Male-biased ADRs	PK vs. ADR
Alimentary tract, metabolism	Liraglutide	CLT	Headache, vomiting, nausea	–	Concordant
	Ranitidine	***AUC*, Tmax**	–	**Duodenal damage**	Concordant
	Rosiglitazone	CLT	Fracture	–	Concordant
Blood and blood forming organs	Heparin	CLT	Blood disorders, lymphatic disorders, bleeding (60 yoa)	–	Concordant
	Aspirin	*AUC*, CIT, $t_{1/2}$	Elevated fibrinogen, CVD in T2D	**Bleeding**	Concordant
	Warfarin	CLT	Bleeding	–	Concordant
	Clopidogrel	*AUC*, Cmax	Fracture, bleeding, GI symptoms, IBD	–	Concordant
	Dabigatran	*AUC*	Bleeding	–	Concordant
Cardiovascular system	Torasemide	*AUC*, Cmax, CIT, $t_{1/2}$	Hospitalization	–	Concordant
	Pravastatin	AUC, Cmax	CHD	–	Concordant
	Amlodipine	**CLT**	Edema, flushing, palpitations	–	Discordant
	Digoxin	CLT	Mortality	–	Concordant
	Verapamil	CLT	Constipation, edema, fatigue, headache	–	Concordant
	Aliskiren	*AUC*, Cmax	Diarrhea	–	Concordant
	Losartan	*AUC*, Cmax	–	**Angina, mortality**	Discordant
	Propranolol			–	Concordant

(continued)

Table 1 (continued)

WHO ATC category	Drug[a]	PK measure[b]	Female-biased ADRs	Male-biased ADRs	PK vs. ADR
		AUC, Cmax, ClT	Dizziness, muscle pain, headache, dry mouth		
	Dofetilide	SysExp	TdP	–	Concordant
Genito-urinary system, sex hormones	Mirabegron	*AUC*, Cmax, SysExp	Treatment discontinuation (CAN), treatment discontinuation (CZE)	**Treatment discontinuation (UK)**	Concordant
	Darifenacin	*AUC*, Cmax, ClT	F > M, ADRs not Specified	–	Concordant
	Trospium	*AUC*, Cmax	Cognitive impairments	–	Concordant
Systemic hormonal Preparations	Prednisone	*AUC*, ClT	Depression, fatigue, hair loss, mood swings, weight gain	–	Concordant
Anti-infectives	Levofloxacin	ClT, SysExp	Fluoroquinolone toxicity	–	Concordant
	Daptomycin	CLT	F requires lower doses		Concordant
	Erythromycin	**CLT**	TdP	–	Discordant
	Voriconazole	*AUC*, Cmax	Cardiac QTc symptoms	–	Concordant
Antineoplastics, Immunomodulators	**Cyclosporin**	**CLT**	–	–	Discordant[c]
	Fluorouracil	*AUC*, ClT	Stomatitis, leukopenia, alopecia, diarrhea, mucositis	–	Concordant
	Paclitaxel	CLT	Myocardial infarction, death, lesion revascularization	–	Concordant
	Capecitabine	*AUC*	Dose-limiting toxicity	–	Concordant

	Infliximab	CLT	Allergic reactions	–	Concordant
	Lenvatinib	*AUC*, ClT	Grade III adverse reactions		Concordant
	Adalimumab	CLT	Allergic reactions	–	Concordant
	Tamoxifen	*AUC*, Cmax	Gastrointestinal problems, cardiovascular events		Concordant
	Mitotane	Cmax	Treatment failure		Concordant
Anesthetics, analgesics	Morphine	CLT	Respiratory depression, hypoxic sensitivity, emesis, nausea	–	Concordant
	Oxycodone	CLT	Nausea, pruritus, negative affect	–	Concordant
	Buprenorphine	*AUC*, Cmax	Sleep disturbance	–	Concordant
	Tramadol	*AUC*, Cmax	Treatment discontinuation	–	Concordant
	Zolmitriptan	*AUC*, Cmax	Face and neck pressure	–	Concordant
	Ketamine	**ClT**	–	**Verbal learning, subjective memory**	Concordant
Anti-epileptics, anti-Parkinson's	**Carbamazepine**	**ClT, $t_{1/2}$**	Cognitive impairment, elevated LDL/HDL	–	Discordant
	Gabapentin	Cmax	Dizziness, somnolescence, nausea	–	Concordant
	Perampanel	*AUC*, ClT	Dizziness, headache, treatment discontinuation	–	Concordant
	Pramipexole	*AUC*, Cmax	Nausea, fatigue	–	Concordant
	Levodopa	*AUC*, Cmax	Motor complications and dyskinesia		Concordant
Psycholeptics	Olanzapine	CLT	Severe weight gain		Concordant
	Clozapine	CLT		**Hypertension, increases in BMI, elevated homocysteine, increased**	Discordant

(continued)

Table 1 (continued)

WHO ATC category	Drug[a]	PK measure[b]	Female-biased ADRs	Male-biased ADRs	PK vs. ADR
			Blood glucose, laxative use, obesity, type II diabetes, neutropenia, leukopenia, weight gain	**basal metabolic rate, increased plasma lipids, QTc symptoms, blood dyscrasias, myocarditis, cardiomyopathy**	
	Risperidone	CLT	Hyperprolactinemia, neurological effects, headache, hypotension	–	Concordant
	Aripiprazole	*AUC*, Cmax	Blood pressure, heart rate, elongated QTc	–	Concordant
	Diazepam	$t_{1/2}$	Psychomotor Impairment	–	Concordant
	Zolpidem	*AUC*, Cmax, ClT	Cognitive impairment, driving impairment	–	Concordant
	Eszopiclone	*AUC*	Dysgeusia	–	Concordant
Psychoanaleptics	Imipramine	CLT	Dry mouth, constipation, sweating, tremor, treatment discontinuation	–	Concordant
	Nortriptyline	CLT	Dry mouth	–	Concordant
	Fluoxetine	CLT	Hypercortisolemia, elevated albumin, elevated tryptophan, suicidal ideation	–	Concordant
	Citalopram	CLT	Elevated ADH	–	Concordant
	Sertraline	*AUC*, ClT, $t_{1/2}$	Cholesterol, nausea, dizziness, delusions	**Dyspepsia, sexual dysfunction, urinary frequency**	Concordant
	Bupropion	*AUC*, Cmax, $t_{1/2}$	EEG abnormalities, seizure	–	Concordant
	Methylphenidate	***AUC***	Anxiety disorder	–	Discordant

Antiparasitics	Primaquine	*AUC*, Cmax	Nausea	–	Concordant
Respiratory	Terfenadine	Cmax	TdP	–	Concordant
	Fexofenadine	*AUC*, Cmax	Visual attention deficits, reaction time deficits, driving impairments	–	Concordant
Miscellaneous	MDMA	CLT	Elevated copeptin, hyponatremia	–	Concordant
	Cannabis	CLT	Increased subjective emotional responses, problematic use, introvertive anhedonia	–	Concordant

AUC area under the curve, *Cmax* maximum circulating concentration, *Tmax* time required to reach *Cmax* value, $t_{1/2}$ elimination half-life, *CIT* clearance time, exposure, or plasma concentration after a fixed time interval, *SysExp* systemic exposure

[a] Font style of drug name indicates direction of PK drug exposure bias: (normal font: F > M; **bold font**: M > F)

[b] Font style of PK measure indicates direction of greater drug exposure (normal: F > M; **bold**: M > F)

[c] No evidence of sex differences in ADRs

patterns of sex differences in ADRs are greatly clarified. Overall, 81 of 91 drugs (89%) had higher PK values in women than in men. And among the 59 drugs for which ADR data were available, 96% of drugs with higher PK values in women also resulted in a higher incidence of ADRs in women (50 of 52 drugs; Zucker and Prendergast (2020); Table 1). Curiously, in 7 drugs male PK values exceeded those of females, however only 2 these 7 drugs (29%) generated male-biased ADRs (4 exhibited female-biased ADRs, 1 yielded no bias). These data do not indicate causality, and it remains possible that sex differences in PKs parallel these sex differences in ADRs but come about via independent processes. However, in the absence of any obvious reason to suspect that our sample is not representative of the thousands of drugs currently approved for human use, these data suggest that elevated drug concentrations and decreased elimination times are substantially more prevalent in women than men and present a quantifiable health risk for women.

3.2 Factors Influencing Sex Differences in Pharmacokinetics

Drug clearance is strongly linked to sex-specific expression of metabolic enzyme systems (Beierle et al. 1999; Cotreau et al. 2005; Greenblatt and von Moltke 2008); renal clearance of drugs is decreased in women because of a relatively lower glomerular filtration rate compared to men (Anderson 2008). Women have a slower gastric emptying time and lower gastric pH, lower plasma volume, body mass index, average organ blood flow, and total body water differences, all of which affect drug distribution and PKs (Islam et al. 2017). Responses to drugs are also affected by physiological changes during the menstrual cycle. The striking hormonal variations across days over the course of the human menstrual cycle is unparalleled in men in which hormonal variations largely occur within rather than across days (Brambilla et al. 2007).

Women, on average, weigh less than men. The amount of body weight adjusted dosing in clinical practice is presently unknown (Arpon et al. 2014). Most drugs are not administered on a mg/kg basis but as a "one-size-fits-all" dose, which can lead to higher exposures in women (Fadiran and Zhang 2015). Under optimal circumstances, the dose should be based on mg/kg body weight, or titrated to the desired clinical effect (Vree et al. 2004). Correction for height, weight, surface area, or body composition eliminates a minority of sex-dependent PK differences (Fadiran and Zhang 2015). The inference that weight-corrected PKs are comparable between men and women is not generally warranted but must be examined on a case-by-case basis, if data on both sexes exist. It would be useful in future research to examine whether, for a drug with a sexually differentiated pattern of ADRs, correction for body weight eliminates the sex differences in PKs. If so, this would underscore the importance of understanding sex differences in PKs. If not, it would suggest that sex differences in PKs may be but one of many sex-related variables that contribute to the manifestation of sex differences in ADRs.

3.3 Selection of the Appropriate Drug Dose

Medications with a low therapeutic index (i.e., where the lowest effective dose approaches toxic concentrations) pose a significant challenge for contending with sex differences in PKs (Fife and Maibach 2005; Polasek et al. 2018), because when a therapeutic index is narrow, such differences may be more clinically significant, and titration of dosage may not be effective. A detailed study of sex differences for drugs with steep dose response curves or narrow therapeutic indices is needed (Panetta and Srinivasan 1998). In contrast, drugs with wider therapeutic indexes may pose less of a challenge. A fixed dosing regimen may be less of an impediment, but even in these instances, selecting the lowest effective dose would be prudent in women, at a minimum to decrease the potential for ADRs and drug–drug interactions due to polypharmacy.

3.4 Limitations in Population PK Studies

Population PK studies commonly rely on sparse blood sampling regimens from subjects in phase II and III clinical trials. Still, PK data are included on only a small minority of FDA-approved drug labels (Fadiran and Zhang 2015): among >2,500 drugs indexed in the Physicians' Desk Reference, < 4% included population PK information in their labelling (Duan 2007). Data on sex differences in PKs are routinely derived from small clinical studies, typically enrolling 12–24 healthy control subjects. Studies with small sample sizes may only be capable of detecting very large sex differences in PKs, and as effect sizes decrease, under-powered experimental designs become less and less capable of identifying real sex differences in PKs.

4 General Conclusions and Future Directions

Sex differences in PK values predict sex differences in ADRs but primarily when biased toward women. Data from our 2020 analysis revealed a striking sex difference in PKs: among patients administered a standard drug dose, females were exposed to higher blood drug concentrations and exhibited longer drug elimination times than males. This likely contributes to the marked increase in ADRs in women, raising the possibility that women are routinely overmedicated. Whether this relation holds for the many drugs for which sex-stratified PK data are not available remains to be determined. The present results support the hypothesis that for drugs with sex differences in PKs and a sufficiently broad therapeutic index, dose reductions in women would yield a reduction in side effects.

Several previous reports have identified links between sex-specific patterns of PK values, PDs (pharmacodynamics), and ADRs (Humphries et al. 2017; Salzano et al. 2017; Tamargo et al. 2017); the present analysis (Zucker and Prendergast 2020) extends this linkage to include multiple categories of FDA-approved medications.

Our results indicate that if a significant, female-biased PK sex difference is identified, then there is a strong likelihood that a female-biased pattern of ADRs will be present. For the drugs identified in this analysis, the pattern of outcomes supports the conjecture that women are overmedicated. The intended efficacy of drugs in relation to sex remains in need of additional, intensive investigation.

Men typically weigh more than women, and evaluating the extent to which sex differences in ADRs can be explained by sex differences in body weight between women and men is warranted. Unfortunately, in the absence of clear and accessible data integrating PKs, PDs, and ADRs in women and men (i.e., data stratified by and evaluated by sex, with comparable statistical power), this is difficult to systematically evaluate. Additional work is necessary to determine how biological sex and body weight interact to drive PKs. A complete understanding of how sex differences in ADRs manifest would also benefit by integrating information on sex differences in PKs and ADRs with gender-related variables and biopsychosocial factors (Richardson et al. 2015).

A limitation in the present analysis arises from deficiencies in the data upon which the analysis is based: the standards of evidence in many clinical reports submitted to and approved by the FDA were not as rigorous as would be desired, given the stakes. Some reports with claims of no statistical differences between the sexes were not supported by F statistics or p values, and in other instances further complicated by small sample sizes and increased risk of Type II error. Estimates of treatment effect size were also largely absent.

Finally, it may not be practical or possible to thoroughly catalog and quantify ADRs prior to FDA approval. Less common ADRs, although no less harmful, may only become apparent after a drug is in widespread use for years. Consequently, the vast majority of data on ADRs are found in post-marketing reports and typically emerge years after a drug appears on the market. In light of the strong association between elevated PKs in women and increased ADRs, if a drug exhibits female-biased PKs, then one strategy for minimizing ADRs in women may be to treat women with lower doses than men initially and increase dosages only if the lower dose fails to achieve the desired therapeutic effect.

References

Anderson GD (2008) Gender differences in pharmacological response. Int Rev Neurobiol 83:1–10. https://doi.org/10.1016/S0074-7742(08)00001-9

Arpon DR, Gandhi MK, Martin JH (2014) A new frontier in haematology – combining pharmacokinetic with pharmacodynamic factors to improve choice and dose of drug. Br J Clin Pharmacol 78:274–281. https://doi.org/10.1111/bcp.12318

Beierle I, Meibohm B, Derendorf H (1999) Gender differences in pharmacokinetics and pharmacodynamics. Int J Clin Pharmacol Ther 37:529–547

Bierer BE, Meloney LG (2022) Strategies to optimize inclusion of women in multi-national clinical trials. Contemp Clin Trials 117:106770. https://doi.org/10.1016/j.cct.2022.106770

Brabete AC, Greaves L, Maximos M, Huber E, Li A, Lê M-L (2022) A sex- and gender-based analysis of adverse drug reactions: a scoping review of pharmacovigilance databases. Pharmaceuticals (Basel) 15:298. https://doi.org/10.3390/ph15030298

Brambilla DJ, O'Donnell AB, Matsumoto AM, McKinlay JB (2007) Intraindividual variation in levels of serum testosterone and other reproductive and adrenal hormones in men. Clin Endocrinol (Oxf) 67:853–862. https://doi.org/10.1111/j.1365-2265.2007.02976.x

Chen ML, Lee SC, Ng MJ, Schuirmann DJ, Lesko LJ, Williams RL (2000) Pharmacokinetic analysis of bioequivalence trials: implications for sex-related issues in clinical pharmacology and biopharmaceutics. Clin Pharmacol Ther 68:510–521. https://doi.org/10.1067/mcp.2000.111184

Cotreau MM, von Moltke LL, Greenblatt DJ (2005) The influence of age and sex on the clearance of cytochrome P450 3A substrates. Clin Pharmacokinet 44:33–60. https://doi.org/10.2165/00003088-200544010-00002

Damien S, Patural H, Trombert-Paviot B, Beyens M-N (2016) Adverse drug reactions in children: 10 years of pharmacovigilance. Arch Pediatr 23:468–476. https://doi.org/10.1016/j.arcped.2016.01.015

de Vries ST, Denig P, Ekhart C, Burgers JS, Kleefstra N, Mol PGM, van Puijenbroek EP (2019) Sex differences in adverse drug reactions reported to the National Pharmacovigilance Centre in The Netherlands: an explorative observational study. Br J Clin Pharmacol 85:1507–1515. https://doi.org/10.1111/bcp.13923

Duan JZ (2007) Applications of population pharmacokinetics in current drug labelling. J Clin Pharm Ther 32:57–79. https://doi.org/10.1111/j.1365-2710.2007.00799.x

Fadiran EO, Zhang L (2015) Effects of sex differences in the pharmacokinetics of drugs and their impact on the safety of medicines in women. Med Women:41–68

Fife DJ, Maibach HI (2005) Gender differences in the pharmacokinetics of Oral dermatologic medications. J Toxicol Cutaneous Ocular Toxicol 23:119–133. https://doi.org/10.1081/CUS-120030169

Franconi F, Campesi I (2014) Pharmacogenomics, pharmacokinetics and pharmacodynamics: interaction with biological differences between men and women. Br J Pharmacol 171:580–594

Franconi F, Campesi I (2017) Sex impact on biomarkers, pharmacokinetics and pharmacodynamics. Curr Med Chem 24:2561–2575. https://doi.org/10.2174/0929867323666161003124616

Gandhi M, Aweeka F, Greenblatt RM, Blaschke TF (2004) Sex differences in pharmacokinetics and pharmacodynamics. Annu Rev Pharmacol Toxicol 44:499–523. https://doi.org/10.1146/annurev.pharmtox.44.101802.121453

Geller SE, Koch AR, Roesch P, Filut A, Hallgren E, Carnes M (2018) The more things change, the more they stay the same: a study to evaluate compliance with inclusion and assessment of women and minorities in randomized controlled trials. Acad Med 93:630–635. https://doi.org/10.1097/ACM.0000000000002027

Greenblatt DJ, von Moltke LL (2008) Gender has a small but statistically significant effect on clearance of CYP3A substrate drugs. J Clin Pharmacol 48:1350–1355. https://doi.org/10.1177/0091270008323754

Greil W, de Bardeci M, Seifert J, Bernegger X, Cattapan K, Stassen H, Wagner AL, Sieberer M, Grohmann R, Toto S (2022) Treatment of depression: are psychotropic drugs appropriately dosed in women and in the elderly? Dosages of psychotropic drugs by sex and age in routine clinical practice. Hum Psychopharmacol Clin Exp 37:e2809

Harris RZ, Benet LZ, Schwartz JB (1995) Gender effects in pharmacokinetics and pharmacodynamics. Drugs 50:222–239. https://doi.org/10.2165/00003495-199550020-00003

Heinrich J (2011) Drug safety: most drugs withdrawn in recent years had greater health risks for women [WWW document]. https://www.gao.gov/products/gao-01-286r. Accessed 30 Jan 23

Humphries KH, Izadnegahdar M, Sedlak T, Saw J, Johnston N, Schenck-Gustafsson K, Shah RU, Regitz-Zagrosek V, Grewal J, Vaccarino V, Wei J, Bairey Merz CN (2017) Sex differences in cardiovascular disease – impact on care and outcomes. Front Neuroendocrinol 46:46–70. https://doi.org/10.1016/j.yfrne.2017.04.001

Islam MM, Iqbal U, Walther BA, Nguyen P-A, Li Y-CJ, Dubey NK, Poly TN, Masud JHB, Atique S, Syed-Abdul S (2017) Gender-based personalized pharmacotherapy: a systematic review. Arch Gynecol Obstet 295:1305–1317. https://doi.org/10.1007/s00404-017-4363-3

Klein SL, Schiebinger L, Stefanick ML, Cahill L, Danska J, de Vries GJ, Kibbe MR, McCarthy MM, Mogil JS, Woodruff TK, Zucker I (2015) Opinion: sex inclusion in basic research drives discovery. Proc Natl Acad Sci U S A 112:5257–5258. https://doi.org/10.1073/pnas.1502843112

Lind LK, von Euler M, Korkmaz S, Gustafsson KS (2017) Sex differences in drugs: the development of a comprehensive knowledge base to improve gender awareness prescribing. Biol Sex Differ 8:32. https://doi.org/10.1186/s13293-017-0155-5

Mamlouk GM, Dorris DM, Barrett LR, Meitzen J (2020) Sex bias and omission in neuroscience research is influenced by research model and journal, but not reported NIH funding. Front Neuroendocrinol 57:100835. https://doi.org/10.1016/j.yfrne.2020.100835

Martin RM, Biswas PN, Freemantle SN, Pearce GL, Mann RD (1998) Age and sex distribution of suspected adverse drug reactions to newly marketed drugs in general practice in England: analysis of 48 cohort studies. Br J Clin Pharmacol 46:505–511. https://doi.org/10.1046/j.1365-2125.1998.00817.x

Meibohm B, Beierle I, Derendorf H (2002) How important are gender differences in pharmacokinetics? Clin Pharmacokinet 41:329–342. https://doi.org/10.2165/00003088-200241050-00002

Nakagawa K, Kajiwara A (2015) Female sex as a risk factor for adverse drug reactions. Nihon Rinsho 73:581–585

Pai M (2012) Drug dosing based on weight and body surface area: mathematical assumptions and limitations in obese adults. Pharmacotherapy 32. https://doi.org/10.1002/j.1875-9114.2012.01108.x

Panetta JA, Srinivasan U (1998) Chapter 33 – gender based medicine. In: Bristol JA (ed) Annual reports in medicinal chemistry. Academic Press, pp 355–363. https://doi.org/10.1016/S0065-7743(08)61098-2

Park H-H, Kim JH, Yoon D, Lee H, Shin J-Y (2021) Gender differences in the adverse events associated with cardiovascular drugs in a spontaneous reporting system in South Korea. Int J Clin Pharmacol 43:1036–1044. https://doi.org/10.1007/s11096-020-01212-z

Polasek TM, Shakib S, Rostami-Hodjegan A (2018) Precision dosing in clinical medicine: present and future. Expert Rev Clin Pharmacol 11:743–746. https://doi.org/10.1080/17512433.2018.1501271

Ramirez FD, Motazedian P, Jung RG, Di Santo P, MacDonald Z, Simard T, Clancy AA, Russo JJ, Welch V, Wells GA, Hibbert B (2017) Sex bias is increasingly prevalent in preclinical cardiovascular research: implications for translational medicine and health equity for women: a systematic assessment of leading cardiovascular journals over a 10-year period. Circulation 135:625–626. https://doi.org/10.1161/CIRCULATIONAHA.116.026668

Rechlin RK, Splinter TFL, Hodges TE, Albert AY, Galea LAM (2022) An analysis of neuroscience and psychiatry papers published from 2009 and 2019 outlines opportunities for increasing discovery of sex differences. Nat Commun 13:2137. https://doi.org/10.1038/s41467-022-29903-3

Richardson SS, Reiches M, Shattuck-Heidorn H, LaBonte ML, Consoli T (2015) Opinion: focus on preclinical sex differences will not address women's and men's health disparities. Proc Natl Acad Sci U S A 112:13419–13420. https://doi.org/10.1073/pnas.1516958112

Salzano A, Demelo-Rodriguez P, Marra AM, Proietti M (2017) A focused review of gender differences in antithrombotic therapy. Curr Med Chem 24:2576–2588. https://doi.org/10.2174/0929867323666161029223512

Schwartz JB (2003) The influence of sex on pharmacokinetics. Clin Pharmacokinet 42:107–121. https://doi.org/10.2165/00003088-200342020-00001

Soldin OP, Mattison DR (2009) Sex differences in pharmacokinetics and pharmacodynamics. Clin Pharmacokinet 48:143–157. https://doi.org/10.2165/00003088-200948030-00001

Tamargo J, Rosano G, Walther T, Duarte J, Niessner A, Kaski JC, Ceconi C, Drexel H, Kjeldsen K, Savarese G, Torp-Pedersen C, Atar D, Lewis BS, Agewall S (2017) Gender differences in the effects of cardiovascular drugs. Eur Heart J Cardiovasc Pharmacother 3:163–182. https://doi.org/10.1093/ehjcvp/pvw042

Tharpe N (2011) Adverse drug reactions in women's health care. J Midwifery Womens Health 56: 205–213. https://doi.org/10.1111/j.1542-2011.2010.00050.x

Vree TB, Dammers E, Valducci R (2004) Sex-related differences in the pharmacokinetics of isosorbide-5-mononitrate (60 mg) after repeated oral administration of two different original prolonged release formulations. Int J Clin Pharmacol Ther 42:463–472. https://doi.org/10.5414/cpp42463

Watson S, Caster O, Rochon PA, den Ruijter H (2019) Reported adverse drug reactions in women and men: aggregated evidence from globally collected individual case reports during half a century. EClinicalMedicine 17:100188. https://doi.org/10.1016/j.eclinm.2019.10.001

Woitowich NC, Beery A, Woodruff T (2020) A 10-year follow-up study of sex inclusion in the biological sciences. Elife 9:e56344. https://doi.org/10.7554/eLife.56344

Yu Y, Chen J, Li D, Wang L, Wang W, Liu H (2016) Systematic analysis of adverse event reports for sex differences in adverse drug events. Sci Rep 6:24955. https://doi.org/10.1038/srep24955

Zucker I, Prendergast BJ (2020) Sex differences in pharmacokinetics predict adverse drug reactions in women. Biol Sex Differ 11:32. https://doi.org/10.1186/s13293-020-00308-5

Zucker I, Prendergast BJ, Beery AK (2022) Pervasive neglect of sex differences in biomedical research. Cold Spring Harb Perspect Biol 14:a039156. https://doi.org/10.1101/cshperspect.a039156

Clinical Pharmacological Considerations in Transgender Medicine

Rene Coig, Victoria Luna Brennan Grieve, and Lauren R. Cirrincione

Contents

R. Coig
Department of Laboratory Medicine and Pathology, University of Washington, Seattle, WA, USA

V. L. B. Grieve
Department of Pharmacy and Therapeutics, University of Pittsburgh, Pittsburgh, PA, USA

L. R. Cirrincione (✉)
Department of Pharmacy, University of Washington, Seattle, WA, USA
e-mail: lc10@uw.edu

S. E. Tsirka, M. Acosta-Martinez (eds.), *Sex and Gender Effects in Pharmacology*, Handbook of Experimental Pharmacology 282,
https://doi.org/10.1007/164_2023_665

Abstract

Transgender medicine is a growing clinical field. Hormone therapy (testosterone or estrogen treatment) is part of the standard of gender-affirming medical care, yet clinical pharmacological knowledge in transgender medicine is lacking. Herein, we summarize available clinical and pharmacologic data for hormone therapy among transgender and gender diverse people.

Keywords

Drug interactions · Drug transport proteins · Drug-metabolizing enzymes · Gender-affirming medical care · Pharmacology · Sex steroid hormones · Transgender

Abbreviations

ATP	Adenosine triphosphate
BCRP	Breast cancer resistance protein
BRFSS	Behavior Risk Factor Surveillance System
CDC	Centers for Disease Control and Prevention
CYP	Cytochrome P450 enzymes
EHR	Electronic health record
OATP	Organic anion transporting polypeptides
SULT	Sulfotransferase
TGD	Transgender and gender diverse
UGT	UDP-glucuronosyltransferase
VSC	Variations in sex characteristics
WPATH	World Professional Association for Transgender Health

1 Introduction

Transgender and gender diverse (TGD) people comprise an increasingly visible population globally. Clinicians may prescribe hormone therapy across the lifespan to support a person's gender expression goals (Coleman et al. 2022), yet TGD people have been underrepresented in most pharmacologic research (Cirrincione et al. 2023). Clinical pharmacological knowledge in transgender medicine is limited.

Sexually dimorphic characteristics may influence the safety and efficacy of certain medications, as described in detail elsewhere in this textbook. Sex steroids affect expression and activity of certain drug-metabolizing enzymes and drug transport proteins based on in vitro and animal model data (Le et al. 2022). It is largely unknown the extent to which sex-specific predictors of drug safety and effectiveness can be generalized to TGD adults undergoing hormone therapy. Herein, we provide an overview of emerging considerations for clinical pharmacology in transgender medicine.

1.1 Terminology

Sex: a culturally defined social construct assigned at birth based on appearance of external genitalia. Commonly referred to as biological factors related to male, female, or intersex characteristics including hormonal expression and genitalia. This assignment carries a set of assumptions regarding the underlying internal genital anatomy and the hormone–tissue interactions that will occur with development and aging. This term is descriptive and not prescriptive.

Gender identity: a social construct related to sex assignment that describes behavioral, psychological, and social traits present in a given culture. Gender identity is an individual's personal understanding of their place in that social construct. Gender expression is the outward manifestation of the intersection of gender identity and environment via behavior and dress. Gender, gender identity, and gender expression are linked but may not be congruent.

Sexual orientation: emotional, romantic, and/or sexual attraction to another individual or individuals of a certain gender or sex. This includes lack of emotional, romantic, and/or sexual attraction as well. Sexual orientation and gender identity are non-interchangeable terms and are independent of each other.

Gender-affirming medical care: medications, surgery, or other medical interventions that a person may or may not choose to meet their gender expression goals.

Transgender: A culturally defined social construct describing people whose gender identities differ from the cultural expectation of their sex assigned at birth. Common examples include transgender men or transmasculine individuals, transgender women or transfeminine individuals, and nonbinary people. May or may not be used by an individual to describe themselves.

Cisgender people: people whose gender aligns with the cultural expectation of their sex assigned at birth; not transgender.

Transgender men/transmasculine person: people identifying as men or along the masculine spectrum and assigned female at birth.

Transgender women/transfeminine person: people identifying as women or along the feminine spectrum and assigned male at birth.

Nonbinary people: people with a gender identity outside of the cultural binary of "man" or "woman." Some labels people may use to describe themselves: nonbinary, genderfluid, genderqueer, agender, pangender, bigender, gender nonconforming.

Intersex people: people born with reproductive or sexual anatomy that does not align with binary definitions of female or male due to any of a variety of variations in sex characteristics (VSC). May or may not be used by a given individual to describe themselves.

1.2 US Demographics

Investigators have estimated at least 25 million people globally are TGD (Winter et al. 2016). Based on US Centers for Disease Control and Prevention (CDC)

Behavioral Risk Factor Surveillance System (BRFSS) data from 2017 to 2020, 1.6 million US people aged ≥13 years were TGD, 38.5% of whom were transgender women, and 35.9% were transgender men (Herman et al. 2022). The remaining respondents (25.6%) were nonbinary (referred to as "gender nonconforming" on BRFSS questionnaires) (Cicero et al. 2020). Respondents identified as straight, lesbian, gay, bisexual, or pansexual (Meyer et al. 2017). TGD people living in the USA are racially and ethnically diverse. TGD adults identified as Asian (5.8%), American Indian or Alaska Native (1.1%), Black (13%), Native Hawaiian, Pacific Islander, biracial, multiracial, or another race or ethnicity (3.8%), and White (54.7%) (Herman et al. 2022). Twenty-one percent of TGD adults identified as Hispanic or Latinx (where "Latinx" was used as a nonbinary form of Latino or Latina) (Herman et al. 2022). Experts anticipate the number of US TGD older adults will increase over the next few decades (Fredriksen-Goldsen 2016). Between 2017 and 2020, 0.3% of US adults ≥65 years of age were TGD (Herman et al. 2022).

1.3 Health Disparities and Co-occurring Medical Conditions

1.3.1 Barriers to Healthcare Access

TGD people face social and structural stigma, discrimination, and barriers to healthcare access (Scheim et al. 2022; James et al. 2016). In a 2015 nonprobability survey of approximately 28,000 US transgender adults, nearly one-quarter of respondents avoided seeking necessary medical care within the year prior to completing the questionnaire, largely because of fear of being disrespected or mistreated (James et al. 2016). Among those who reported receiving medical care, many respondents experienced verbal harassment from healthcare providers, encountered clinical providers who refused to offer gender-affirming medical treatment, or needed to teach clinical providers about transgender people to receive appropriate medical care (James et al. 2016).

Anti-transgender stigma and discrimination are associated with poor health outcomes for TGD people (Coleman et al. 2022). Among >400 TGD adult respondents in a statewide US survey, investigators observed that delaying healthcare due to fear of discrimination was predictive of lower self-reported general health relative to respondents who did not delay seeking healthcare ($\beta = -0.26$, $P < 0.05$) (Seelman et al. 2017). In a US probability survey of 271 TGD adults and 1,162 cisgender adults, TGD respondents had significantly higher age-adjusted odds of reporting poor to fair general health (adjusted odds ratio: 2.50, $P < 0.001$), reporting days per month of poor physical health (adjusted odds ratio: 3.87, $P < 0.001$), and reporting days per month of poor mental health relative to cisgender respondents (adjusted odds ratio: 7.09, $P < 0.001$) (Feldman et al. 2021). Finally, in a separate cohort of approximately 2,500 US lesbian, gay, bisexual, and transgender adults ≥50 years of age, transgender people had significantly lower odds of utilizing preventive health screenings relative to cisgender adults, including mammogram, Papanicolaou (Pap) smear, osteoporosis test, and prostate-specific antigen tests

(Hoy-Ellis et al. 2022). These factors contribute to highly individualized medical experiences for all TGD people.

1.3.2 Chronic Disease Burden

Knowledge about the chronic disease burden among TGD people is limited (Rich et al. 2020). Transgender women have at least 49 times higher odds of HIV globally compared with the general population (aged 15–49 years) (Baral et al. 2013). Transgender men have 6.8 times higher odds of HIV relative to the general population (Stutterheim et al. 2021). HIV prevalence among nonbinary people is currently unknown. Several observational studies have characterized cardiovascular disease risk and metabolic disorders among TGD people undergoing hormone therapy (Rich et al. 2020; Defreyne et al. 2019). One retrospective cohort study in a large US-based healthcare system observed two times higher venous thromboembolism incidence among transgender women than cisgender men or cisgender women (Getahun et al. 2018). Limited clinical data suggest type 2 diabetes incidence may be higher among transgender women than cisgender women (hazard ratio: 1.4, 95% confidence interval: 1.1–1.8), although an association with estrogen treatment appears unlikely (Islam et al. 2021). Testosterone treatment is associated with decreased high-density lipoprotein concentrations, but researchers observed mixed effects of testosterone on low-density lipoprotein and triglyceride concentrations for TGD people (Coleman et al. 2022). Hormone therapy is associated with increased quality of life for TGD people (Baker et al. 2021), and it is a key part of the standard of gender-affirming medical care. Thus, experts typically recommend a harm-reduction approach when prescribing hormone therapy in the context of modifiable and non-modifiable cardiovascular risk factors (Deutsch 2016; Ramsay and Safer 2022).

Investigators have documented several sex-related and gender-related differences in chronic disease risk and outcomes in the general adult population, ranging from autoimmune disorders and infectious diseases (Klein and Flanagan 2016), cardiovascular disease (Colafella and Denton 2018), diabetes (Tramunt et al. 2020), to some neurodegenerative disorders (Ferretti et al. 2018; Gillies et al. 2014). Complex interactions between sex-specific genetic and hormonal factors, gender-specific behaviors, and environmental factors contribute to these differences (F. Mauvais-Jarvis et al. 2020; Khramtsova et al. 2019). Further research is needed to understand how these factors may influence the health and well-being of TGD people.

1.3.3 Considerations Across the Lifespan

TGD older adults are an increasingly visible population with unmet gaps in medical care. Although social support and having feelings of belonging within the lesbian, gay, bisexual, and transgender community were positively associated with perceived physical health among transgender older adults, social support and belonging were lower for TGD older adults than cisgender counterparts (Fredriksen-Goldsen et al. 2014). Several observational studies have suggested TGD older adults may have a higher prevalence of cognitive impairment than the general older adult population (Cheung et al. 2023). For example, in a cross-sectional survey of TGD adults ≥50 years of age, respondents who experienced discrimination in medical settings because of their gender identity had significantly higher odds of subjective cognitive decline compared with TGD older adults who did not (odds ratio: 7.49, 95% confidence interval: 1.71 to 32.79, $P = 0.008$) (Lambrou et al. 2022). In an analysis of Medicare fee-for-service data from 2009 to 2017, the predicted probability of dementia was higher for TGD older adult beneficiaries than cisgender older adult beneficiaries after adjusting for age, race, and ethnicity, census region, and the number of months of enrollment (transgender women vs. cisgender women: 21.3% vs. 13.6%, respectively, $P < 0.0001$; transgender men vs. cisgender men: 20.2% vs. 12.3%, respectively, $P < 0.0001$) (Hughto et al. 2023). Multiple chronic conditions often translate into increased prescription medication use, polypharmacy, and potential drug–drug interactions among older adults (Cerreta et al. 2023). Studies characterizing the scope of these medication-related issues for TGD older adults are lacking (Gamble et al. 2020). Research addressing this topic is needed.

TGD older adults have diverse gender-affirming medical care experiences across the life course. For example, TGD older adults may start hormone therapy later in life, including 50 years or older (see Sect. 2.2) (Gooren and T'Sjoen 2018; Cheung et al. 2023). Among >200 TGD people who presented for gender-affirming surgery at a large US-based academic medical center, patients ≥40 years of age self-reported longer timeframes before starting hormone therapy and other types of gender-affirming care over their lifetime than patients <40 years of age (average timeframes: 37 years vs. 16 years, respectively, $P < 0.001$) (Zaliznyak et al. 2021). Because TGD people may continue hormone therapy long-term (Cheung et al. 2023), increased knowledge on managing hormone therapy for TGD older adults is needed (Gooren and T'Sjoen 2018). Effects of physiologic changes among cisgender older adults on drug safety, including changes in body composition, kidney or liver, are well characterized (Cerreta et al. 2023), but pharmacologic considerations for transgender older adults are an unmet knowledge gap.

2 Pharmacologic Considerations for TGD Adults Undergoing Hormone Therapy

Scientists have characterized differences in medication safety and effectiveness for cisgender women and cisgender men (Cirrincione and Huang 2021), but implications for TGD people undergoing hormone therapy are unknown. The remainder of this chapter focuses on hormone therapy for TGD adults. Specifically, we focus on the role of hormone therapy in gender-affirming medical care, its physiologic and pharmacologic effects, and its potential contribution to interindividual variability in pharmacokinetic processes for TGD people.

2.1 TGD-Inclusive Pharmacologic Research

TGD people face certain barriers related to clinical research participation. These barriers may include concerns about privacy and exploitive or opportunistic research (Asquith et al. 2021) and mistrust of medical and research communities (Owen-Smith et al. 2016). TGD and cisgender scientists in HIV research have made progress in engaging TGD communities in Phase 3 clinical trials (Cirrincione et al. 2023) and conducting drug–hormone interaction studies for HIV pharmacologic prevention interventions (Yager and Anderson 2020). As transgender medicine grows in scope, investigators should prioritize including TGD people in pharmacologic studies in phase 1, 2, and 3 clinical trials across all therapeutic areas (Yager and Anderson 2020). The effects of hormone therapy on drug metabolism and drug transport of other medications among TGD people are unknown. Clinical mechanistic studies in vivo are required to establish the pharmacologic effects of hormone therapy on major drug-handling pathways among TGD people (Cirrincione and Huang 2021).

2.2 Overview of Hormone Therapy

The World Professional Association for Transgender Health (WPATH) issued standards of care for the health of TGD people over the past 40 years and published Standards of Care version 8 in 2022 (Coleman et al. 2022). WPATH recommended hormone therapy as part of the standard of medical care for TGD people (Hembree et al. 2017; Coleman et al. 2022). WPATH also endorsed the Endocrine Society professional guidelines, which provided specific clinical guidance for hormone therapy management (including administration routes and dosing) and clinical laboratory monitoring for TGD people taking hormone therapy (Hembree et al. 2017). Broadly, hormone therapy includes either testosterone or estrogen treatment and aligns a person's secondary sex characteristics with their gender identity (Coleman et al. 2022). Clinicians individualize hormone regimen dosing, agents, and administration routes based on a person's gender expression goals and the safety profiles for specific agents (Table 1) (Hembree et al. 2017).

Clinical laboratory values change markedly during hormone therapy (Hembree et al. 2017). For TGD adults undergoing 12 months of testosterone treatment, investigators have observed 15- to 20-fold increased average serum testosterone concentrations (total and free) and 40% decreased serum estradiol concentrations (Cirrincione and Huang 2021). For TGD adults undergoing estrogen treatment, investigators have observed up to ninefold increased average serum estradiol concentrations and 93–98% decreased testosterone concentrations (total and free) (Cirrincione and Huang 2021).

Changes in sex steroid concentrations have direct effects on interpreting other clinical laboratory values. For example, in a longitudinal electronic health record study of hematological changes among nearly 1,000 transgender adults, investigators observed markedly increased hemoglobin and hematocrit values for

Table 1 Typical agents recommended for TGD adults undergoing hormone therapy

Regimen	Typical medication classes	Prescribed agents
Testosterone treatment		
	• Androgenic agent	• Testosterone (gel, compounded cream, or injection)
Estrogen treatment[a]		
	• Estrogenic agent • Antiandrogenic agent	• 17β-estradiol (tablet, patch, or injection) • Cyproterone acetate[b], spironolactone, or gonadotropin agonist (e.g., leuprolide acetate)

Table modified from Hembree et al. (2017), Coleman et al. (2022). This table provides an overview of hormone therapies that may be recommended for TGD people. It is not a comprehensive list of all agents that might be prescribed in clinical practice

[a] Clinical providers may add-on oral progestogens (e.g., micronized progesterone) or 5α-reductase inhibitors (e.g., finasteride) to support a person's gender expression goals

[b] Not approved in the USA

patients undergoing testosterone treatment and markedly decreased values among patients undergoing estrogen treatment (Antun et al. 2020). Based on these findings, investigators proposed using hematologic reference intervals aligned with an individual's gender identity for TGD people undergoing hormone therapy (Antun et al. 2020). These findings highlight the effect of sex steroids on clinical laboratory values, specifically those with sex-specific reference ranges for the general adult population.

2.3 Drug Absorption

No clinical studies have examined gastric transit times or changes in drug absorption for TGD people undergoing hormone therapy. As discussed in other chapters, gastric processes differ between cisgender women and cisgender men (Vinarov et al. 2021). Examples include slower gastric emptying time and lower gastric acid secretion among cisgender women (Vinarov et al. 2021). Evidence for sex-related differences in nonoral drug disposition is limited, but data suggest cisgender women may have slower intramuscular absorption of certain medications than cisgender men (Franck Mauvais-Jarvis et al. 2021). Clinical and animal model data suggest estrogens and progestogens, but not androgens, contribute to slow gastric emptying times (Jiang et al. 2019). Investigators have yet to characterize the effects of hormone therapy on oral or nonoral drug absorption for TGD people (Yager and Anderson 2020).

2.4 Drug Distribution

Hormone therapy causes marked body composition changes within the first year of treatment. A meta-analysis of 10 prospective European cohorts (approximately 500 transgender adults total with baseline average body mass indices between 20 and 25 kg/m^2) reported increased total body weight within the first 12 months of either testosterone or estrogen treatment relative to baseline (up to +1.8 kg compared with measured body weight before hormone therapy) (Klaver et al. 2017). For transgender adults undergoing testosterone treatment (average age 30 years), total body fat decreased significantly from baseline (−2.6 kg, 95% confidence interval: −3.9 to −1.4; $P < 0.0001$), whereas lean body weight increased significantly from baseline (+3.9 kg, 95% confidence interval: 3.2 to 4.5; $P < 0.00001$). Conversely, transgender adults undergoing estrogen treatment (average age 33 years) had significantly increased total body fat from baseline (+3.0 kg, 95% confidence interval: 2.0 to 3.9; $P < 0.00001$) and significantly decreased lean body weight from baseline (−2.4 kg, 95% confidence interval: −2.8 to −2.1; $P < 0.00001$) (Klaver et al. 2017). Increased total body fat may increase the volume of distribution for certain fat-soluble medications (e.g., neuromuscular blocking agents vecuronium and rocuronium and the benzodiazepine diazepam) (Soldin and Mattison 2009).

Limited clinical data for TGD people observed unchanged serum albumin and corticosteroid-binding globulin concentrations during hormone therapy (Cirrincione and Huang 2021). Sex hormone binding globulin concentrations increased modestly for TGD adults undergoing estrogen treatment (1.3-fold) and decreased markedly for TGD adults undergoing testosterone treatment (51–54%) (Cirrincione and Huang 2021). These findings have implications for pharmacokinetic modeling (Cirrincione and Huang 2021).

2.5 Drug Metabolism

No clinical studies have investigated the effects of hormone therapy on the apparent activities of major drug-metabolizing enzymes among TGD adults. Several drug-metabolizing enzymes in the cytochrome P450 (CYP) enzyme superfamily exhibit differences in apparent activities between cisgender women and cisgender men (Vo and Paine 2022). A comprehensive review of sex-related differences in CYP activity and expression is covered elsewhere in this textbook. As one example among phase I drug-metabolizing enzymes, investigators observed higher (~35%) apparent CYP3A activity for cisgender women than cisgender men (Cirrincione and Huang 2021). Supraphysiologic estradiol concentrations increased CYP3A4 protein levels in human hepatocytes in vitro (Le et al. 2022). Apparent CYP1A2 activity is lower among cisgender women than cisgender men (Cirrincione and Huang 2021). Clinical and in vitro data suggested estrogen has an inhibitory effect on CYP1A2 activity (Le et al. 2022). The clinical relevance of these findings for TGD people undergoing estrogen treatment remains to be determined. Sex-related differences for other major CYPs (CYP2B6, 2C9, 2C19, 2D6, 2E1) are mixed (Franck Mauvais-Jarvis et al. 2021). Several phase II conjugation enzymes have sex-related differences in expression and activity, including uridine diphosphate-glucuronosyltransferase (UGT) 2B17 and 2B15, glutathione S-transferase A1/A2, and sulfotransferase (SULT) 1A1 and 1E1 (Franck Mauvais-Jarvis et al. 2021). Clinical implications for TGD people, particularly those undergoing testosterone treatment, remain to be determined.

2.6 Drug Elimination

The effects of hormone therapy on kidney function is an ongoing area of investigation for TGD people (Krupka et al. 2022). Based on findings from clinical pharmacokinetic studies, plasma concentrations of tenofovir (as tenofovir disoproxil fumarate) and emtricitabine, two anti-HIV agents that are predominantly renally eliminated as unchanged drugs, are 12–27% lower among transgender women undergoing estrogen treatment relative to cisgender men and transgender women not yet taking estrogen treatment (Yager and Anderson 2020). In a separate analysis, investigators observed that estimated creatinine clearance was 60% higher among transgender women than cisgender men ($P = 0.04$), and estimated creatinine clearance influenced tenofovir and emtricitabine clearance based on population pharmacokinetic modeling (Tanaudommongkon et al. 2022).

In a meta-analysis of nine clinical cohorts of TGD adults taking hormone therapy, adults undergoing testosterone treatment had markedly increased serum creatinine concentrations after 12 months of treatment (+0.15 mg/dL, 95% confidence interval: 0.00 to 0.29), whereas adults undergoing estrogen treatment had no significant change in serum creatinine concentrations (−0.05 mg/dL, 95% confidence interval: −0.16 to +0.05) (Krupka et al. 2022). Blood urea nitrogen concentrations did not change markedly during either testosterone or estrogen treatment. Researchers have yet to characterize potential changes in other kidney function biomarkers before and during hormone therapy (e.g., cystatin C, albuminuria, proteinuria) (Krupka et al. 2022).

In one small longitudinal clinical cohort study, investigators observed an 18% apparent decrease in estimated glomerular filtration rate among transgender adults after 12 months of testosterone treatment (using creatinine-based estimating equations with a female modifier for both pre-testosterone and post-testosterone estimates) (Fadich et al. 2021). Median serum creatinine increased by 0.12 mg/dL from baseline to follow-up ($P = 0.0006$). However, investigators did not assess changes in lean muscle mass, which may have contributed to increased serum creatinine concentrations (see Sect. 2.4). Because creatinine-based kidney function estimating equations require the use of stable serum creatinine concentrations and a binary sex modifier (male or female) (Fadich et al. 2021), prospective, longitudinal studies using a gold-standard indicator of glomerular filtration (e.g., iohexol) are needed to characterize potential changes in kidney function and to address altered drug elimination among TGD people undergoing hormone therapy.

2.7 Drug Transport

No studies have examined the clinical effects of hormone therapy on drug transporter activities for TGD adults. Sex-related effects on drug transport protein expression are mixed (Vo and Paine 2022). For example, investigators observed threefold higher hepatic expression of P-glycoprotein, an adenosine triphosphate (ATP)-binding cassette efflux transporter, among cisgender men versus cisgender women but no difference in intestinal P-glycoprotein expression (Vo and Paine 2022). Investigators observed no sex-related differences in the expression of hepatic breast cancer resistance protein (BCRP), an efflux transporter, or organic anion transporting polypeptides (OATP) 1B1, 1B3, 2B1, uptake transporters (Vo and Paine 2022). Animal model data suggest testosterone treatment activated protein expression of kidney organic anion transporter 1 and organic cation transporter 2 (Le et al. 2022). The clinical effects of hormone therapy on drug transport proteins for TGD people remain to be determined.

3 Limitations of Sex/Gender as Binary Variable in Biomedical and Pharmacologic Research

All sex-related and gender-related pharmacological knowledge relies on a binary male–female framework (Bhargava et al. 2021; Franck Mauvais-Jarvis et al. 2021). However, experts recognize the binary male–female framework fails to capture the spectrum of sex and its associated physiological and behavioral phenotypes, with unclear implications for growing fields, including nanomedicine (Sharifi et al. 2021). As one example, variations in sex characteristics (also described as "intersex") include several biologic underpinnings such as genetic and hormonal factors (Conway 2022). Additionally, investigators have noted gaps in how sex-related differences are studied and reported in the literature (Garcia-Sifuentes and Maney 2021). Appropriately designed studies are needed in pharmacologic research to identify and characterize sex-specific outcomes.

4 Conclusions and Clinical Implications

TGD people may undergo testosterone or estrogen treatment as part of their medical care. Hormone therapy is part of the standard of gender-affirming medical care. Yet, the effects of hormone therapy on the safety and effectiveness of other prescribed medications among TGD people have not been established (Cirrincione and Huang 2021). Although experimental and animal model data suggest potential hormone-mediated changes in major drug-handling proteins may exist for TGD adults undergoing hormone therapy, empirical clinical data for drug–hormone interactions are lacking due to TGD people facing significant barriers and stigma accessing healthcare and participating in clinical research.

•Take Home Messages

- TGD people are a diverse and increasingly visible population, and transgender medicine is a growing clinical field.
- Clinical pharmacological data from the general adult population suggest medication safety and efficacy may differ between cisgender women and cisgender men. Yet, the implications for TGD adults, and the role of sex steroids in these findings, are unknown.
- TGD populations are underrepresented in clinical research, and pharmacologic knowledge for TGD people undergoing hormone therapy is lacking.
- Increased pharmacological studies specific to TGD populations or enriched for TGD priority populations are warranted.

Acknowledgment RC is supported by the National Institute of Health Biological Mechanisms for Healthy Aging Training Grant under Award Number T32AG066574. LRC is supported by the National Institute of General Medical Sciences of the National Institutes of Health under Award Number K23GM147350. The opinions expressed in this manuscript are those of the authors and should not be interpreted as the position of the National Institutes of Health.

References

Antun A, Zhang Q, Bhasin S, Bradlyn A, Flanders WD, Getahun D et al (2020) Longitudinal changes in hematologic parameters among transgender people receiving hormone therapy. Journal of the Endocrine Society 4(11):bvaa119

Asquith A, Sava L, Harris AB, Radix AE, Pardee DJ, Reisner SL (2021) Patient-centered practices for engaging transgender and gender diverse patients in clinical research studies. BMC Med Res Methodol 21(1):202. https://doi.org/10.1186/s12874-021-01328-4

Baker KE, Wilson LM, Sharma R, Dukhanin V, McArthur K, Robinson KA (2021) Hormone therapy, mental health, and quality of life among transgender people: a systematic review. J Endocr Soc 5(4):bvab011

Baral SD, Poteat T, Stromdahl S, Wirtz AL, Guadamuz TE, Beyrer C (2013) Worldwide burden of HIV in transgender women: a systematic review and meta-analysis. Lancet Infect Dis 13(3): 214–222. https://doi.org/10.1016/s1473-3099(12)70315-8

Bhargava A, Arnold AP, Bangasser DA, Denton KM, Gupta A, Hilliard Krause LM et al (2021) Considering sex as a biological variable in basic and clinical studies: an endocrine society scientific statement. Endocr Rev 42:219. https://doi.org/10.1210/endrev/bnaa034

Cerreta F, Vučić K, Laslop A (2023) Assessing medicines for use in the geriatric population. Clin Pharmacol Ther 113(3):536–540. https://doi.org/10.1002/cpt.2793

Cheung AS, Nolan BJ, Zwickl S (2023) Transgender health and the impact of aging and menopause. Climacteric 1-7. https://doi.org/10.1080/13697137.2023.2176217

Cicero EC, Reisner SL, Merwin EI, Humphreys JC, Silva SG (2020) The health status of transgender and gender nonbinary adults in the United States. PloS One 15(2):e0228765. https://doi.org/10.1371/journal.pone.0228765

Cirrincione LR, Huang KJ (2021) Sex and gender differences in clinical pharmacology: implications for transgender medicine. Clin Pharmacol Ther 110(4):897–908. https://doi.org/10.1002/cpt.2234

Cirrincione LR, Grieve VLB, Holloway J, Marzinke MA (2023) Inclusion of transgender and gender diverse people in phase III trials: examples from HIV pharmacologic prevention studies. Clin Pharmacol Ther 113(3):557–564. https://doi.org/10.1002/cpt.2801

Colafella KMM, Denton KM (2018) Sex-specific differences in hypertension and associated cardiovascular disease. Nat Rev Nephrol 14(3):185–201. https://doi.org/10.1038/nrneph.2017.189

Coleman E, Radix A, Bouman W, Brown G, Vries A, Deutsch M et al (2022) Standards of care for the health of transgender and gender diverse people, version 8. Int J Transgender Health 23:S1–S259. https://doi.org/10.1080/26895269.2022.2100644

Conway GS (2022) Differences in sex development (DSD) and related conditions: mechanisms, prevalences and changing practice. Int J Impot Res. https://doi.org/10.1038/s41443-022-00606-z

Defreyne J, Van de Bruaene LDL, Rietzschel E, Van Schuylenbergh J, T'Sjoen GGR (2019) Effects of gender-affirming hormones on lipid, metabolic, and cardiac surrogate blood markers in transgender persons. Clin Chem 65(1):119–134. https://doi.org/10.1373/clinchem.2018.288241

Deutsch MB (2016) Guidelines for the primary and gender-affirming care of transgender and gender nonbinary people. University of California, San Francisco

Fadich SK, Kalayjian A, Greene DN, Cirrincione LR (2021) A retrospective analysis of creatinine-based kidney function with and without sex assigned at birth among transgender adults. Ann Pharmacother 56(7):791–799. https://doi.org/10.1177/10600280211050120

Feldman JL, Luhur WE, Herman JL, Poteat T, Meyer IH (2021) Health and health care access in the US transgender population health (TransPop) survey. Andrology 9(6):1707–1718

Ferretti MT, Iulita MF, Cavedo E, Chiesa PA, Schumacher Dimech A, Santuccione Chadha A et al (2018) Sex differences in Alzheimer disease - the gateway to precision medicine. Nat Rev Neurol 14(8):457–469. https://doi.org/10.1038/s41582-018-0032-9

Fredriksen-Goldsen KI (2016) The future of LGBT+ aging: a blueprint for action in services, policies, and research. Generations 40(2):6–15

Fredriksen-Goldsen KI, Cook-Daniels L, Kim H-J, Erosheva EA, Emlet CA, Hoy-Ellis CP et al (2014) Physical and mental health of transgender older adults: an at-risk and underserved population. Gerontologist 54(3):488–500

Gamble RM, Taylor SS, Huggins AD, Ehrenfeld JM (2020) Trans-specific geriatric health assessment (TGHA): an inclusive clinical guideline for the geriatric transgender patient in a primary care setting. Maturitas 132:70–75. https://doi.org/10.1016/j.maturitas.2019.12.005

Garcia-Sifuentes Y, Maney DL (2021) Reporting and misreporting of sex differences in the biological sciences. Elife 10. https://doi.org/10.7554/eLife.70817

Getahun D, Nash R, Flanders WD, Baird TC, Becerra-Culqui TA, Cromwell L et al (2018) Cross-sex hormones and acute cardiovascular events in transgender persons: a cohort study. Ann Intern Med 169(4):205–213

Gillies GE, Pienaar IS, Vohra S, Qamhawi Z (2014) Sex differences in Parkinson's disease. Front Neuroendocrinol 35(3):370–384. https://doi.org/10.1016/j.yfrne.2014.02.002

Gooren LJ, T'Sjoen G (2018) Endocrine treatment of aging transgender people. Rev Endocr Metab Disord 19(3):253–262. https://doi.org/10.1007/s11154-018-9449-0

Hembree WC, Cohen-Kettenis PT, Gooren L, Hannema SE, Meyer WJ, Murad MH et al (2017) Endocrine treatment of gender-dysphoric/gender-incongruent persons: an endocrine society clinical practice guideline. J Clin Endocrinol Metab 102(11):3869–3903. https://doi.org/10.1210/jc.2017-01658

Herman JL, Flores AR, O'Neill KK (2022) How many adults and youth identify as transgender in the United States? https://williamsinstitute.law.ucla.edu/wp-content/uploads/Trans-Pop-Update-Jun-2022.pdf. Accessed 1 Sept 2022

Hoy-Ellis CP, Fredriksen-Goldsen KI, Kim H-J (2022) Utilization of recommended preventive health screenings between transgender and cisgender older adults in sexual and gender minority communities. J Aging Health 34(6–8):844–857. https://doi.org/10.1177/08982643211068557

Hughto JM, Varma H, Babbs G, Yee K, Alpert A, Hughes L et al (2023) Disparities in health condition diagnoses among aging transgender and cisgender medicare beneficiaries, 2008-2017. Front Endocrinol 14, 1102348. https://doi.org/10.3389/fendo.2023.1102348

Islam N, Nash R, Zhang Q, Panagiotakopoulos L, Daley T, Bhasin S et al (2021) Is there a link between hormone use and diabetes incidence in transgender people? Data from the STRONG cohort. J Clin Endocrinol Metabol 107(4):e1549–e1557. https://doi.org/10.1210/clinem/dgab832

James S, Herman J, Rankin S, Keisling M, Mottet L, Anafi MA (2016) The report of the 2015 US transgender survey

Jiang Y, Greenwood-Van Meerveld B, Johnson AC, Travagli RA (2019) Role of estrogen and stress on the brain-gut axis. Am J Physiol Gastrointest Liver Physiol 317(2):G203–G209. https://doi.org/10.1152/ajpgi.00144.2019

Khramtsova EA, Davis LK, Stranger BE (2019) The role of sex in the genomics of human complex traits. Nat Rev Genet 20(3):173–190. https://doi.org/10.1038/s41576-018-0083-1

Klaver M, Dekker M, de Mutsert R, Twisk JWR, den Heijer M (2017) Cross-sex hormone therapy in transgender persons affects total body weight, body fat and lean body mass: a meta-analysis. Andrologia 49(5). https://doi.org/10.1111/and.12660

Klein SL, Flanagan KL (2016) Sex differences in immune responses. Nat Rev Immunol 16(10): 626–638. https://doi.org/10.1038/nri.2016.90

Krupka E, Curtis S, Ferguson T, Whitlock R, Askin N, Millar AC et al (2022) The effect of gender-affirming hormone therapy on measures of kidney function: a systematic review and meta-analysis. Clin J Am Soc Nephrol 17(9):1305–1315

Lambrou NH, Gleason CE, Obedin-Maliver J, Lunn MR, Flentje A, Lubensky ME et al (2022) Subjective cognitive decline associated with discrimination in medical settings among transgender and nonbinary older adults. Int J Environ Res Public Health 19(15). https://doi.org/10.3390/ijerph19159168

Le A, Huang KJ, Cirrincione LR (2022) Regulation of drug-metabolizing enzymes by sex-related hormones: clinical implications for transgender medicine. Trends Pharmacol Sci 43(7): 582–592. https://doi.org/10.1016/j.tips.2022.03.006

Mauvais-Jarvis F, Bairey Merz N, Barnes PJ, Brinton RD, Carrero JJ, DeMeo DL et al (2020) Sex and gender: modifiers of health, disease, and medicine. Lancet 396(10250):565–582. https://doi.org/10.1016/s0140-6736(20)31561-0

Mauvais-Jarvis F, Berthold HK, Campesi I, Carrero J-J, Dhakal S, Franconi F et al (2021) Sex- and gender-based pharmacological response to drugs. Pharmacol Rev 73(2):730. https://doi.org/10.1124/pharmrev.120.000206

Meyer IH, Brown TNT, Herman JL, Reisner SL, Bockting WO (2017) Demographic characteristics and health status of transgender adults in select US regions: behavioral risk factor surveillance system, 2014. Am J Public Health 107(4):582–589. https://doi.org/10.2105/AJPH.2016.303648

Owen-Smith AA, Woodyatt C, Sineath RC, Hunkeler EM, Barnwell T, Graham A et al (2016) Perceptions of barriers to and facilitators of participation in health research among transgender people. Transgend Health 1(1):187–196. https://doi.org/10.1089/trgh.2016.0023

Ramsay A, Safer JD (2022) Update in adult transgender medicine. Annu Rev Med 74:117. https://doi.org/10.1146/annurev-med-020222-121106

Rich AJ, Scheim AI, Koehoorn M, Poteat T (2020) Non-HIV chronic disease burden among transgender populations globally: a systematic review and narrative synthesis. Prev Med Rep 20:101259. https://doi.org/10.1016/j.pmedr.2020.101259

Scheim AI, Baker KE, Restar AJ, Sell RL (2022) Health and health care among transgender adults in the United States. Annu Rev Public Health 43:503–523

Seelman KL, Colón-Diaz MJP, LeCroix RH, Xavier-Brier M, Kattari L (2017) Transgender noninclusive healthcare and delaying care because of fear: connections to general health and mental health among transgender adults. Transgender Health 2(1):17–28. https://doi.org/10.1089/trgh.2016.0024

Sharifi S, Caracciolo G, Pozzi D, Digiacomo L, Swann J, Daldrup-Link HE et al (2021) The role of sex as a biological variable in the efficacy and toxicity of therapeutic nanomedicine. Adv Drug Deliv Rev 174:337–347. https://doi.org/10.1016/j.addr.2021.04.028

Soldin OP, Mattison DR (2009) Sex differences in pharmacokinetics and pharmacodynamics. Clin Pharmacokinet 48(3):143–157. https://doi.org/10.2165/00003088-200948030-00001

Stutterheim SE, van Dijk M, Wang H, Jonas KJ (2021) The worldwide burden of HIV in transgender individuals: an updated systematic review and meta-analysis. PloS One 16(12): e0260063. https://doi.org/10.1371/journal.pone.0260063

Tanaudommongkon A, Chaturvedula A, Hendrix CW, Fuchs EJ, Shieh E, Bakshi RP et al (2022) Population pharmacokinetics of tenofovir, emtricitabine and intracellular metabolites in transgender women. Br J Clin Pharmacol 88(8):3674–3682. https://doi.org/10.1111/bcp.15310

Tramunt B, Smati S, Grandgeorge N, Lenfant F, Arnal JF, Montagner A et al (2020) Sex differences in metabolic regulation and diabetes susceptibility. Diabetologia 63(3):453–461. https://doi.org/10.1007/s00125-019-05040-3

Vinarov Z, Abdallah M, Agundez JAG, Allegaert K, Basit AW, Braeckmans M et al (2021) Impact of gastrointestinal tract variability on oral drug absorption and pharmacokinetics: an UNGAP review. Eur J Pharm Sci 162:105812. https://doi.org/10.1016/j.ejps.2021.105812

Vo KD, Paine MF (2022) Sex-specific pharmacological differences. In: Atkinson's principles of clinical pharmacology. Elsevier, pp 405–424

Winter S, Diamond M, Green J, Karasic D, Reed T, Whittle S et al (2016) Transgender people: health at the margins of society. Lancet 388(10042):390–400

Yager JL, Anderson PL (2020) Pharmacology and drug interactions with HIV PrEP in transgender persons receiving gender affirming hormone therapy. Expert Opin Drug Metab Toxicol 16(6): 463–474. https://doi.org/10.1080/17425255.2020.1752662

Zaliznyak M, Yuan N, Bresee C, Freedman A, Garcia MM (2021) How early in life do transgender adults begin to experience gender dysphoria? Why this matters for patients, providers, and for our healthcare system. Sexual Med 9(6):100448–100448. https://doi.org/10.1016/j.esxm.2021.100448

Sex and Gender Differences in the Pharmacology of the Overactive Urinary Bladder

Andrea Pautz and Martin C. Michel

Contents

Abstract

Dysfunction of the lower urinary tract in general and the overactive bladder syndrome (OAB) in particular are prevalent and have major impact on the quality of life of the afflicted patients and their partners. We concisely review sex and gender differences in patients and animal models in physiological bladder function, its alterations in disease (mostly OAB), and its responses to treatment. Women appear to have a smaller functional bladder capacity and, therefore, must void more often than men. On the other hand, men have a greater bladder outlet resistance, which is partly attributed to a longer urethra and partly to the

A. Pautz · M. C. Michel (✉)
Department of Pharmacology, University Medical Center, Johannes Gutenberg University, Mainz, Germany
e-mail: marmiche@uni-mainz.de

S. E. Tsirka, M. Acosta-Martinez (eds.), *Sex and Gender Effects in Pharmacology*, Handbook of Experimental Pharmacology 282,
https://doi.org/10.1007/164_2023_667

presence of the prostate. Sex and gender differences in bladder contractility appear small and were not found consistently. The ability of bladder smooth muscle to relax may be somewhat smaller in females. However, females are heavily underrepresented in experimental studies on bladder function. Stress urinary incontinence is found predominantly in women (particularly those after childbirth). OAB is similarly prevalent in men and women. Females seek treatment much more often and are overrepresented in clinical trials. Treatment responses in OAB patients are similar in both genders for oral medications, but improvements upon injections of onabotulinum toxin type A appear smaller in men. We conclude that there is no evidence for major sex and gender differences in bladder dysfunction as related to OAB and its treatment responses, but female animals are heavily underrepresented in experimental studies.

Keywords

Muscarinic receptor antagonists · Onabotulinum toxin type A · Overactive bladder syndrome · Treatment · Urinary bladder

1 Introduction

The urinary bladder stores the urine continuously produced by the kidneys to enable intermittent voiding under appropriate settings, which includes socially acceptable situations in humans. To enable this, urine storage and voiding are regulated by a complex network consisting of sensors in the bladder wall that activate afferent pathways (Kanai and Wyndaele 2011), of neuronal networks in the spinal cord and brain that process and coordinate such incoming signals (Fowler et al. 2008; Ikeda 2021), and of efferent pathways that lead to bladder smooth muscle relaxation during the storage and to contraction during the voiding phase (Beckel and Holstege 2011).

Disturbances of bladder functions can be grouped into those of storage and those of voiding. The former can involve too much or too little contraction of the detrusor smooth muscle, whereas the latter can involve too much or too little bladder outlet resistance. Disturbances of the storage function can lead to clinical conditions such as the overactive bladder syndrome (OAB) typically attributed to detrusor overactivity (DO), or stress urinary incontinence if there is too little outlet resistance. Stress urinary incontinence is mostly found in women, particularly in those having given vaginal childbirth (Hampel et al. 2004; Padmanabhan and Dmochowski 2014); its presence in men is largely limited to post-prostatectomy. Disturbances in voiding function can occur if the detrusor contracts too little (underactive bladder syndrome) (Cho and Kim 2020) or if the bladder outlet resistance is too high, e.g., in elderly men with an enlarged prostate (Bosch et al. 2019). As stress urinary incontinence is predominantly found in women and increased bladder outlet resistance manifesting as lower urinary tract symptoms suggestive of benign prostatic hyperplasia exclusively in men, these will not be covered in this chapter on sex and gender differences.

Possible gender differences related to bladder cancer will also not be discussed, although this is a condition occurring more frequently in men.

This chapter will focus on sex and gender differences in bladder physiology and pathology, particularly as related to OAB, and differences in response to OAB-related medications. OAB has been defined by the International Continence Society by the presence of urgency, with or without incontinence, usually accompanied by frequency and nocturia (Abrams et al. 2002). Within each section, we will initially discuss clinical findings and then experimental data that can provide possible mechanistic explanations for the clinical data.

2 Healthy Bladder and Its Physiology

2.1 Clinical Data

In a matched pairs analysis, men had a greater daily fluid intake and greater mean voided volume than women; accordingly, females had more micturition than males, which became even more pronounced when number of voids were adjusted for differences in fluid intake (Mueller et al. 2005). Such differences were not explained by those of body mass index, urine output during daytime or nighttime. Recent data indicate that women are more likely to experience nocturia than men (Yoon et al. 2022; Yow et al. 2021). Other studies indicate that this may be explained by a greater prevalence of nocturnal polyuria in women (Weiss et al. 2022). However, a greater prevalence of nocturia in females was not found in all studies (Clemens et al. 2020).

2.2 Gross Anatomy and Histology

The male and female lower urinary tract differ fundamentally anatomically, which is accompanied by physiological differences (Abelson et al. 2018). The male urethra is partly surrounded by the prostate and due to the presence of the penis is longer than in women; a longer urethra intrinsically can cause a greater bladder outlet resistance, a difference that can get accentuated by compression of the urethra by the surrounding prostate. As a consequence, the detrusor is thicker in men than in women, apparently because greater pressure is needed to overcome the greater resistance from the longer urethra.

2.3 Experimental Data

A small number of studies compared bladder weight in male and female rodents. One study in Sprague-Dawley rats found that female animals had a smaller bladder but a much smaller body weight, resulting into an increased bladder/body weight ratio (284 ± 11 vs. 355 ± 8 mg/kg) (Longhurst and Levendusky 2000). Among the female animals, bladder weight and bladder/body weight ratio were comparable in

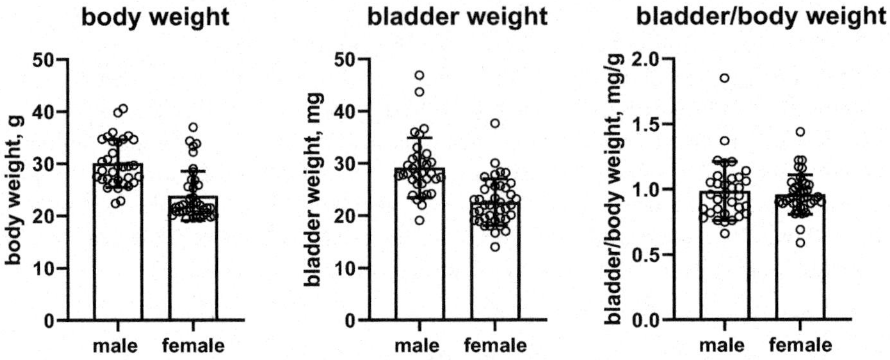

Fig. 1 Body weight, bladder weight, and bladder/body weight in male and female mice. Each datapoint represents one mouse from a total of 39 male and 33 female mice). Reproduced with permission from (Erdogan et al. 2023)

metestrus, diestrus, proestrus, and estrous. Similar observations were made in two other studies in Wistar rats (Frazier et al. 2006; Kories et al. 2003). A recent paper reported on the pooled data from the control groups of five distinct studies in C57BL/6J and C57BL/6N mice (Erdogan et al. 2023): based on 33 male and 39 female animals, female mice had a smaller bladder weight (22.6 vs. 29.2 mg, mean difference 6.6 mg [95% confidence interval 4.2; 9.0]) and a lower body weight, resulting in a similar bladder/body weight ratio in both sexes (0.957 vs. 0.986 mg/g, mean difference 0.029 [−0.06; 0.118]; Fig. 1).

While increased bladder outlet resistance in men is mostly attributed to prostatic enlargement, some data indicate that the sympathetic innervation of the bladder neck is denser in men (Gosling et al. 1999), a factor potentially contributing to bladder outlet resistance by stimulating contraction in the trigone. On the other hand, higher expression of α_{1A}-adrenoceptors at the mRNA and protein level was reported in the bladder trigone of women (Sigala et al. 2004).

Within the bladder, sex differences have been reported not only for smooth muscle but also for other elements including the urothelium. For instance, uroplakin II and IIIa knock-out mice exhibited sex differences of moderate effect sizes (Aboushwareb et al. 2009). Several ion channels relevant for the sensing function or the urothelium such as acid-sensitive ion channels 1 and 2, or the vanilloid receptor TRPV1 are differentially expressed in male and female animals (Kobayashi et al. 2009).

2.3.1 Contraction Studies

The density and affinity of muscarinic acetylcholine receptors were similar in males and female pigs (B_{max} 113 ± 16 vs. 125 ± 19 fmol/mg protein) (Goepel et al. 1998) and in Wistar rats (B_{max} 144 ± 5 vs. 140 ± 6 fmol/mg protein) measured by [^{3}H]-l-quinuclidinyl benzylate binding (Kories et al. 2003) (Fig. 2). Based on competition binding with the M_3-selective antagonist darifenacin both sexes had about 30% M_3 and 70% M_2 receptors. M_2 and M_3 receptors primarily couple G_i and G_q proteins,

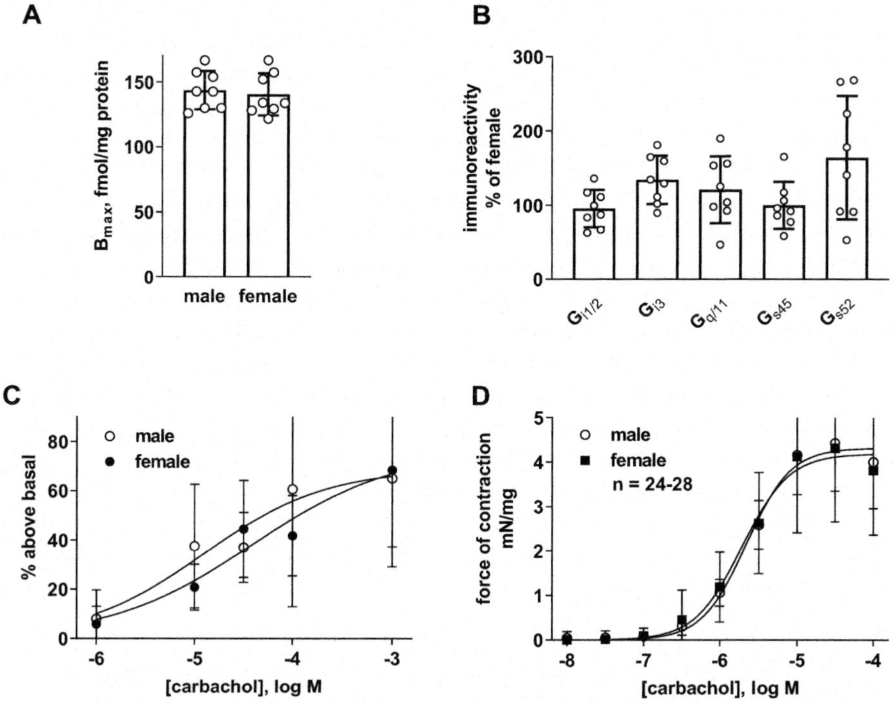

Fig. 2 Muscarinic receptor density (panel **a**), G protein α-subunit expression (panel **b**), and carbachol-induced inositol phosphate formation (panel **c**) and contraction in male and female rat bladder (panel **d**). Al data shown as means ± SD of 8 animals per group unless otherwise noted. Adapted with permission from (Kories et al. 2003)

respectively, and male and female rats also had similar protein levels of the α subunits of $G_{q/11}$, G_{i2}, and G_{i3} based on immunoblotting (Kories et al. 2003) (Fig. 2). Similarly, the potency and efficacy of the muscarinic agonist carbachol to stimulate inositol phosphate formation were comparable in male and female bladders, as was the inhibition by the M_2-preferring antagonist methoctramine and by darifenacin.

A rat study had reported that the contractile responses to electrical field stimulation but not to carbachol were smaller in females than in males; responses to both were smaller in estrus as compared to metestrus and diestrus (Longhurst and Levendusky 2000). The potency of pirenzepine, methoctramine, and the M_3-preferring antagonist 4-diphenylacetoxy-N-methylpiperidine methiodide was similar in both sexes. A later study confirmed that the potency and efficacy of carbachol to stimulate contraction of isolated rat bladder strips were similar in both sexes (E_{max} 4.3 ± 0.1 vs. 4.2 ± 0.2 mN/mg wet weight) and, based on Schild analysis, to the potency of atropine, the M_1-selective pirenzepine, methoctramine and darifenacin to inhibit the carbachol response (Kories et al. 2003). A study in three different mouse strains using five distinct muscarinic receptor agonists found that maximum contractile responses were considerably smaller in female compared to male animals in C57BL/6 mice but smaller or non-existent differences were observed in 129/SvJ and N1F2 mice; the potency of the agonist did not exhibit consistent sex differences in either strain (Choppin 2002). A study using cat isolated detrusor smooth muscle cells found similar contraction (assessed as shortening in response to a maximally effective concentration of acetylcholine) in both sexes (21.3 ± 0.2% vs. 21.7 ± 0.3%) (An et al. 2002). In pig bladder strips, contractile responses to electrical field stimulation, acetylcholine and KCl were similar in female samples and those from castrated male animals; within that study, micromolar concentrations of estradiol caused detrusor relaxation that was similar in strips from female and male castrated animals and was not substantially affected by the estrogen receptor antagonist ICI 182-780 (Dambros et al. 2004). We are aware of two studies comparing contractile responses to carbachol and other stimulants in human isolated bladder strips. Based on 25 consecutive patients (20 males, 5 females), the two groups were of similar age and exhibited a similar E_{max} (4.4 ± 0.6 vs. 4.4 ± 2.2 mN/mg) and pEC_{50} of carbachol (6.07 ± 0.05 vs. 6.32 ± 0.14) (Kories et al. 2003). A later study, also with few female samples, did not detect major gender differences in contractile responses (Fry et al. 2011).

Although the female human trigone was reported to have a greater α_{1A}-adrenoceptor mRNA expression than the male (Sigala et al. 2004), the α_1-adrenoceptor agonist phenylephrine enhanced the contraction induced by carbachol in male but not female trigone (Walther et al. 2018).

While most of these in vitro studies did not detect relevant sex differences in contractile responses or in antagonist potency, an in vivo study reported that female rats imbibed more water (adjusted for body weight) than males, and that tolterodine reduced water intake and urine output in female but not male animals; moreover, tolterodine decreased voided volume per micturition in females but not in males (Yoshimura et al. 2000).

2.3.2 Relaxation Studies

Radioligand binding studies to detect and quantify β-adrenoceptors have been performed using [^{3}H]-dihydroalprenolol or [^{125}I]-iodocyanopindolol as the radioligands; both detect β_1- and β_2-adrenoceptors but fail to label β_3-adrenoceptors unless excessive concentrations of the radioligand are used (Niclauß et al. 2006). This has implications for the interpretation of the reported findings as relaxant responses are mediated at least partly in some species such as rats and almost exclusively in others such as humans by β_3-adrenoceptors (Michel and Vrydag 2006). With these caveats, β-adrenoceptor density was reported to be greater in young female than male rabbits in the bladder base, whereas no such differences were seen in older rabbits or in the bladder dome of either age group (Latifpour et al. 1990). Another study confirmed a greater β-adrenoceptor density in the trigone of young female rabbits (Morita et al. 1998). In contrast, experiments in pigs failed to observe sex differences in either bladder region for both β- and α_2-adrenoceptors

(Goepel et al. 1997). β_3-Adrenoceptor mRNA was detected in intact and ovariectomized female detrusor but no quantification was reported (Matsubara et al. 2002).

β-Adrenoceptors primarily couple to G_s, although G_i protein coupling has been observed for β_3-adrenoceptors (Alexander et al. 2021). Male and female rats had a similar protein expression of the α subunits of G_s proteins based on immunoblotting (Kories et al. 2003). Basal and forskolin-stimulated cAMP formation were also similar in both sexes.

An early study using rabbit detrusor and trigone strips reported similar relaxation by isoprenaline in both sexes in the detrusor whereas relaxation in the trigone was considerably stronger in female than male samples; relaxation in response to forskolin was similar in both bladder regions and in male and female animals (Morita et al. 1998). In rats, relaxation by isoprenaline was similar in intact, ovariectomized, and ovariectomized animals having received estrogen supplementation (Matsubara et al. 2002). Relaxation by BRL 37344 within the same study was similarly effective in all three groups but less potent in the ovariectomized compared to the other two groups, pointing to a possible role of estrogen in facilitating relaxation. However, these data are difficult to interpret because relaxation in rat bladder is a mixed β_2/β_3-adrenoceptor response (Michel and Vrydag 2006); isoprenaline is similarly potent at both subtypes, whereas BRL 37344 has only little if any selectivity for β_3-adrenoceptors (Cernecka et al. 2014), making it unclear why the responses to the two agonists should differentially be affected by ovariectomy. Another study compared relaxant responses of isolated rat bladder strips in response to noradrenaline, the general β-adrenoceptor agonist isoprenaline, the mixed $\beta_{2/3}$-adrenoceptor agonist BRL 37344, and to CGP 12177, which is a partial β_3-agonist in low and a non-orthotopic β_1-agonist in high concentrations (Frazier et al. 2006). While the potency was similar in male and female rats for all four agonists, the E_{max} was smaller in the female than the male rats; while these differences were qualitatively consistent across the four agonists, the quantitative differences ranged from $<10\%$ to $>50\%$ (Fig. 3). The relaxation response to 10 μM of the direct adenylyl cyclase stimulator forskolin was also somewhat smaller in female than in male bladders ($61 \pm 3\%$ vs. $68 \pm 2\%$).

2.3.3 Proposed Factors of Bladder Pathophysiology

Various factors have been proposed to be involved in the pathophysiology of bladder enlargement, such as nerve growth factor and its receptor tropomyosin receptor kinase A (Ochodnicky et al. 2011) and angiotensin II type 1 and 2 receptors (Yamada et al. 2009), or in that of fibrosis and inflammation, such as collagens (Ochodnicky et al. 2011; Shen et al. 2015) and/or inflammation indicated by markers such as monocyte chemoattractant protein-1 (Sukumaran et al. 2012) or interleukin-6 (Shen et al. 2015). A recent study compared the mRNA expression of such factors in the pooled control groups of three mouse studies (combined $n = 17$–19 in each sex) (Erdogan et al. 2023). While expression of nerve growth factor and angiotensin type 2 receptors did not differ between sexes, that of angiotensin type 1 receptors (+30.3% [1.7; 58.9]) and collagen I (+63.4% [4.0; 122.7]) was greater in female mice. Numeric differences in collagen II, monocyte chemoattractant protein-1, or

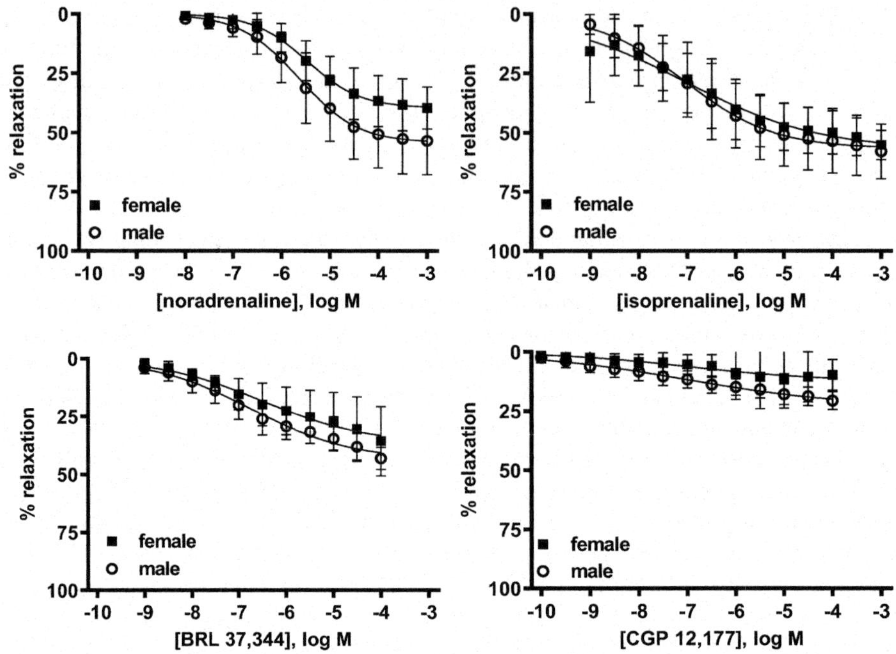

Fig. 3 Relaxation of male and female rat bladder by different β-adrenoceptor agonists. Data are shown as means ± SD of 6 animals each. Adapted with permission from (Frazier et al. 2006)

transforming growth factor-β were observed but were difficult to interpret based on very wide confidence intervals; tropomyosin receptor kinase A and interleukin-6 had too low expression in both sexes to allow interpretation.

Taken together these data indicate that females have a smaller urinary bladder, but this difference is largely explained by the difference in body weight. Based on limited data, there are no major differences in the presence of muscarinic receptors, G protein α subunits, cAMP and inositol phosphate formation. Contractile and relaxant responses are largely similar in both sexes, although some investigators have reported sex differences under certain conditions. While most of these data are based on rats and mice, limited data indicate that they may also be applicable to other mammalian species including rabbits, pigs, cats, and humans.

3 Pathophysiology in OAB

3.1 Clinical Data

Epidemiological studies on OAB differed in design and applied definition of the condition but have consistently reported that it occurs with comparable prevalence in men and women (Coyne et al. 2009; Goepel et al. 2002; Lapitan and Chye 2001;

Milsom et al. 2001; Norby et al. 2005; Stewart et al. 2003). Perhaps most relevant is a very large, population-based survey (19,165 participants aged ≥18 years from Canada, Germany, Italy, Sweden, and the UK) applying the definition of OAB provided by the International Continence Society (Irwin et al. 2006); the prevalence of OAB was 10.8% in men and 12.8% in women with increasing values by age in both genders. An even larger study (211,648 participants) was performed in patients visiting a physician (general practitioner, gynecologist, urologist) for any reason, i.e., not specifically related to bladder problems, in Germany (Goepel et al. 2002). Urgency, the defining symptom of OAB (Abrams et al. 2002), was similarly prevalent in both genders (21.4% vs. 25.4%), but urgency incontinence was reported considerably more often in females (14.3% vs. 22.8%). The odds ratio for reporting urgency relative to males was 1.575 [1.538; 1.162] and for urgency incontinence 2.336 [2.275; 2.399] based on these data; for comparison, the odds ratio for reporting stress urinary incontinence, known to occur primarily in women, was 6.578 [6.400; 6.762]. However, like healthcare seeking behavior related to OAB (see below), the latter data are not easy to interpret because they may at least partly reflect that women experiencing urinary or other health problems may be more likely to see a physician.

3.2 Experimental Data

More robust data on sex differences in bladder dysfunction comes from animal models of disease. The largest number of studies describe bladder dysfunction related to diabetes mellitus (Arioglu-Inan et al. 2018; Ellenbroek et al. 2018; Yesilyurt et al. 2022). Diabetic patients are reported to exhibit bladder dysfunction in 43–87% of patients with type 1 and 25% of patients with type 2 diabetes (Kempler et al. 2011). Glucose homeostasis is known to differ between genders (Basu et al. 2017; Diaf et al. 2014; Mauvais-Jarvis 2017), as well as the prevalence of diabetes and its risk factors (Seghieri et al. 2022). Insulin receptor substrate-2 knock-out mice exhibit a known sexual dimorphism regarding extent of glucose elevation (Kubota et al. 2000; Masaki et al. 2004) that is associated with a differential survival (Withers et al. 1998), i.e., the male animals are diabetic whereas the females are not.

Bladder weight appears to be the most frequently reported outcome parameter in studies of the lower urinary tract in animal models of diabetes and was reported in more than 150 studies (Arioglu-Inan et al. 2018; Ellenbroek et al. 2018; Yesilyurt et al. 2022). An enlarged bladder was observed in all models of type 1 diabetes, whereas this was less consistently observed in those of type 2 diabetes. However, female animals are vastly underrepresented in those studies with only 12 cohorts of female as compared to 59 cohorts of male rats in the streptozotocin-induced model of type 1 diabetes (Arioglu-Inan et al. 2018); they are similarly underrepresented in studies in animal models of type 2 diabetes (Ellenbroek et al. 2018), and only a single study has reported on a direct sex comparison (Erdogan et al. 2023). An indirect comparison across studies in the streptozotocin model in rats using the 12 female and 59 male cohorts found that bladder weight increased somewhat more in female than male rats, but due to large variability in either sex and the indirect comparison across studies this could not easily be interpreted (Arioglu-Inan et al. 2018). Bladder enlargement has been reported to be present in male but not female Bartter's mice (Kim et al. 2018).

We have recently reported on bladder and bladder/body weight data from 16 studies across nine different rat and mice models of diabetes and obesity (Yesilyurt et al. 2022). Five of these studies had included both male and female mice and enabled a direct sex comparison (Erdogan et al. 2023). This included models of type 1 diabetes (RIP-LCMV mice), type 2 diabetes (db/db mice, two studies in ob/ob mice, insulin receptor substrate-2 knock-out mice) and of obesity (mice on a high-fat diet); it included models in which bladder weight in the diabetic/obese groups was increased (RIP-LCMV and ob/ob mice) or not (IRS2 knock-out and db/db mice and mice on a high-fat diet). Based on the sex differences in body weight, data were mainly analyzed for bladder/body weight ratio with the pooled control mice (see above) and with the diabetic/obese mice within each study. The bladder/body weight ratio did not differ substantially between sexes in RIP-LCMV mice and db/db mice. It was numerically greater in females in two studies in ob/ob mice, but that reached statistical significance in only one of the two studies; it was also greater in mice on a high-fat diet. Female insulin receptor substrate-2 knock-out mice had a smaller bladder/body weight ratio.

Taken together, only very limited direct sex comparisons were reported in animal models of disease. These limited data indicate that sex differences may exist for some outcome parameters but are not consistent across models.

4 Treatment Responses

Differences in treatment responses can conceptually be related to multiple, not mutually exclusive factors including those in tissue responsiveness (see above). Other contributing factors include pharmacokinetic differences, e.g., women having an ~40% greater exposure than men after ingesting mirabegron that declined to ~20% after adjusting for body weight differences (Krauwinkel et al. 2012). A key factor in therapeutic outcomes is also adherence to treatment, although a greater adherence was reported sometimes in men (Goodson et al. 2018) and sometimes in women (Kalder et al. 2014).

Despite a comparable prevalence in both genders, women were consistently overrepresented in randomized clinical studies of OAB medications (Chapple et al. 2014; Novara et al. 2008), except for those that were specifically designed to test effects in one gender. This occurred irrespective of drug group (e.g., muscarinic antagonists and β_3-adrenoceptor agonists) and to specific drugs within a drug group. The randomized clinical trials with OAB medications recruiting both genders typically were neither designed nor with sample sizes in the hundreds powered to explore gender differences. While data comparing efficacy and tolerability in males vs. females have been reported, they were typically based on secondary and underpowered analyses.

In contrast, non-interventional studies typically included >1,000 OAB patients. While these also were not designed to compare drug effects between genders, their much larger sample sizes at least had statistical power to detect possible gender differences. Such non-interventional studies have been reported for multiple muscarinic receptor antagonists. While non-interventional studies intrinsically are unsuitable to demonstrate the efficacy of a drug in absolute terms because of the absence of a control group, they should be suitable for analyses of potential gender differences. We focus here on six such studies reported in five papers that included explicit gender comparisons.

One non-interventional study included 2,250 OAB patients treated for ≈12 weeks with tolterodine in its immediate release formulation and applied logistic regression analysis for urgency, incontinence, and pollakiuria outcomes as well as global tolerability (Michel et al. 2002). After adjustment for age and baseline symptom intensity, gender was not associated with statistically significant differences in symptom improvement except for incontinence (odds ratio urgency 0.764 [0.583; 1.001], incontinence 1.453 [1.062; 1.990], frequency 0.745 [0.552; 1.004]). Similarly, global tolerability was similar in both genders (0.993 [0.790; 1.249]).

Another non-interventional study was primarily designed to study cardiovascular safety in 4,450 OAB patients treated for 12–14 weeks with solifenacin (Michel et al. 2008). In a multiple regression analysis with adjustment for age, body mass index, and presence of comedication, coronary heart disease/myocardial infarction, heart failure and diabetes, treatment-emergent adverse events were similar in both genders (odds ratio 0.840 [0.559; 1.265]). A preplanned secondary analysis of this study compared the efficacy of solifenacin in men, nulliparous women and those with 1, 2 or >2 previous vaginal child deliveries (Witte et al. 2009). Improvements upon treatment were comparable across all five groups for urgency, incontinence, urinary frequency, nocturia, pad use, and several patient-reported outcome scales including those for quality of life, although some small group differences reached statistical significance with large patient numbers.

A third non-interventional study included 3,766 OAB patients treated with darifenacin for ≈12 weeks and also applied multiple regression analysis (Schneider et al. 2010). After adjustment for age, body mass index, past and present smoking, alcohol and caffeine consumption, and baseline symptom intensity, women exhibited slightly greater improvements of urgency, urinary frequency and nocturia, but not for incontinence. However, these gender differences were small relative to the overall therapeutic response: women improved 0.4416, 0.3316, and 0.1638 episodes more in urgency, micturition and nocturia, respectively, as compared to an improvement of 4.1, 4.7, and 1.4 episodes, respectively, in the overall study cohort. The global tolerability rating did not differ between genders.

A fourth study included 773 OAB patients treated with fesoterodine for ≈4 months (Schneider et al. 2014). While it was not designed to compare men and women and did not analyze numerical differences in outcome parameters statistically, both genders reported a similar degree of satisfaction with treatment (76.0% vs. 74.4% reporting to be satisfied or very satisfied).

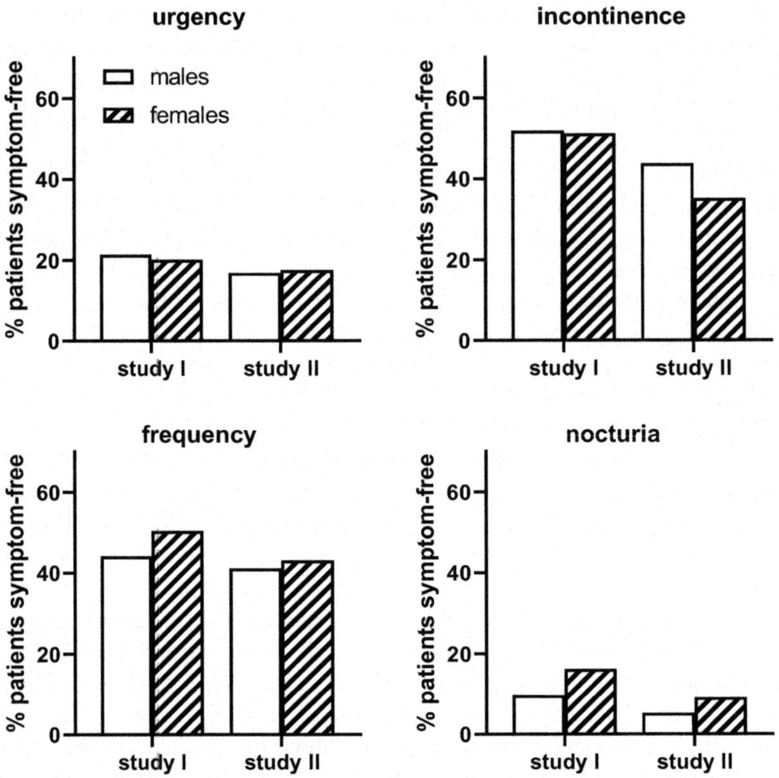

Fig. 4 Percentage of men (open bars) and women (hatched bars) becoming free of urgency, incontinence, frequency and nocturia in two studies (cohort I 1335 patients, cohort II 745 patients. Adapted with permission from (Müderrisoglu et al. 2022)

Finally, two studies of similar design including 1,335 and 745 OAB patients treated with propiverine in its extended release formulation for $\approx$12 weeks were reported in one publication (Amiri et al. 2021). In a logistic regression analysis adjusting for age, body weight, height, body mass index, duration of OAB symptoms and baseline symptom intensity, gender was not associated with the decision for a starting dose of 30 vs. 45 mg. Small differences in urgency improvement reached statistical significance in favor of women in the first but not the second study; improvement in incontinence, urinary frequency, and nocturia were similar between men and women in both studies. While most non-interventional studies have focused on mean or median symptom improvement, a secondary analysis of the two propiverine studies explored the probability to become free of a given symptom (Müderrisoglu et al. 2022). In these analyses, men and women similarly often became free of urgency and incontinence, whereas women had a slightly greater chance to become free of pollakiuria and nocturia (Fig. 4).

OAB patients that have proven resistant to treatment with oral medication and patients with neurogenic voiding dysfunction often benefit from intra-detrusor injections of onabotulinum toxin type A (BoNT/A) (Michel et al. 2023). Some original studies recruiting both men and women and some meta-analyses compared the responsiveness to BoNT/A between genders. In a retrospective analysis of 24 patients with Parkinson's disease and OAB symptoms, men were less likely to experience symptom improvement (Vurture et al. 2018). In another retrospective analysis of 125 adults with myelomeningocele receiving BoNT/A, male gender was also associated with a less success rate (Peyronnet et al. 2018). A systematic review of 17 studies of BoNT/A in OAB studies reporting predictive factors for therapeutic success, male gender was also associated with a smaller success (Abrar et al. 2021).

Taken together treatment responses to muscarinic receptor antagonists if anything show only minor if any differences in therapeutic improvements of bladder function. Studies with BoNT/A in neurogenic voiding dysfunction and in OAB have reported more consistently that men were less likely to experience substantial symptom improvement than women.

5 Conclusions and Research Directions

Some anatomical differences exist between males and females in the urinary tract, most importantly a longer urethra and the presence of a prostate in men. These have implications for bladder outlet resistance. As the vast majority of experimental studies on bladder physiology have been performed in males only, our knowledge on possible sex and gender differences is limited. This limited evidence does not suggest major differences. Some conditions of the lower urinary tract are highly gender-related including stress urinary incontinence in women and benign prostate hyperplasia in men. However, OAB occurs with comparable prevalence in both genders. Treatment responses to oral OAB medications are also similar between genders, but several studies indicate that those to the injectable onabotulinum toxin type A are smaller in men than in women. A better understanding of possible sex and gender differences in bladder physiology, particularly at the experimental level is a major knowledge gap.

Declarations Work in the authors' lab in the bladder field is funded by the Deutsche Forschungsgemeinschaft (Mi 294/10-1) and Apogepha Arzneimittel GmbH.

AP does not report a conflict of interest. MCM is an investigator, consultant, and/or speaker in the bladder field for Apogepha, Astellas, Dr. Willmar Schwabe; he is a former shareholder of Velicept.

References

Abelson B, Sun D, Que L, Nebel RA, Baker D, Popiel P, Amundsen CL, Chai T, Close C, DiSanto M, Fraser MO, Kielb SJ, Kuchel G, Mueller ER, Palmer MH, Parker-Autry C, Wolfe AJ, Damaser MS (2018) Sex differences in lower urinary tract biology and physiology. Biol Sex Differ 9:45

Aboushwareb T, Zhou G, Deng FM, Turner C, Andersson KE, Tar M, Zhao W, Melman A, D'Agostino R Jr, Sun TT, Christ GJ (2009) Alterations in bladder function associated with urothelial defects in uroplakin II and IIIa knockout mice. Neurourol Urodyn 28:1028–1033

Abrams P, Cardozo L, Fall M, Griffiths D, Rosier P, Ulmsten U, van Kerrebroeck P, Victor A, Wein A (2002) The standardisation of terminology of lower urinary tract function: report from the standardisation sub-committee of the International Continence Society. Neurourol Urodyn 21: 167–178

Abrar M, Pindoria N, Malde S, Chancellor M, DeRidder D, Sahai A (2021) Predictors of poor response and adverse events following botulinum toxin a for refractory idiopathic overactive bladder: a systematic review. Eur Urol Focus 7:1448–1467

Alexander SP, Christopoulos A, Davenport AP, Kelly E, Mathie A, Peters JA, Veale EL, Armstrong JF, Faccenda E, Harding SD, Pawson AJ, Southan C, Davies JA, Abbracchio MP, Alexander W, Al-Hosaini K, Bäck M, Barnes NM, Bathgate R, Beaulieu JM, Bernstein KE, Bettler B, Birdsall NJM, Blaho V, Boulay F, Bousquet C, Bräuner-Osborne H, Burnstock G, Caló G, Castaño JP, Catt KJ, Ceruti S, Chazot P, Chiang N, Chini B, Chun J, Cianciulli A, Civelli O, Clapp LH, Couture R, Csaba Z, Dahlgren C, Dent G, Singh KD, Douglas SD, Dournaud P, Eguchi S, Escher E, Filardo EJ, Fong T, Fumagalli M, Gainetdinov RR, Gasparo M, Gerard C, Gershengorn M, Gobeil F, Goodfriend TL, Goudet C, Gregory KJ, Gundlach AL, Hamann J, Hanson J, Hauger RL, Hay DL, Heinemann A, Hollenberg MD, Holliday ND, Horiuchi M, Hoyer D, Hunyady L, Husain A, AP IJ, Inagami T, Jacobson KA, Jensen RT, Jockers R, Jonnalagadda D, Karnik S, Kaupmann K, Kemp J, Kennedy C, Kihara Y, Kitazawa T, Kozielewicz P, Kreienkamp HJ, Kukkonen JP, Langenhan T, Leach K, Lecca D, Lee JD, Leeman SE, Leprince J, Li XX, Williams TL, Lolait SJ, Lupp A, Macrae R, Maguire J, Mazella J, McArdle CA, Melmed S, Michel MC, Miller LJ, Mitolo V, Mouillac B, Müller CE, Murphy P, Nahon JL, Ngo T, Norel X, Nyimanu D, O'Carroll AM, Offermanns S, Panaro MA, Parmentier M, Pertwee RG, Pin JP, Prossnitz ER, Quinn M, Ramachandran R, Ray M, Reinscheid RK, Rondard P, Rovati GE, Ruzza C, Sanger GJ, Schöneberg T, Schulte G, Schulz S, Segaloff DL, Serhan CN, Stoddart LA, Sugimoto Y, Summers R, Tan VP, Thal D, Thomas WW, Timmermans P, Tirupula K, Tulipano G, Unal H, Unger T, Valant C, Vanderheyden P, Vaudry D, Vaudry H, Vilardaga JP, Walker CS, Wang JM, Ward DT, Wester HJ, Willars GB, Woodruff TM, Yao C, Ye RD (2021) THE CONCISE GUIDE TO PHARMACOLOGY 2021/22: G protein-coupled receptors. Br J Pharmacol 178(Suppl 1):S27–s156

Amiri M, Schneider T, Oelke M, Murgas S, Michel MC (2021) Factors associated with decisions for initial dosing, up-titration of propiverine and treatment outcomes in overactive bladder syndrome patients in a non-interventional setting. J Clin Med 10:311

An JY, Yun HS, Lee YP, Yang SJ, Shim JO, Jeong JH, Shin CY, Kim JH, Kim DS, Sohn UD (2002) The intracellular pathway of the acetylcholine-induced contraction in cat detrusor muscle cells. Br J Pharmacol 137:1001–1010

Arioglu-Inan E, Ellenbroek JH, Michel MC (2018) A systematic review of urinary bladder hypertrophy in experimental diabetes: part I. Streptozotocin-induced rat models. Neurourol Urodyn 37:1212–1219

Basu A, Dube S, Basu R (2017) Men are from Mars, women are from Venus: sex differences in insulin action and secretion. In: Mauvais-Jarvis F (ed) Sex and gender factors affecting metabolic homeostasis, diabetes and obesity. Springer, Cham, pp 53–64

Beckel JM, Holstege G (2011) Neuroanatomy of the lower urinary tract. Handb Exp Pharmacol:99–116

Bosch R, Abrams P, Averbeck MA, Finazzi Agró E, Gammie A, Marcelissen T, Solomon E (2019) Do functional changes occur in the bladder due to bladder outlet obstruction? – ICI-RS 2018. Neurourol Urodyn 38(Suppl 5):S56–s65

Cernecka H, Sand C, Michel MC (2014) The odd sibling: features of β_3-adrenoceptor pharmacology. Mol Pharmacol 86:479–484

Chapple CR, Cardozo L, Nitti VW, Siddiqui E, Michel MC (2014) Mirabegron in overactive bladder: a review of efficacy, safety, and tolerability. Neurourol Urodyn 33:17–30

Cho KJ, Kim JC (2020) Management of urinary incontinence with underactive bladder: a review. Int Neurourol J 24:111–117

Choppin A (2002) Muscarinic receptors in isolated urinary bladder smooth muscle from different mouse strains. Br J Pharmacol 137:522–528

Clemens JQ, Wiseman JB, Smith AR, Amundsen CL, Yang CC, Bradley MS, Kirkali Z, Agochukwu NQ, Cameron AP (2020) Prevalence, subtypes, and correlates of nocturia in the symptoms of lower urinary tract dysfunction research network cohort. Neurourol Urodyn 39: 1098–1107

Coyne KS, Sexton CC, Thompson CL, Milsom I, Irwin D, Kopp ZS, Chapple CR, Kaplan S, Tubaro A, Aiyer LP, Wein AJ (2009) The prevalence of lower urinary tract symptoms (LUTS) in the USA, the UK and Sweden: results from the epidemiology of LUTS (EpiLUTS) study. BJU Int 104:352–360

Dambros M, van Koeveringe GA, Bast A, van Kerrebroeck PEV (2004) Relaxant effects of estradiol through non-genomic pathways in male and female pig bladder smooth muscle. Pharmacology 72:121–127

Diaf M, Khaled BM, Habib HH, Belbraoued S (2014) Effect of gender and body weight on postprandial glucose and lipid metabolism in adults with type 2 diabetes. J Nepal Med Assoc 52:866–877

Ellenbroek JH, Arioglu-Inan E, Michel MC (2018) A systematic review of urinary bladder hypertrophy in experimental diabetes: part 2. Comparison of animal models and functional consequences. Neurourol Urodyn 37:2346–2360

Erdogan BR, Michel MB, Matthes J, Castañeda TR, Christen U, Arioglu-Inan E, Michel MC, Pautz A (2023) A comparison of urinary bladder weight in male and female mice across five models of diabetes and obesity. Front Pharmacol 14

Fowler CJ, Griffiths D, De Groat WC (2008) The neural control of micturition. Nat Rev Neurosci 9: 453–466

Frazier EP, Schneider T, Michel MC (2006) Effects of gender, age and hypertension on ß-adrenergic receptor function in rat urinary bladder. Naunyn Schmiedeberg's Arch Pharmacol 373:300–309

Fry CH, Bayliss M, Young JS, Hussain M (2011) Influence of age and bladder dysfunction on the contractile properties of isolated human detrusor. BJU Int 108:E91–E96

Goepel M, Gronewald A, Krege S, Michel MC (1998) Muscarinic receptor subtypes in porcine detrusor: comparison with humans and regulation by bladder augmentation. Urol Res 26:149–154

Goepel M, Hoffmann J, Piro M, Rübben H, Michel MC (2002) Prevalence and physician awareness of symptoms of urinary bladder dysfunction. Eur Urol 41:234–239

Goepel M, Wittmann A, Rübben H, Michel MC (1997) Comparison of adrenoceptor subtype expression in porcine and human bladder and prostate. Urol Res 25:199–206

Goodson AB, Cantrell MA, Shaw RF, Lund BC (2018) Comparative effectiveness of anticholinergic agents for lower urinary tract symptoms. J Manag Care Spec Pharm 24:65–72

Gosling JA, Dixon JS, Jen PYP (1999) The distribution of noradrenergic nerves in the human lower urinary tract. Eur Urol 36(Suppl 1):23–30

Hampel C, Artibani W, Espuna Pons M, Haab F, Jackson S, Romero J, Gavart S, Papanicolaou S (2004) Understanding the burden of stress urinary incontinence in Europe: a qualitative review of the literature. Eur Urol 46:15–27

Ikeda Y (2021) Neurophysiological control of urinary bladder storage and voiding-functional changes through development and pathology. Pediatr Nephrol 36:1041–1052

Irwin DE, Milsom I, Hunskaar S, Reillly K, Kopp Z, Herschorn S, Coyne K, Kelleher C, Hampel C, Artibani W, Abrams P (2006) Population-based survey of urinary incontinence, overactive bladder, and other lower urinary tract symptoms in five countries: results of the EPIC study. Eur Urol 50:1306–1315

Kalder M, Pantazis K, Dinas K, Albert US, Heilmaier C, Kostev K (2014) Discontinuation of treatment using anticholinergic medications in patients with urinary incontinence. Obstet Gynecol 124:794–800

Kanai A, Wyndaele JJ (2011) Researching bladder afferents – determining the effects of $ß_3$-adrenergic receptor agonists and botulinum toxin type-A. Neurourol Urodyn 30:684–691

Kempler P, Amarenco G, Freeman R, Frontoni S, Horowitz M, Stevens M, Low P, Pop-Busui R, Tahrani AA, Tesfaye S, Várkonyi T, Ziegler D, Valensi P (2011) Management strategies for gastrointestinal, erectile, bladder, and sudomotor dysfunction in patients with diabetes. Diabetes Metab Res Rev 27:665–677

Kim JM, Xu S, Guo X, Hu H, Dong K, Wang T (2018) Urinary bladder hypertrophy characteristic of male ROMK Bartter's mice does not occur in female mice. Am J Physiol Regul Integr Comp Physiol 314:R334–r341

Kobayashi H, Yoshiyama M, Zakoji H, Takeda M, Araki I (2009) Sex differences in the expression profile of acid-sensing ion channels in the mouse urinary bladder: a possible involvement in irritative bladder symptoms. BJU Int 104:1746–1751

Kories C, Czyborra C, Fetscher C, Schneider T, Krege S, Michel MC (2003) Gender comparison of muscarinic receptor expression and function in rat and human urinary bladder: differential regulation of M_2 and M3? Naunyn Schmiedeberg's Arch Pharmacol 367:524–531

Krauwinkel W, van Dijk J, Schaddelee M, Eltink C, Meijer J, Strabach G, van Marle S, Kerbusch V, van Gelderen M (2012) Pharmacokinetic properties of mirabegron, a ß3-adrenoceptor agonist: results from two phase I, randomized, multiple-dose studies in healthy young and elderly men and women. Clin Ther 34:2144–2160

Kubota N, Tobe K, Terauchi Y, Eto K, Yamauchi T, Suzuki R, Tsubamoto Y, Komeda K, Nakano R, Miki H, Satoh S, Sekihara H, Sciacchitano S, Lesniak M, Aizawa S, Nagai R, Kimura S, Akanuma Y, Taylor SI, Kadowaki T (2000) Disruption of insulin receptor substrate 2 causes type 2 diabetes because of liver insulin resistance and lack of compensatory beta-cell hyperplasia. Diabetes 49:1880–1889

Lapitan MC, Chye PLH (2001) The epidemiology of overactive bladder among females in Asia: a questionnaire study. Int Urogynecol J 12:226–231

Latifpour J, Kondo S, O'Hollaren B, Morita T, Weiss RM (1990) Autonomic receptors in urinary tract: sex and age differences. J Pharmacol Exp Ther 253:661–667

Longhurst PA, Levendusky M (2000) Influence of gender and the oestrous cycle on in vitro contractile responses of the rat urinary bladder to cholinergic stimulation. Br J Pharmacol 131:177–184

Masaki T, Chiba S, Noguchi H, Yasuda T, Tobe K, Suzuki R, Kadowaki T, Yoshimatsu H (2004) Obesity in insulin receptor substrate-2-deficient mice: disrupted control of arcuate nucleus neuropeptides. Obes Res 12:878–885

Matsubara S, Okada H, Shirakawa T, Gotoh A, Kuno T, Kamidono S (2002) Estrogen levels influence beta-3-adrenoceptor-mediated relaxation of the female rat detrusor muscle. Urology 59:621–625

Mauvais-Jarvis F (2017) Epidemiology of gender differences in diabetes and obesity. In: Mauvais-Jarvis F (ed) Sex and gender factors affecting metabolic homeostasis, diabetes and obesity. Springer, Cham, pp 3–8

Michel MC, Cardozo L, Chermanksy CJ, Cruz F, Igawa Y, Lee K-S, Sahai A, Wein AJ, Andersson KE (2023) Current and emerging pharmacological targets and treatments of urinary incontinence and related disorders. Pharmacol Rev 75(4):554–674

Michel MC, Schneider T, Krege S, Goepel M (2002) Do gender or age affect the efficacy and safety of tolterodine? J Urol 168:1027–1031

Michel MC, Vrydag W (2006) α_1-, α_2- and ß-adrenoceptors in the urinary bladder, urethra and prostate. Br J Pharmacol 147:S88–S119

Michel MC, Wetterauer U, Vogel M, de la Rosette JJMCH (2008) Cardiovascular safety and overall tolerability of solifenacin in routine clinical use. Drug Saf 31:505–514

Milsom I, Abrams P, Cardozo L, Roberts RG, Thüroff JW, Wein AJ (2001) How widespread are the symptoms of an overactive bladder and how are they managed? A population-based prevalence study. BJU Int 87:760–766

Morita T, Masuda H, Tosaka A, Ishizaka K, Tsuhii T, Kondo S (1998) Sex differences in function and distribution of ß-adrenoceptors in rabbit urinary bladder. J Urol 159:555–558

Müderrisoglu AE, Oelke M, Schneider T, Murgas S, de la Rosette J, Michel MC (2022) What are realistic expectations to become free of overactive bladder symptoms? Experience from non-interventional studies with propiverine. Adv Ther 39:2489–2501

Mueller E, Latini J, Lux M, Stablein U, Brubaker L, Kreder K, Fitzgerald MP (2005) Gender differences in 24-hour urinary diaries of asymptomatic north American adults. J Urol 173:490–492

Niclauß N, Michel-Reher MB, Alewijnse AE, Michel MC (2006) Comparison of three radioligands for the labelling of human ß-adrenoceptor subtypes. Naunyn Schmiedeberg's Arch Pharmacol 374:99–105

Norby B, Nordling J, Mortensen S (2005) Lower urinary tract symptoms in the Danish population: a population-based study of symptom prevalence, health-care seeking behavior and prevalence of treatment in elderly males and females. Eur Urol 47:817–823

Novara G, Galfano A, Secco S, D'Elia C, Cavalleri S, Ficarra V, Artibani W (2008) A systematic review and meta-analysis of randomized controlled trials with antimuscarinic drugs for overactive bladder. Eur Urol 54:740–764

Ochodnicky P, Cruz CD, Yoshimura N, Michel MC (2011) Nerve growth factor in bladder dysfunction: contributing factor, biomarker and therapeutic target. Neurourol Urodyn 30: 1227–1241

Padmanabhan P, Dmochowski R (2014) Urinary incontinence in women: a comprehensive review of the pathophysiology, diagnosis and treatment. Minerva Ginecol 66:469–478

Peyronnet B, Even A, Capon G, De Seze M, Hascoet J, Biardeau X, Baron M, Perrouin-Verbe MA, Boutin JM, Saussine C, Phé V, Lenormand L, Chartier-Kastler E, Cornu JN, Karsenty G, Manunta A, Schurch B, Denys P, Amarenco G, Game X (2018) Intradetrusor injections of botulinum toxin A in adults with spinal dysraphism. J Urol 200:875–880

Schneider T, Arumi D, Crook TJ, Sun F, Michel MC (2014) An observational study of patient satisfaction with fesoterodine in the treatment of overactive bladder: effects of additional educational material. Int J Clin Pract 68:1074–1080

Schneider T, Marschall-Kehrel D, Hanisch JU, Michel MC (2010) Do gender, age or life style factors affect responses to anti-muscarinic treatment in overactive bladder patients? Int J Clin Pract 64:1287–1293

Seghieri G, Franconi F, Campesi I (2022) Why we need sex-gender medicine: the striking example of type 2 diabetes. Diabetology 3:460–469

Shen S, C-m X, Qiao L-Y (2015) The urinary bladder of spontaneously hypertensive rat demonstrates bladder hypertrophy, inflammation, and fibrosis but not hyperplasia. Life Sci 121:22–27

Sigala S, Peroni A, Mirabella G, Fornari S, Palazzolo F, Pezzotti G, Simeone C, Cunico SC, Spano P (2004) Alpha1 adrenoceptor subtypes in human urinary bladder: sex and regional comparison. Life Sci 76:417–427

Stewart WF, van Rooyen JB, Cundiff GW, Abrams P, Herzog AR, Corey R, Hunt TL, Wein AJ (2003) Prevalence and burden of overactive bladder in the United States. World J Urol 20:327–336

Sukumaran V, Veeraveedu PT, Gurusamy N, Lakshmanan AP, Yamaguchi K, Ma M, Suzuki K, Kodama M, Watanabe K (2012) Telmisartan acts through the modulation of ACE-2/ANG 1-7/ mas receptor in rats with dilated cardiomyopathy induced by experimental autoimmune myocarditis. Life Sci 90:289–300

Vurture G, Peyronnet B, Feigin A, Biagioni MC, Gilbert R, Rosenblum N, Frucht S, Di Rocco A, Nitti VW, Brucker BM (2018) Outcomes of intradetrusor onabotulinum toxin A injection in patients with Parkinson's disease. Neurourol Urodyn 37:2669–2677

Walther S, Strittmatter F, Hennenberg M, Gratzke C, Stief CG, Roosen A (2018) Adreno-muscarinic synergy in the male human urinary outflow tract. Neurourol Urodyn 37:2128–2134

Weiss JP, Bosch JLHR, Chapple CR, Bacci ED, Simeone JC, Rosenberg MT, Mueller ER, Andersson FL, Juul K, Chughtai B, Coyne KS (2022) The prevalence of nocturnal polyuria in the United States: results from the epidemiology of nocturnal polyuria study. Eur Urol Focus 8(5):1415–1423

Withers DJ, Gutierrez JS, Towery H, Burks DJ, Ren J-M, Previs S, Zhang Y, Bernal D, Pons S, Shulman GI, Bonner-Weir S, White MF (1998) Disruption of IRS-2 causes type 2 diabetes in mice. Nature 391:900–904

Witte LPW, Peschers U, Vogel M, de la Rosette JJMCH, Michel MC (2009) Does the number of previous vaginal deliveries affect overactive bladder symptoms or their response to treatment? LUTS 1:82–87

Yamada S, Takeuchi C, Oyunzul L, Ito Y (2009) Bladder angiotensin-II receptors: characterization and alteration in bladder outlet obstruction. Eur Urol 55:482–490

Yesilyurt ZE, Matthes J, Hintermann E, Castañeda TR, Elvert R, Beltran-Ornelas JH, Silva-Velasco DL, Xia N, Kannt A, Christen U, Centurión D, Li H, Pautz A, Arioglu-Inan E, Michel MC (2022) Analysis of 16 studies in nine rodent models does not support the hypothesis that diabetic polyuria is a main reason of urinary bladder enlargement. Front Physiol 13:923555

Yoon JH, Lee K, Park EJ, Kwon T, Park S, Moon KH, Kim SC (2022) Analysis of changes in the pathophysiology of nocturia according to the number of nocturia episode, age, and gender using frequency volume charts: a retrospective observational study. Medicine (Baltimore) 101:e31295

Yoshimura Y, Schmidt F, Constantinou CE (2000) Gender specificity of tolterodine on micturition and the diurnal variation of urine production of the conscious rat. BJU Int 87:879–885

Yow HY, Tiong JJL, Mai CW, van der Werf E, Zainuddin ZM, Toh CC, Ngoo KS, Goh EH, Fadzli AN, Lok SH, Ong TA (2021) Prevalence of nocturia among community-dwelling adults: a population-based study in Malaysia. BMC Urol 21:95

Part II

Pathologies of the Brain

Sex Differences in the Evaluation and Treatment of Stroke

Sonia K. Singh and Louise McCullough

Contents

Abstract

There are differences in the prevalence and strength of risk factors in women, along with sex-specific risk factors such as pregnancy. Women have a higher lifetime risk of stroke compared to men, with worse outcomes including higher rates of death and disability. We have made strides in the identification of sex-specific risk factors but with the paucity of sex-specific end points in clinical trials, stroke treatment and research are hindered.

S. K. Singh · L. McCullough (✉)
McGovern Medical School, UTHealth Houston, Houston, TX, USA
e-mail: sonia.k.singh@uth.tmc.edu; louise.d.mccullough@uth.tmc.edu

S. E. Tsirka, M. Acosta-Martinez (eds.), *Sex and Gender Effects in Pharmacology*,
Handbook of Experimental Pharmacology 282,
https://doi.org/10.1007/164_2023_682

Keywords

Differences · Disability · Pregnancy · Sex · Stroke

1 Sex Differences in Stroke

Sex refers to the biological characteristics of individuals. This encompasses the genetic, biologic, and physiological factors that influence pathophysiology, clinical manifestations, and the response to treatment of disease. In contrast, gender is a social construct that includes gender identity and societal roles that influence lifestyle, nutritional habits, exercise, disease perception, and use of healthcare. Both sex and gender are intricately connected, impacting both the behavior of patients and doctors and culminate in our knowledge of "sex and gender differences in health, disease and medicine" (Mauvais-Jarvis et al. 2020).

2 Epidemiology

As of 2019, stroke was the second leading cause of death worldwide, and the second leading contributor to disability adjusted life years (Vyas et al. 2021). In 2019, stroke was the third leading cause of death in women in the USA, and fifth in men (Heron 2021). Of these stroke deaths, 57.1% were women (Heron 2021). Although men have a higher incidence of stroke throughout most of their lifespan, women have a higher stroke prevalence, largely driven by their longer life expectancy. Women have a higher lifetime risk of stroke compared to men as demonstrated in the Framingham Heart Study (FHS) wherein lifetime risk of stroke among those 55–75 years of age was 1 in 5 for females (95% CI, 20–21%) and $\approx$1 in 6 for males (95% CI, 14–17%) (Seshadri et al. 2006). While the etiology of the majority of strokes is attributed to traditional vascular risk factors that occur in both men and women, such as hypertension, hyperlipidemia, diabetes mellitus, smoking, and atrial fibrillation, it is known that each of these confers a higher stroke risk or has higher incidence in one sex versus the other. Stroke risk factors unique to females includes oral contraceptive pill use (OCPs), pregnancy, menopause, and hormone therapy (HT) (Bushnell et al. 2018). A Swedish study found that the risk of stroke recurrence has decreased in both men and women between 2012 and 2020, but there is a higher rate of recurrent stroke in women, likely driven by older age of women at the time of their first stroke (Eriksson et al. 2023; Tsao et al. 2022).

3 Stroke Symptoms

While the traditional symptoms of stroke such as hemiparesis, hemi-body numbness, aphasia, dysarthria, facial weakness, vertigo, and imbalance immediately beckon stroke alerts in the emergency room, non-traditional symptoms such as face or hemi-body pain, lightheadedness, headaches, or reduced level of consciousness can also be secondary to cerebrovascular events. Multiple studies have demonstrated that while women are more likely than men to report non-traditional symptoms, they are often less likely to be diagnosed with an ischemic event even in the presence of traditional stroke symptoms (Lisabeth et al. 2009; Yu et al. 2019, 2021; Shajahan et al. 2023; Ali et al. 2022a). In addition to a higher likelihood of being diagnosed with a stroke mimic, women were also less likely than men to have their diagnosis revised to minor stroke or TIA despite being equally likely to have ischemic changes on MRI (Table 1) (Yu et al. 2021).

4 Outcomes

Data from the Greater Cincinnati Northern Kentucky Stroke Study (GCNKSS) suggest that reduced rates of stroke in males have not been equally experienced by women (Madsen et al. 2017). Additionally, a decline in stroke incidence and mortality over time in the USA has been observed in the White population, but not in other racial or ethnic groups. These social determinants of health and their intersectionality impact both stroke risk and outcome and stand to confound conclusions around changes in stroke risk and sex differences (Bushnell et al. 2018). A population-based cohort study in Canada did not find an overall sex difference in hazard of death for death within 90 days but the hazard of death was higher in female than male patients between the ages of 50–70 years with the most extreme difference occurring around age 57 (hazard ratio 95% CI 1.25 [1.10–1.40] at 90 days, *p*-interaction 0.002; 1.15 [1.10–1.20] at 365 days, *p*-interaction 0.002) (Yu et al. 2023). Other than women being at higher odds of receiving endovascular thrombectomy (OR 1.35, 95% CI [1.19–1.54]), possibly due to the higher rates of cardioembolic stroke, care was found to be similar in both sexes (Yu et al. 2023).

Female sex has also been found to be a risk factor for post-stroke depression (Lyu et al. 2022). In the weeks immediately after a stroke, women reported a higher prevalence of depression, however the persistence of these symptoms did not differ between men and women (Volz et al. 2021). This was also found to be true of cognitive impairment after stroke, which is more common in females especially during the early post-stroke period (Bako et al. 2022).

There are also sex/gender differences in health-related quality of life after ischemic stroke. Analysis of the participants of the Brain Attack Surveillance in Corpus Christie (BASIC) Project, a population-based stroke study found that women had poorer HRQoL (health-related quality of life) compared with men at 90 days post-stroke (Phan et al. 2022). Contributing factors included sociodemographic (race and ethnicity, marital status, educational level) and pre-stroke factors like physical function before stroke, in addition to stroke severity (Phan et al. 2022). Tracking the functional status for 5 years among survivors of acute ischemic stroke in Japan, female sex was associated with a higher risk of functional dependency at 5 years post-stroke despite correction for confounding factors such as age and 3-month modified Rankin score (Irie et al. 2023).

Table 1 Studies on sex differences in stroke presentation

Study name	Study type	Total patients	Percentage female	Median age	Key findings
Lisabeth et al. (2009)	Prospective observational study	461	48.6% (224)	68	1. 51.8% of women reported a non-traditional stroke or TIA symptom compared to 43.9% of men ($p = 0.09$) 2. Mental status change was more prevalent in women (23.2% in women versus 15.2% in men, $p = 0.03$) 3. The odds of reporting at least 1 non-traditional stroke/TIA symptom were 1.42 times (95% CI, 0.97–2.06) greater in women than in men
Yu et al. Spectrometry for transient ischemic attack rapid assessment (SpecTRA) (Yu et al. 2019)	Prospective cohort	1,648	46.7% (770)	70	1. Women (522 of 770 [67.8%]) were less likely than men (674 of 878 [76.8%]) to receive a diagnosis of cerebral ischemia (adjusted risk ratio [aRR], 0.88; 95% CI, 0.82–0.95) 2. 90-day stroke recurrence outcome (aRR, 0.90; 95% CI, 0.48–1.66) and 90-day composite outcome (aRR, 0.86; 95% CI, 0.54–1.32) were similar for men and women

(continued)

Table 1 (continued)

Study name	Study type	Total patients	Percentage female	Median age	Key findings
Yu et al. Diagnosis of Uncertain-Origin Benign Transient Neurological Symptoms (DOUBT) Study Group (Yu et al. 2021)	Post-hoc analysis of data from multicenter international prospective cohort study	1,028	51 (552)	63	1. Women are more likely to be initially diagnosed with a stroke mimic (54% female versus 42% men, adjusted OR 1.60 95% CI 1.24–2.07) 2. Women are less likely than men to have their diagnosis revised to minor stroke or TIA (13% versus 20%, OR 0.53, 95% CI 0.32–0.88) 3. Women were equally likely to have ischemia on MRI compared to men (5% versus 8%, OR 0.56, 95% CI 0.26–1.21)
Shajahan et al. (2023)	Systematic review and meta-analysis of 21 articles	36,636	47% (17,143)	62–79 (mean)	1. Women and men presented with similar mean percentage of a motor deficit (56% women and men) or a speech deficit (41% versus 40% 2. Women were more likely than men to present with generalized weakness (49% versus 36%), mental status change (31% versus 21%), and confusion (37% versus 28%) 3. Women had higher risk than

(continued)

Table 1 (continued)

Study name	Study type	Total patients	Percentage female	Median age	Key findings
					men of presenting with generalized weakness (RR 0.49, 95% CI 1.09–2.03), mental status change (RR 1.44, 95% CI 1.22–1.71), fatigue (RR 1.42, 95% CI 1.05–1.92), and loss of consciousness (RR 1.30, 95% CI 1.12–1.51) 4. Women had a lower risk of presenting with dysarthria (RR 0.89, 95% CI 0.82–0.95), dizziness (RR 0.87, 95% CI 0.80–0.95), gait disturbance (RR 0.79, 95% CI 0.65–0.97), and imbalance (RR 0.68, 95% CI 0.57–0.81)
Ali et al. (2022a)	Systematic review and meta-analysis	582, 844	50%	74	1. Headache (pooled odds ratio [OR], 1.24 [95% CI, 1.11–1.39]; $I^2 = 75.2\%$; 30 studies), changes in mental status (OR, 1.38 [95% CI, 1.19–1.61]; $I^2 = 95.0\%$; 17 studies) and stupor/coma (OR, 1.39 [95% CI, 1.25–1.55]; $I^2 = 27.0\%$; 13 studies) were more frequent in women with any

(continued)

Table 1 (continued)

Study name	Study type	Total patients	Percentage female	Median age	Key findings
					type of stroke compared to men 2. Dysarthria (OR, 1.14 [95% CI, 1.04–1.24]; $I^2 = 48.6\%$; 11 studies) and vertigo (OR, 1.23 [95% CI, 1.13–1.34]; $I^2 = 44.0\%$; eight studies) occurred more frequently in women compared to men 3. Paresis/hemiparesis (OR, 0.73 [95% CI, 0.54–0.97]; $I^2 = 72.6\%$; seven studies) and focal visual disturbances (OR, 0.83 [95% CI, 0.70–0.99]; $I^2 = 62.8\%$; 16 studies) occurred less frequently in women compared with men with any type of stroke
Irie et al. (2023)	Longitudinal observational study	8,446	40% (3,377)	71.9	1. Female sex was associated with a higher risk of functional dependency at 5 years post-stroke even when adjusting for age, 3-month mRS score, and other confounding factors (multivariable-adjusted OR vs. men, 1.56 [95% confidence interval, 1.26–

(continued)

Table 1 (continued)

Study name	Study type	Total patients	Percentage female	Median age	Key findings
					1.93]) 2. Increased risk of functional dependency in female patients was even more marked in patients aged ≥75 years than in those aged <75 years ($p = 0.02$) 3. Female sex was associated with a lower risk of death 4. No sex differences were observed in stroke recurrence during the 5 years post-stroke

Women have worse outcomes after ischemic stroke, including objective measures of functional disability and in patient-reported outcomes (Table 2) (Oliveira et al. 2023; Phan et al. 2019; Carcel et al. 2019). While the modified Rankin scale is commonly used to measure functional disability, women have also been found to have higher scores on Patient-Reported Outcome Measures (PROMs), and incorporating PROMs into ischemic stroke outcome measures may offer additional insight into sex-specific differences in stroke recovery (Figs. 1 and 2) (Oliveira et al. 2023).

5 Estrogen and Stroke

The three major types of estrogen are estriol, estradiol, and estrol. A meta-analysis of available literature found no association between estradiol levels and risk of ischemic stroke (Holmegard et al. 2016). While low testosterone levels have been associated with increased stroke risk in men, there is no clear relationship between testosterone levels and risk of stroke in women. The adrenal hormone, dehydroepiandrosterone, can be used to synthesize both estrogen and testosterone. Low DHEA levels have been associated with an increased risk of ischemic stroke and were found to be inversely related with stroke severity in post-menopausal women (Pappa et al. 2012). One small study found that estradiol levels correlated with functional

Table 2 Differences between ischemic and hemorrhagic strokes. Adapted from Vyas et al. (2021)

Ischemic stroke	Hemorrhagic stroke
• Risk of ischemic stroke and TIA is higher for women than men <30	• Women have higher prevalence and incidence of intracranial aneuryms
• Risk of ischemic stroke and TIA is higher in men for midlife (age 40–80)	• Women have higher incidence of subarachnoid hemorrhage compared to men
• Risk of ischemic stroke and TIA is equal in those >80 years	• Men have higher incidence of intracerebral hemorrhage

Fig. 1 Stroke subtypes pie chart (Heron 2021)

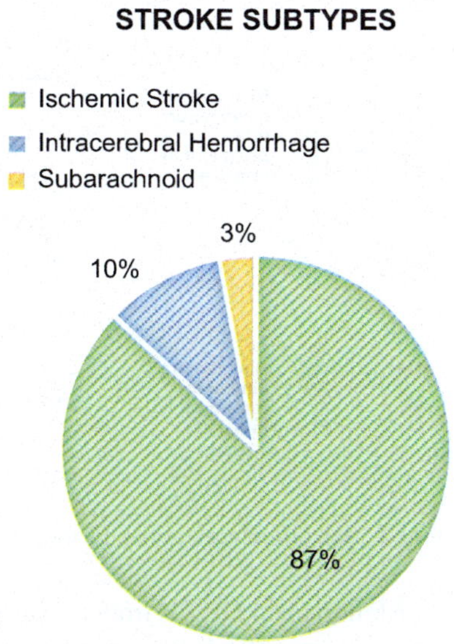

outcomes (change in mRS) in both men and women in the acute phase (24 h) of stroke. However, no significant difference in estradiol levels was seen 24 h post-stroke in men or women. Testosterone levels decreased at 24 h after stroke in men. The enzyme P450 aromatase actively converts testosterone to estradiol (Manwani et al. 2021). Aromatase levels increased after acute ischemic stroke, but this was only true for women, suggesting an active aromatization process in post-menopausal women after acute ischemic stroke (Manwani et al. 2021).

In the reproductive age group, stroke incidence is low but this risk is significantly increased with the use of OCPs, especially those containing high amounts of estrogen. Oral estrogens have a dose-response association with risk, and since their introduction and recognition of thrombotic risk, their doses have declined (Gillum et al. 2000; Sheikh et al. 2018). To explain this, we must recall that the physiology of estrogen as a hormone – it has positive cardiovascular effects, but can also enhance coagulation thereby increasing the risk of clotting in a woman on estrogen containing OCPs. Both oral contraceptive use and hormone replacement therapy have been associated with an increased risk of stroke, particularly during the first year of use (Johansson et al. 2022).

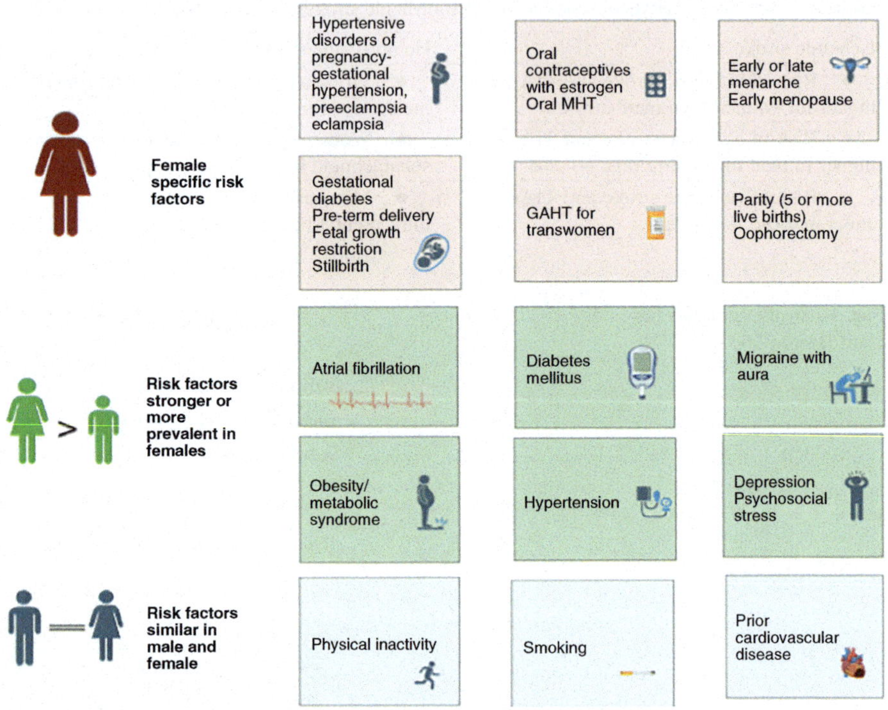

Fig. 2 Sex differences in risk factors (Yu et al. 2019; Poorthuis et al. 2017; Rexrode et al. 2022)

Menopausal HRT's impacts on stroke are dependent on the timing of initiation as most aging-related diseases manifest 10 years after menopause. Menopausal HRT specifically reduced all-cause mortality and cardiovascular disease when started in women under 60 years of age and/or less than 10 years since menopause (Islam et al. 2022).

6 Stroke Etiology

Stroke etiology dictates secondary prevention strategies. Of strokes in women, a higher percentage is due to atrial fibrillation compared to men who are more likely to have strokes due to large or small vessel disease (Förster et al. 2009). Studies have found that women have significantly higher percentages of cardioembolic stroke and lower rates of thromboembolic and lacunar strokes, which concurred with imaging analysis that showed that women have higher rates of territorial and lower rates of border zone and lacunar infarcts.

7 Atrial Fibrillation

There are a number of risk factors for the development of atrial fibrillation including genetic, vascular risk factors and the more recently described atrial cardiomyopathy. The American Heart Association, American College of Cardiology and Heart Rhythm Society recommends using the CHA2DS2-VASc score to predict stroke risk and need for anticoagulation in patients with atrial fibrillation. Oral anticoagulation therapy reduces the risk of stroke from atrial fibrillation. Despite this, it was found that in the care of newly diagnosed atrial fibrillation in the USA, women are less likely to receive oral anticoagulation compared to men (Yong et al. 2020).

A Canadian study of 28,886 patients with incident non-valvular atrial fibrillation who presented to ED found that among patients discharged home, the incidence of stroke at 1 year was higher in females than in males (2.9 versus 2.3%, difference 0.01, 95% CI 0.002–0.01) and that among admitted patients, there was a 48% higher risk of stroke in females compared to males (adjusted hazard ratio 1.14–1.92) (Yong et al. 2020). Among women who were discharged home, there was a 5% lower rate of oral anticoagulants use in 1 year compared to males (adjusted hazard ratio 0.95, 95% CI 0.91–0.99). When anticoagulation was initiated, women were found to have higher adherence to direct anticoagulants, though both sexes had poor warfarin control (Table 3) (Yong et al. 2020).

Novel anticoagulants (dabigatran, rivaroxaban, apixaban, and edoxaban) are now recommended over warfarin for stroke prevention in patients with non-valvular atrial fibrillation. While NOACs are as effective as warfarin and have improved safety in both males and females, meta-analysis indicated that the risk of bleeding is lower in females (Pancholy et al. 2014).

Percutaneous left atrial appendage occlusion (LAAO) has been used as an alternative to anticoagulation in patients with non-valvular atrial fibrillation who have contraindications to anticoagulation. No sex differences were found in the reduced risk of death, stroke, and long-term bleeding among men and women but women have been found to have higher rates of peri-procedural complications (all-cause mortality, stroke, major bleeding, pericardial effusion) (Zeitler et al. 2023; Alkhouli et al. 2022; Mathai et al. 2023).

8 Treatment of Acute Ischemic Strokes

8.1 Thrombolysis

Acute strokes presenting within 4.5 h of symptom onset might be eligible for thrombolytic agents given intravenously. The three factors that have been found to modify the effects of rtTPA are time from symptom onset to treatment, presence of ApoE2 phenotype, and female gender (Kent et al. 2005; Broderick et al. 2001). Multiple studies have found that intra-arterial thrombolysis resulted in improved outcomes for females relative to males (Broderick et al. 2001). However, the

Table 3 CHAD2DS2VAS score

	Risk factor	Score
C	Congestive heart failure/LV dysfunction	1
H	Hypertension	1
A2	Age > 75	2
D	Diabetes mellitus	1
S2	Stroke/TIA/thromboembolism	2
V	Vascular disease (prior myocardial infarction, peripheral artery disease, aortic plaque)	1
A	Age 65–74	1
S	Female sex	1

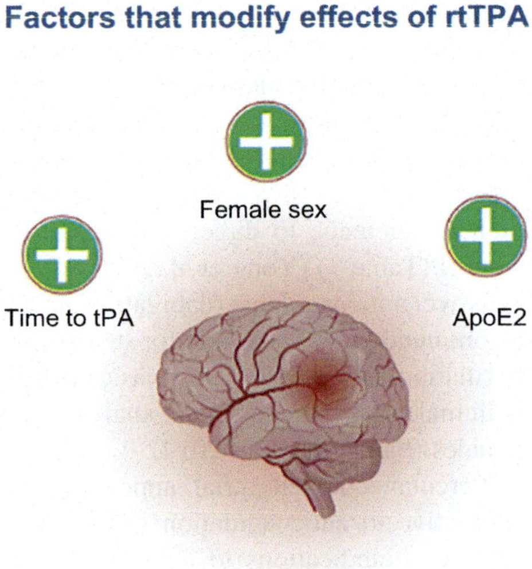

Fig. 3 Factors that modify effects of rtPA

Efficacy and Safety of MRI-Based Thrombolysis in Wake-Up Stroke (WAKE-UP) Trial found that sex did not modify the treatment effect of alteplase but it is important to note that of the 503 randomized patients, only 35.4% were women (Wouters et al. 2023).

The mechanisms of this relationship between sex and rtTPA have been hypothesized to be due to the higher levels of plasminogen activator inhibitor-1 in females with acute ischemic stroke compared to males, the neuroprotective effects of estrogen, differences in vascular anatomy, and the stroke etiology itself (better recanalization of fibrin-rich embolic occlusion in cardioembolism compared to platelet-rich occlusion in thromboembolism and atherosclerosis) (Fig. 3) (Kent et al. 2005).

Earlier studies consistently showed that women with acute stroke were less likely to be treated with IV thrombolysis compared with men, although this gap has closed in more recent years (Strong et al. 2020). These disparities in tPA administration may be due to the fact that women may be more likely to live alone before stroke and atypical symptoms of stroke leading to inappropriate triage and ineligibility for thrombolysis (Bushnell et al. 2018).

The analysis of sex differences in the Norwegian Tenecteplase Trial (NOR-TEST), found although only 40% of those enrolled were women, there were no significant differences in clinical outcome between males and females. Similar to other studies, enrolled women had a lower burden of cardiovascular risk factors like diabetes mellitus and higher mean high density lipoprotein cholesterol level. Thrombolysis, irrespective of agent (tenecteplase/alteplase), was equally effective and safe in both women and men (Ihle-Hansen et al. 2022).

9 Carotid Intervention

Carotid artery stenosis is typically measured with duplex ultrasound or CTA/angiography. Patients are stratified based on degree of stenosis and the presence of symptoms (symptomatic or asymptomatic). Management includes optimal medical therapy (applicable to extracranial stenosis including vertebral artery as listed in Table 4), carotid endarterectomy (CEA), and carotid artery stenting (CAS).

Clinically, it has been observed that women with carotid stenosis have better outcomes when treated with drug/medical therapy compared to carotid intervention (see Table 4 for optimal medical therapy). In a pooled analysis of patients with symptomatic 50–99% carotid stenosis, medical therapy (aspirin 1,300 mg/day along with risk reduction i.e., smoking cessation and control of hypertension/diabetes mellitus) was associated with a lower stroke rate in women but not men. Furthermore, one in nine carotid procedures prevented strokes in males compared to only 1 procedure in 36 in females. In a combined analysis of two clinical trials related to asymptomatic carotid stenosis, CEA reduced the stroke risk in men with no definite benefit in women (Rothwell and Goldstein 2004; Rothwell et al. 2004; Dansey et al. 2020). Symptomatic females were found to have a slightly higher 30-day mortality rate following CEA and asymptomatic females had twice as many in hospital strokes following carotid artery stenting (CAS) when compared to their male counterparts (Rothwell et al. 2004). However, in a study evaluating patients with both asymptomatic and symptomatic carotid stenosis that underwent CEA, no differences in outcomes were found between sexes in the USA and Canada despite differences in clinical and procedural characteristics (Li et al. 2023). It has also been found that there is a significant discrepancy in the proportion of females compared to males receiving pre-operative best medical therapy (see Table 4) for stroke prevention prior to carotid artery revascularization, and in-hospital outcomes were worse in patients without this best medical therapy (Bose et al. 2023). Despite this, the Society for Vascular Surgery continues to recommend that low-risk surgical patients with asymptomatic carotid stenosis of >70%, carotid endarterectomy with best medical therapy is favored over maximal medical therapy alone in the long-term prevention of stroke and death (grade IB) and carotid endarterectomy (CEA) is recommended

Table 4 Optimal medical management of carotid stenosis adapted from European Society for Vascular Surgery (ESVS) 2023 (Hackam 2021; Naylor et al. 2023)

Modality	Recommendations	2023 ESVS practice guidelines for asymptomatic carotid stenosis	2023 ESVS practice guidelines for symptomatic carotid stenosis
Diet	Mediterranean diet	Level of evidence I / level B	Same as asymptomatic
Exercise	Moderate intensity at least 150 min per week	Level of evidence I / level B	Same as asymptomatic
Smoking	Smoking cessation with varenicline, bupropion	Level of evidence IB	Same as asymptomatic
Antithrombotic therapy	Aspirin 75–325 mg per day	Class IIa/level C II a for >50% asymptomatic carotid stenosis Class I/level B for aspirin 75–325 mg daily rather than >325 mg aspirin daily if undergoing carotid endarterectomy	
	Aspirin daily + rivaroxaban 2.5 mg twice daily		
	Clopidogrel 75 mg daily or ticagrelor 90 mg BID (if ASA intolerant or allergic)	Class IIa/level C II a for >50% asymptomatic carotid stenosis if intolerant or allergic to aspirin	
	Aspirin 75–325 mg daily + clopidogrel 75 mg daily	Class I/level B for asymptomatic carotid stenosis undergoing carotid stenting: – Clopidogrel 75 mg to be started 3 days prior to stenting, and single load of clopidogrel 300 mg in urgent cases. – Continue aspirin and clopidogrel for at least 4 weeks after stenting and then antiplatelet to be continued indefinitely	1. Class I/level A for symptomatic carotid stenosis patients who are not being considered for CEA or CAS following TIA or minor ischemic stroke to get short-term aspirin plus clopidogrel for 21 days followed by clopidogrel monotherapy, or long-term aspirin therapy plus modified release dipyridamole 2. Class I/level B for recently symptomatic carotid stenosis patients who are not being considered for

(continued)

Table 4 (continued)

Modality	Recommendations	2023 ESVS practice guidelines for asymptomatic carotid stenosis	2023 ESVS practice guidelines for symptomatic carotid stenosis
			CEA/CAS who are intolerant or allergic to aspirin and clopidogrel, dipyridamole monotherapy or ticagrelor monotherapy is recommended 3. Class I/level A for recently symptomatic carotid stenosis patients scheduled to undergo CEA, antiplatelet therapy is to be prescribed throughout the perioperative period and long-term 4. Class IIa/level C for recently symptomatic patients with a 50–99% carotid stenosis who are to undergo CEA, perioperative combination antiplatelet therapy should be considered, and should be started after imaging excludes intracranial hemorrhage 5. Class IIa/level B in recently symptomatic patients with 50–99% stenosis who are undergoing CEA and aspirin monotherapy is preferred over combination therapy, aspirin 300–325 mg daily to be given for 14 days followed by 75–162 mg daily 6. Class I/level B for recently symptomatic patients undergoing CEA on aspirin monotherapy, lower dose of 75–325 mg is

(continued)

Table 4 (continued)

Modality	Recommendations	2023 ESVS practice guidelines for asymptomatic carotid stenosis	2023 ESVS practice guidelines for symptomatic carotid stenosis
			preferred rather than >325 mg aspirin daily. Class I/level C use of dipyridamole modified release monotherapy (200 mg twice daily) if intolerant to aspirin or clopidogrel 7. Class I/level C for recently symptomatic patients undergoing CAS to get combination of aspirin (75–325 mg daily) and clopidogrel. Clopidogrel 75 mg should be started 3 days prior, and 300 mg loading dose in urgent cases. Aspirin and clopidogrel to be continued for at least 4 weeks after stenting and then long-term monotherapy with clopidogrel indefinitely
Lipid-lowering therapy for goal LDL <1.8 mmol/L (70 mg/dl)	High-dose statin	Class I/level B for long-term prevention of stroke, MI, and other cardiovascular events	Class I/level B for long-term prevention of stroke, MI, and other cardiovascular events Class I/level A for commencement of statin therapy pre-operatively if patient is scheduled to undergo CEA or CAS
	Add ezetimibe or PCSK9 inhibitor	Class IIa/level C for dyslipidemic patients who are intolerant to statins, with or without ezetimibe, therapy with PCSK9 inhibitors to be considered	Class I/level B for addition to ezetimibe 10 mg daily in those with symptomatic carotid stenosis who do not reach lipid targets on maximum doses or maximum tolerated doses of statins Class IIa/level B for additional treatment

(continued)

Table 4 (continued)

Modality	Recommendations	2023 ESVS practice guidelines for asymptomatic carotid stenosis	2023 ESVS practice guidelines for symptomatic carotid stenosis
			with PCSK9 inhibitors in symptomatic carotid stenosis patients who are intolerant of or unable to achieve target LDL on statins with or without ezetimibe
	Icosapent ethyl (high-dose EPA) if fasting triglyceride elevated		
Antihypertensive therapy	Goal blood pressure < 130/80 mmHg	Class I/level A	
	ACE inhibitor or ARB (high prevalence of renovascular hypertension)		
Glucose lowering therapy	HbA1c <7 Metformin, GLP-1 agonist, SGLT-2 antagonist	Class I/level B	

over transfemoral carotid artery stenting in low and standard risk patients with >50% carotid stenosis (grade I, level A) (AbuRahma et al. 2022).

These differences are thought to relate to histopathological finding that carotid artery plaques in women have a more stable and less inflammatory phenotype (fewer macrophages) compared to men (Hellings et al. 2007). MRI analysis has shown that the carotid plaques in men have thin fibrous caps on the plaques with a lipid-rich necrotic core, making them more prone to rupture, possibly explaining why CEA is more effective in reducing subsequent stroke in asymptomatic men with carotid stenosis (Ota et al. 2010).

9.1 Endovascular Interventions

In recent years, endovascular thrombectomy (EVT) has dramatically improved outcomes for eligible patients with large vessel occlusions. Women with atrial fibrillation are less often treated with anticoagulation, which may then lead to a greater number of large vessel cardioembolic strokes in women, and thereby a higher need for thrombectomy (Rexrode et al. 2022). A study of almost 400 patients who underwent endovascular stent placement for large vessel occlusions found that women had higher rates of atrial fibrillation and were older. However, despite these differences, females experienced comparable functional outcomes (90-day clinical outcome) and greater years of optimal life after intervention compared to males (Sheth et al. 2019). Recanalization success and treatment effect on mRS do not differ between men and women (Sheth et al. 2019; Dmytriw et al. 2021; Sun et al. 2023). The ANGEL-ACT registry showed similar clinical outcomes in men and women with anterior circulation LVO treated with EVT but analysis of the subgroup of patients with lower NIHSS (<15) showed that women tended to have better outcomes (Sun et al. 2023). After EVT however, they found that women were more likely to be disabled at discharge but were less likely to experience in-hospital death compared to men (Demel et al. 2022).

The differences in post-stroke outcomes of patients undergoing EVT are largely explained by differences in baseline epidemiological variables such as age and that the stroke is due to a cardioembolic event. Women are more likely to live alone and have more pre-stroke disability, thereby creating a potential delay between symptom onset and activation of emergency response (Ospel et al. 2022; Ali et al. 2022b). The proportion of women living alone is close to double that of men after the age of 75, 45% of women versus 23% of men (PRB 2000). There is a direct association between social isolation, loneliness, and coronary heart disease and stroke mortality, which may contribute to poor recovery in women (Cené et al. 2022). Analysis of data from the Multicentre Randomized Controlled Trial of Endovascular Treatment for Acute Ischaemic Stroke in The Netherlands (MR CLEAN) Registry found that the mean onset-to-door time was longer in women which contributed to longer onset-to-groin times in women (Ali et al. 2022b).

10 Treatment of Intracerebral Hemorrhage

There are currently no medical treatments that improve outcomes for ICH in randomized controlled trials. The primary goal is to ensure that blood pressure is lowered, anticoagulants are reversed, and neurosurgical intervention is performed, if indicated. The Intensive Blood Pressure Reduction in Acute Cerebral Hemorrhage trials 1 and 2 randomized patients into an intensive target of less than 140 mmHg within 1 h, or the guideline-recommended blood pressure treatment (>160 mmHg) (Sandset et al. 2020). There were no differences in outcome in patients with more intensive blood pressure lowering. Notably, there was no effect of sex on the combined end point of death or major disability, hematoma growth, or effect of randomized blood pressure lowering treatment (Sandset et al. 2020). In those intracerebral hemorrhages associated with anticoagulant use, discontinuation of the offending agent and reversing anticoagulation is key to improving outcomes.

11 Pregnancy

Stroke can occur any time during pregnancy but the post-partum period confers the highest per day risk of stroke, with the highest risk being in the immediate post-partum period up to 2 weeks post-partum (Bushnell et al. 2018). The risks for all types of strokes (ischemic stroke, intracerebral hemorrhage, and subarachnoid hemorrhage) increase (Swartz et al. 2017). However, in contrast to the general population in whom ischemic strokes are more common, up to half of maternal strokes are due to subarachnoid hemorrhage or ICH. The USA has the highest maternal mortality rates among developed countries, and cardiovascular disease is the leading cause (Mehta et al. 2021). Pregnancy-related mortality rates for non-Hispanic Black and American Indian/Alaska Native women are up to 2–3 times that of White women, and these disparities persist independently of socioeconomic variables (Petersen et al. 2019).

The hypertensive disorders of pregnancy including chronic or gestational hypertension, pre-eclampsia, eclampsia, or the HELLP (hemolysis, elevated liver enzymes, low platelet) syndrome are important risk factors for stroke in pregnancy. Other risk factors include migraine, thrombophilia, congenital or acquired heart disease, and infections. Pregnancy-related strokes are most commonly due to pre-eclampsia, eclampsia, reversible cerebral vasospasm syndrome (RCVS), and posterior reversible vasospasm (PRES), all of which share features of endothelial dysfunction and failure of cerebrovascular autoregulation (Bushnell et al. 2018; Swartz et al. 2017; Mehta et al. 2021; Miller and Leffert 2020).

tPA is safe in pregnancy and should be considered when appropriate as the large molecular size makes it incapable of crossing the placenta. Current guidelines dictate that tPA is standard of care for acute ischemic stroke in pregnancy, and thrombolytic therapy should be considered while weighing the maternal and fetal risks and benefits. Management of hypertension guidelines shared between the 2018 AHA guidelines for acute hypertension in stroke and the American College of Obstetrics and Gynecology recommend the use of IV labetalol, hydralazine, and nicardipine. Oral therapies include labetalol (first line per ACOG) and nifedipine, though the latter is not amongst those listed by the AHA for acute hypertension management in acute ischemic stroke (Miller and Leffert 2020; Mehta et al. 2021).

Hemorrhagic strokes can lead to life-threatening complications like hematoma expansion, cerebral edema, raised intracranial pressure, hydrocephalus, and brain herniation. Hyperosmolar therapy is the mainstay of management of raised ICP along with elevation of head end of bed, minimization of pain with analgesics and anxiolytics, and normothermia maintenance. Mannitol and hypertonic saline are used as life-saving measures in impeding brain herniation, and while they can decrease amniotic fluid volume, the maternal therapeutic benefits would likely outweigh fetal risks (Mehta et al. 2021; Miller and Leffert 2020).

Subarachnoid hemorrhages can be complicated by delayed cerebral ischemia due to vasospasm, and nimodipine is safe to use during pregnancy (Mehta et al. 2021). Warfarin, unfractionated heparin, and low-molecular-weight heparin can be used if needed for secondary stroke prevention while breastfeeding (Mehta et al. 2021; Miller and Leffert 2020).

12 Secondary Stroke Prevention

12.1 Antiplatelets

It has been found that prophylactic low-dose aspirin is helpful in reducing the risk of both ischemic strokes and TIAs in women for primary prevention, although the net value is uncertain. There is no significant reduction of risk of myocardial infarction or death from cardiovascular causes in women and leads to an increase in major bleeds (gastrointestinal and other extracranial sites) (Ridker et al. 2005; Antithrombotic Trialists' (ATT) Collaboration et al. 2009). A meta-analysis of randomized controlled trials of cardiovascular events in women and men found that aspirin therapy reduced the risk of a composite of cardiovascular events due to its effect on reducing the risk of ischemic stroke in women and myocardial infarction in men (Berger et al. 2006). These differences are likely due to differences in aspirin metabolism, increased prevalence of aspirin resistance in women, and the fact that women have a greater risk of stroke compared to myocardial infarction, whereas the converse is true for men who have a greater risk of myocardial infarction (Berger et al. 2006). The major side effect of aspirin therapy is the risk of major bleeding, which was increased by 70% in both men and women (Berger et al. 2006).

The data studying various combinations of aspirin and clopidogrel have varied results with some showing benefits of aspirin and DAPT for secondary stroke prevention in men, but not women as elaborated upon in Table 4 (Antithrombotic Trialists' (ATT) Collaboration et al. 2009; Hoshino et al. 2022; CAPRIE Steering Committee 1996; SPS3 Investigators et al. 2012; Bhatt et al. 2006; Diener et al. 2004; Sacco et al. 2008; Shinohara and Huang 2012).

There are sex differences at the platelet-vascular interface that might explain these differences. Women have higher platelet responsiveness and retain more platelet reactivity even after the initial decrement caused by aspirin initiation in both sexes. P2Y12 inhibition reduces fibrinogen in both sexes, but P-selectin is less inhibited in women, thereby women may have a lower ability to inhibit platelet proinflammatory functions (Table 5) (Sabetta et al. 2022).

Table 5 Sex differences in the effectiveness of antiplatelets for stroke prevention

Study	Drug tested	Outcome
Antithrombotic Trialists' (ATT) Collaboration et al. (2009)	Aspirin	Aspirin significantly reduced stroke incidence in women but not men
Clopidogrel versus Aspirin in Patients at Risk of Ischemic Events (CAPRIE) (1996)	Clopidogrel versus aspirin	Only 28% of patients enrolled were female No sub-analysis of sex-related side effects
Secondary Prevention of Small Subcortical Strokes (SPS3) Trial (SPS3 Investigators et al. 2012)	Aspirin and clopidogrel versus aspirin alone	No clear difference between secondary prevention in male and female patients
Clopidogrel for High Atherothrombotic Risk and Ischemic Stabilization, Management and Avoidance (CHARISMA) Trial (Bhatt et al. 2006)	Aspirin and clopidogrel versus aspirin alone	No difference between male and female patients but the combination of aspirin and clopidogrel was more effective in males
Management of ATherothrombosis with Clopidogrel in High-risk patients (MATCH) study (Diener et al. 2004)	Aspirin and clopidogrel combination versus clopidogrel alone	Better treatment effect in men patients compared to women
The Prevention Regimen for Effectively Avoiding Second Strokes (PRoFESS) trial (Sacco et al. 2008)	Clopidogrel versus fixed dose combination of aspirin and dipyridamole	Only 36% of enrolled patients were female No clear sex difference
The Cilostazol Stroke Prevention Study 2 (CSPS2) and Cilostazol versus Aspirin for Secondary Ischaemic Stroke Prevention (CASISP) (Shinohara and Huang 2012)	Cilostazol versus aspirin	Annual incidences of stroke (cilostazol 2.89%, aspirin 4.50%; $p = 0.0032$) and intracranial hemorrhage (0.25 vs. 1.22%; $p<0.001$) were significantly lower in male patients in the cilostazol group, with no difference between the two treatment groups in females
The Cilostazol Stroke Prevention Study combination trial – subgroup analysis (Hoshino et al. 2022)	Monotherapy (aspirin or clopidogrel) versus dual antiplatelet (aspirin and cilostazol or clopidogrel and cilostazol)	Long-term DAPT using cilostazol reduced the recurrence of ischemic stroke and prolonged the recurrence-free time in male patients, but not in female patients

13 Pitfalls in Research and the Way Forward

Despite ample evidence to suggest that the pathophysiology of stroke is sex specific, there is a paucity of sex-specific endpoints in clinical trials, hindering stroke treatment and research (Carcel et al. 2021). Minocycline, which is anti-inflammatory and an inhibitor of cell death, improved functional outcome after ischemic stroke in men, but had no benefit in women, although the trial was relatively small (Amiri-Nikpour et al. 2015). However, this male-specific benefit was also seen in an experimental mouse model of ischemic stroke, illustrating the importance of assessing sex as a variable in both clinical and experimental research (Li and McCullough 2009). The Systolic Blood Pressure Improvement Trial (SPRINT) reported that aggressive blood pressure control improved composite cardiovascular risk, including stroke, however, only 36% of those enrolled this study were female (Wenger et al. 2016; SPRINT Research Group et al. 2015; Gillis and Sullivan 2016). The study was terminated because of improved outcomes in men (HR 0.72, 95% CI, 0.59–0.88) before statistical significance was reached in females (HR 0.84, CI 95%, 0.62–1.14) casting doubt over the generalizability of SPRINT to females. A recent Cochrane review of seven randomized clinical trials (including SPRINT) found there was little to no difference in total mortality and cardiovascular mortality between people with hypertension and cardiovascular disease treated to a lower compared to a standard blood pressure target (Saiz et al. 2022).

Not all trials have shown exclusive benefits to men, and fortunately there has been a slow but steady increase in the female representation in clinical trials. The PARAGON-HF trial (Angiotensin Receptor Neprilysin Inhibitor with Angiotensin Receptor Blocker Global Outcomes in Heart Failure and Preserved Left Ventricular Ejection Fraction) recruited more women ($n = 2,479$; 52%) than previous heart failure trials (McMurray et al. 2020). They found that compared with valsartan, sacubitril-valsartan seemed to reduce the risk of heart failure hospitalization more in women than in men. In the Efficacy Study of Combined Treatment With Uric Acid and rtPA in Acute Ischemic Stroke (URICO-ICTUS) trial which enrolled an equal number of men and women, women with acute ischemic stroke treated with alteplase had excellent outcomes with reduction in infarct growth with the administration of uric acid, which was not significant in men (Chamorro et al. 2014; Llull et al. 2015).

While we have made strides in the identification of sex differences in stroke, there are still many areas that need improvement, especially in Black and Hispanic women. Though gender parity is favorable in neurology faculty over the past several years, fewer women serve as a principal investigator in clinical trials (Rawlley et al. 2023). Research in the future must focus on bridging gaps in our knowledge base in order to be able to be adequately equipped to provide the best care for patients of both sexes (Fig. 4).

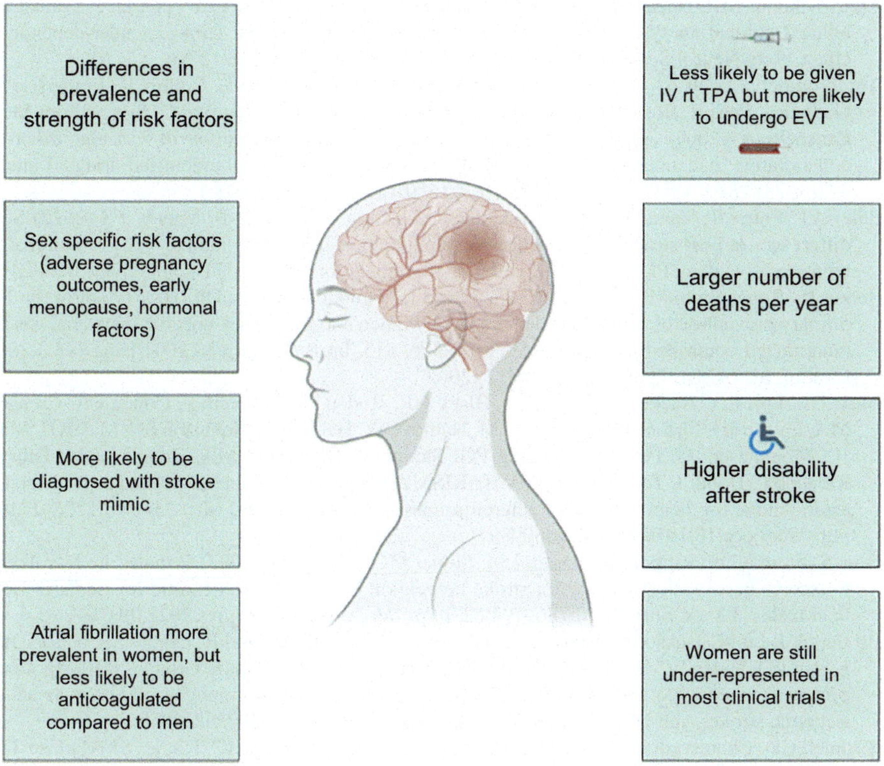

Fig. 4 Highlights (Adapted from 66)

References

AbuRahma AF, Avgerinos ED, Chang RW, Darling RC III, Duncan AA, Forbes TL, Malas MB, Murad MH, Perler BA, Powell RJ, Rockman CB, Zhou W (2022) Society for vascular surgery clinical practice guidelines for management of extracranial cerebrovascular disease. J Vasc Surg 75(1S):4S–22S. https://doi.org/10.1016/j.jvs.2021.04.073

Ali M, van Os HJA, van der Weerd N, Schoones JW, Heymans MW, Kruyt ND, Visser MC, Wermer MJH (2022a) Sex differences in presentation of stroke: a systematic review and meta-analysis. Stroke 53(2):345–354. https://doi.org/10.1161/STROKEAHA.120.034040

Ali M, van der Meij A, van Os HJA, Ali M, Van Zwet EW, Spaander FHM, Hofmeijer J, Nederkoorn PJ, van den Wijngaard IR, Majoie CBLM, van Es ACGM, Schonewille WJ, van Walderveen MAA, Dippel DWJ, Visser MC, Kruyt ND, Wermer MJH, Registry Investigators MRCLEAN (2022b) Sex differences in onset to hospital arrival time, prestroke disability, and clinical symptoms in patients with a large vessel occlusion: a MR CLEAN Registry substudy. J Neurointerv Surg:jnis-2022-019670. https://doi.org/10.1136/jnis-2022-019670

Alkhouli M, Russo AM, Thaler D, Windecker S, Anderson JA, Gage R, Lakkireddy D (2022) Sex differences in safety and effectiveness of LAAO: insights from the amulet IDE trial. JACC Cardiovasc Interv 15(21):2143–2155. https://doi.org/10.1016/j.jcin.2022.06.037

Amiri-Nikpour MR, Nazarbaghi S, Hamdi-Holasou M, Rezaei Y (2015) An open-label evaluator-blinded clinical study of minocycline neuroprotection in ischemic stroke: gender-dependent effect. Acta Neurol Scand 131(1):45–50. https://doi.org/10.1111/ane.12296

Antithrombotic Trialists' (ATT) Collaboration, Baigent C, Blackwell L, Collins R, Emberson J, Godwin J, Peto R, Buring J, Hennekens C, Kearney P, Meade T, Patrono C, Roncaglioni MC, Zanchetti A (2009) Aspirin in the primary and secondary prevention of vascular disease: collaborative meta-analysis of individual participant data from randomised trials. Lancet 373(9678):1849–1860. https://doi.org/10.1016/S0140-6736(09)60503-1

Bako AT, Potter T, Tannous J, Pan AP, Johnson C, Baig E, Downer B, Vahidy FS (2022) Sex differences in post-stroke cognitive decline: a population-based longitudinal study of nationally representative data. PLoS One 17(5):e0268249. https://doi.org/10.1371/journal.pone.0268249

Berger JS, Roncaglioni MC, Avanzini F, Pangrazzi I, Tognoni G, Brown DL (2006) Aspirin for the primary prevention of cardiovascular events in women and men: a sex-specific meta-analysis of randomized controlled trials. JAMA 295(3):306–313. https://doi.org/10.1001/jama.295.3.306. Erratum in: JAMA. 2006 May 3;295(17):2002

Bhatt DL, Fox KA, Hacke W, Berger PB, Black HR, Boden WE, Cacoub P, Cohen EA, Creager MA, Easton JD, Flather MD, Haffner SM, Hamm CW, Hankey GJ, Johnston SC, Mak KH, Mas JL, Montalescot G, Pearson TA, Steg PG, Steinhubl SR, Weber MA, Brennan DM, Fabry-Ribaudo L, Booth J, Topol EJ (2006) CHARISMA Investigators. Clopidogrel and aspirin versus aspirin alone for the prevention of atherothrombotic events. N Engl J Med 354(16):1706–1717. https://doi.org/10.1056/NEJMoa060989

Bose S, Stonko DP, Pappas GM, Drudi LM, Stoner MC, Hicks CW (2023) Females are less likely to receive best medical therapy for stroke prevention before and after carotid revascularization than males. J Vasc Surg 77(3):786–794.e2. https://doi.org/10.1016/j.jvs.2022.09.028

Broderick J, Lu M, Jackson C, Pancioli A, Tilley BC, Fagan SC, Kothari R, Levine SR, Marler JR, Lyden PD, Haley EC Jr, Brott T, Grotta JC, NINDS t-PA Stroke Study Group (2001) Apolipoprotein E phenotype and the efficacy of intravenous tissue plasminogen activator in acute ischemic stroke. Ann Neurol 49(6):736–744. https://doi.org/10.1002/ana.1058

Bushnell CD, Chaturvedi S, Gage KR, Herson PS, Hurn PD, Jiménez MC, Kittner SJ, Madsen TE, McCullough LD, McDermott M, Reeves MJ, Rundek T (2018) Sex differences in stroke: challenges and opportunities. J Cereb Blood Flow Metab 38(12):2179–2191. https://doi.org/10.1177/0271678X18793324

CAPRIE Steering Committee (1996) A randomised, blinded, trial of clopidogrel versus aspirin in patients at risk of ischaemic events (CAPRIE). CAPRIE Steering Committee. Lancet 348(9038):1329–1339. https://doi.org/10.1016/s0140-6736(96)09457-3

Carcel C, Wang X, Sandset EC, Delcourt C, Arima H, Lindley R, Hackett ML, Lavados P, Robinson TG, Muñoz Venturelli P, Olavarría VV, Brunser A, Berge E, Chalmers J, Woodward M, Anderson CS (2019) Sex differences in treatment and outcome after stroke: pooled analysis including 19,000 participants. Neurology 93(24):e2170–e2180. https://doi.org/10.1212/WNL.0000000000008615. Erratum in: Neurology. 2021 Jun 8;96(23):1106

Carcel C, Harris K, Peters SAE, Sandset EC, Balicki G, Bushnell CD, Howard VJ, Reeves MJ, Anderson CS, Kelly PJ, Woodward M (2021) Representation of women in stroke clinical trials: a review of 281 trials involving more than 500,000 participants. Neurology 97(18):e1768–e1774. https://doi.org/10.1212/WNL.0000000000012767

Cené CW, Beckie TM, Sims M, Suglia SF, Aggarwal B, Moise N, Jiménez MC, Gaye B, McCullough LD, American Heart Association Social Determinants of Health Committee of the Council on Epidemiology and Prevention and Council on Quality of Care and Outcomes Research, Prevention Science Committee of the Council on Epidemiology and Prevention and Council on Cardiovascular and Stroke Nursing, Council on Arteriosclerosis, Thrombosis and Vascular Biology; and Stroke Council (2022) Effects of objective and perceived social isolation on cardiovascular and brain health: a scientific statement from the American Heart Association. J Am Heart Assoc 11(16):e026493. https://doi.org/10.1161/JAHA.122.026493

Chamorro A, Amaro S, Castellanos M, Segura T, Arenillas J, Martí-Fábregas J, Gállego J, Krupinski J, Gomis M, Cánovas D, Carné X, Deulofeu R, Román LS, Oleaga L, Torres F, Planas AM, URICO-ICTUS Investigators (2014) Safety and efficacy of uric acid in patients with acute stroke (URICO-ICTUS): a randomised, double-blind phase 2b/3 trial. Lancet Neurol 13(5):453–460. https://doi.org/10.1016/S1474-4422(14)70054-7

Dansey KD, Pothof AB, Zettervall SL, Swerdlow NJ, Liang P, Schneider JR, Nolan BW, Schermerhorn ML (2020) Clinical impact of sex on carotid revascularization. J Vasc Surg 71(5):1587–1594.e2. https://doi.org/10.1016/j.jvs.2019.07.088

Demel SL, Reeves M, Xu H, Xian Y, Mac Grory B, Fonarow GC, Matsouaka R, Smith EE, Saver J, Schwamm L (2022) Sex differences in endovascular therapy for ischemic stroke: results from the get with the guidelines-stroke registry. Stroke 53(10):3099–3106. https://doi.org/10.1161/STROKEAHA.122.038491

Diener HC, Bogousslavsky J, Brass LM, Cimminiello C, Csiba L, Kaste M, Leys D, Matias-Guiu J, Rupprecht HJ, MATCH investigators (2004) Aspirin and clopidogrel compared with clopidogrel alone after recent ischaemic stroke or transient ischaemic attack in high-risk patients (MATCH): randomised, double-blind, placebo-controlled trial. Lancet 364(9431):331–337. https://doi.org/10.1016/S0140-6736(04)16721-4

Dmytriw AA, Ku JC, Yang VXD, Hui N, Uchida K, Morimoto T, Spears J, Marotta TR, Diestro JDB (2021) Do outcomes between women and men differ after endovascular thrombectomy? A meta-analysis. AJNR Am J Neuroradiol 42(5):910–915. https://doi.org/10.3174/ajnr.A7075

Eriksson M, Grundberg A, Inge E, von Euler M (2023) Stroke recurrence following 28 days after first stroke in men and women 2012 to 2020: observations from the Swedish Stroke Register. J Am Heart Assoc 12(3):e028222. https://doi.org/10.1161/JAHA.122.028222

Förster A, Gass A, Kern R, Wolf ME, Ottomeyer C, Zohsel K, Hennerici M, Szabo K (2009) Gender differences in acute ischemic stroke: etiology, stroke patterns and response to thrombolysis. Stroke 40(7):2428–2432. https://doi.org/10.1161/STROKEAHA.109.548750

Gillis EE, Sullivan JC (2016) Sex differences in hypertension: recent advances. Hypertension 68(6): 1322–1327. https://doi.org/10.1161/HYPERTENSIONAHA.116.06602

Gillum LA, Mamidipudi SK, Johnston SC (2000) Ischemic stroke risk with oral contraceptives: a meta-analysis. JAMA 284(1):72–78. https://doi.org/10.1001/jama.284.1.72

Hackam DG (2021) Optimal medical management of asymptomatic carotid stenosis. Stroke 52(6): 2191–2198. https://doi.org/10.1161/STROKEAHA.120.033994

Hellings WE, Pasterkamp G, Verhoeven BA, De Kleijn DP, De Vries JP, Seldenrijk KA, van den Broek T, Moll FL (2007) Gender-associated differences in plaque phenotype of patients undergoing carotid endarterectomy. J Vasc Surg 45(2):289–296.; discussion 296–297. https://doi.org/10.1016/j.jvs.2006.09.051

Heron M (2021) Deaths: leading causes for 2019. Natl Vital Stat Rep 70(9):1–114

Holmegard HN, Nordestgaard BG, Jensen GB, Tybjærg-Hansen A, Benn M (2016) Sex hormones and ischemic stroke: a prospective cohort study and meta-analyses. J Clin Endocrinol Metab 101(1):69–78. https://doi.org/10.1210/jc.2015-2687

Hoshino H, Toyoda K, Omae K, Takahashi K, Uchiyama S, Kimura K, Yamaguchi K, Minematsu K, Origasa H, Yamaguchi T, CSPS.com Trial Investigators (2022) Sex difference in the impact of dual antiplatelet therapy using cilostazol for secondary stroke prevention: a sub-analysis of CSPS.com. J Atheroscler Thromb. https://doi.org/10.5551/jat.63660

Ihle-Hansen H, Sandset EC, Ihle-Hansen H, Hagberg G, Thommessen B, Rønning OM, Kvistad CE, Novotny V, Naess H, Waje-Andreassen U, Thomassen L, Logallo N (2022) Sex differences in the Norwegian tenecteplase trial (NOR-TEST). Eur J Neurol 29(2):609–614. https://doi.org/10.1111/ene.15126

Irie F, Matsuo R, Nakamura K, Wakisaka Y, Ago T, Kitazono T, Kamouchi M, Fukuoka Stroke Registry Investigators (2023) Sex differences in long-term functional decline after ischemic stroke: a longitudinal observational study from the Fukuoka Stroke Registry. Cerebrovasc Dis:1–8. https://doi.org/10.1159/000526940

Islam S, Dover DC, Daniele P, Hawkins NM, Humphries KH, Kaul P, Sandhu RK (2022) Sex differences in the management of oral anticoagulation and outcomes for emergency department presentation of incident atrial fibrillation. Ann Emerg Med 80(2):97–107. https://doi.org/10.1016/j.annemergmed.2022.03.010

Johansson T, Fowler P, Ek WE, Skalkidou A, Karlsson T, Johansson Å (2022) Oral contraceptives, hormone replacement therapy, and stroke risk. Stroke 53(10):3107–3115. https://doi.org/10.1161/STROKEAHA.121.038659

Kent DM, Price LL, Ringleb P, Hill MD, Selker HP (2005) Sex-based differences in response to recombinant tissue plasminogen activator in acute ischemic stroke: a pooled analysis of randomized clinical trials. Stroke 36(1):62–65. https://doi.org/10.1161/01.STR.0000150515.15576.29

Li J, McCullough LD (2009) Sex differences in minocycline-induced neuroprotection after experimental stroke. J Cereb Blood Flow Metab 29(4):670–674. https://doi.org/10.1038/jcbfm.2009.3

Li B, Eisenberg N, Howe KL, Forbes TL, Roche-Nagle G (2023) The impact of sex on outcomes following carotid endarterectomy. Ann Vasc Surg 88:210–217. https://doi.org/10.1016/j.avsg.2022.08.003

Lisabeth LD, Brown DL, Hughes R, Majersik JJ, Morgenstern LB (2009) Acute stroke symptoms: comparing women and men. Stroke 40(6):2031–2036. https://doi.org/10.1161/STROKEAHA.109.546812

Llull L, Laredo C, Renú A, Pérez B, Vila E, Obach V, Urra X, Planas A, Amaro S, Chamorro Á (2015) Uric acid therapy improves clinical outcome in women with acute ischemic stroke. Stroke 46(8):2162–2167. https://doi.org/10.1161/STROKEAHA.115.009960

Lyu Y, Li W, Tang T (2022) Prevalence trends and influencing factors of post-stroke depression: a study based on the national health and nutrition examination survey. Med Sci Monit 28: e933367. https://doi.org/10.12659/MSM.933367

Madsen TE, Khoury J, Alwell K, Moomaw CJ, Rademacher E, Flaherty ML, Woo D, Mackey J, La Rosa DLR, F, Martini S, Ferioli S, Adeoye O, Khatri P, Broderick JP, Kissela BM, Kleindorfer D. (2017) Sex-specific stroke incidence over time in the Greater Cincinnati/Northern Kentucky Stroke Study. Neurology 89(10):990–996. https://doi.org/10.1212/WNL.0000000000004325

Manwani B, Fall P, Zhu L, O'Reilly MR, Conway S, Staff I, McCullough LD (2021) Increased P450 aromatase levels in post-menopausal women after acute ischemic stroke. Biol Sex Differ 12(1):8. https://doi.org/10.1186/s13293-020-00357-w

Mathai SV, Sohal S, Flatow E, Nagaraj S, Hajra A, Chugh Y, Palaiodimos L, Lee HJ, Ansari J, Cohen M, Volgman AS, Faillace R (2023) Sex differences in periprocedural and long-term outcomes following transcatheter left atrial appendage occlusion: a systematic review and meta-analysis. Cardiovasc Revasc Med 48:23–31. https://doi.org/10.1016/j.carrev.2022.10.002

Mauvais-Jarvis F, Bairey Merz N, Barnes PJ, Brinton RD, Carrero JJ, DeMeo DL, De Vries GJ, Epperson CN, Govindan R, Klein SL, Lonardo A, Maki PM, McCullough LD, Regitz-Zagrosek V, Regensteiner JG, Rubin JB, Sandberg K, Suzuki A (2020) Sex and gender: modifiers of health, disease, and medicine. Lancet 396(10250):565–582. https://doi.org/10.1016/S0140-6736(20)31561-0. Erratum in: Lancet. 2020 Sep 5;396(10252):668

McMurray JJV, Jackson AM, Lam CSP, Redfield MM, Anand IS, Ge J, Lefkowitz MP, Maggioni AP, Martinez F, Packer M, Pfeffer MA, Pieske B, Rizkala AR, Sabarwal SV, Shah AM, Shah SJ, Shi VC, van Veldhuisen DJ, Zannad F, Zile MR, Cikes M, Goncalvesova E, Katova T, Kosztin A, Lelonek M, Sweitzer N, Vardeny O, Claggett B, Jhund PS, Solomon SD (2020) Effects of sacubitril-valsartan versus valsartan in women compared with men with heart failure and preserved ejection fraction: insights from PARAGON-HF. Circulation 141(5):338–351. https://doi.org/10.1161/CIRCULATIONAHA.119.044491

Mehta LS, Sharma G, Creanga AA, Hameed AB, Hollier LM, Johnson JC, Leffert L, McCullough LD, Mujahid MS, Watson K, White CJ, American Heart Association Advocacy Coordinating Committee (2021) Call to action: maternal health and saving mothers: a policy statement from the American Heart Association. Circulation 144(15):e251–e269. https://doi.org/10.1161/CIR.0000000000001000

Miller EC, Leffert L (2020) Stroke in pregnancy: a focused update. Anesth Analg 130(4): 1085–1096. https://doi.org/10.1213/ANE.0000000000004203

Naylor R, Rantner B, Ancetti S, de Borst GJ, De Carlo M, Halliday A, Kakkos SK, Markus HS, DJH MC, Sillesen H, van den Berg JC, Vega de Ceniga M, Venermo MA, FEG V, Committee EG, Antoniou GA, Bastos Goncalves F, Bjorck M, Chakfe N, Coscas R, Dias NV, Dick F, Hinchliffe RJ, Kolh P, Koncar IB, Lindholt JS, BME M, Resch TA, Trimarchi S, Tulamo R, Twine CP, Wanhainen A, Reviewers D, Bellmunt-Montoya S, Bulbulia R, Darling RC 3rd, Eckstein HH, Giannoukas A, MJW K, Lindström D, Schermerhorn M, Stone DH (2023) Editor's choice – European Society for vascular surgery (ESVS) 2023 clinical practice guidelines on the management of atherosclerotic carotid and vertebral artery disease. Eur J Vasc Endovasc Surg 65(1):7–111. https://doi.org/10.1016/j.ejvs.2022.04.011

Oliveira LC, Ponciano A, Tuozzo C, Viswanathan A, Rost NS, Etherton MR (2023) Poststroke disability: association between sex and patient-reported outcomes. Stroke 54(2):345–353. https://doi.org/10.1161/STROKEAHA.122.041502

Ospel JM, Schaafsma JD, Leslie-Mazwi TM, Amin-Hanjani S, Asdaghi N, Gordon-Perue GL, Couillard P, Hadidi NN, Bushnell C, McCullough LD, Goyal M, American Heart Association Stroke Council, Council on Cardiovascular Radiology and Intervention, Council on Epidemiology and Prevention (2022) Toward a better understanding of sex- and gender-related differences in endovascular stroke treatment: a scientific statement from the American Heart Association/American Stroke Association. Stroke 53(8):e396–e406. https://doi.org/10.1161/STR.0000000000000411

Ota H, Reeves MJ, Zhu DC, Majid A, Collar A, Yuan C, DeMarco JK (2010) Sex differences in patients with asymptomatic carotid atherosclerotic plaque: in vivo 3.0-T magnetic resonance study. Stroke 41(8):1630–1635. https://doi.org/10.1161/STROKEAHA.110.581306

Pancholy SB, Sharma PS, Pancholy DS, Patel TM, Callans DJ, Marchlinski FE (2014) Meta-analysis of gender differences in residual stroke risk and major bleeding in patients with nonvalvular atrial fibrillation treated with oral anticoagulants. Am J Cardiol 113(3):485–490. https://doi.org/10.1016/j.amjcard.2013.10.035

Pappa T, Vemmos K, Saltiki K, Mantzou E, Stamatelopoulos K, Alevizaki M (2012) Severity and outcome of acute stroke in women: relation to adrenal sex steroid levels. Metabolism 61(1): 84–91. https://doi.org/10.1016/j.metabol.2011.06.003

Petersen EE, Davis NL, Goodman D, Cox S, Syverson C, Seed K, Shapiro-Mendoza C, Callaghan WM, Barfield W (2019) Racial/ethnic disparities in pregnancy-related deaths – United States, 2007–2016. MMWR Morb Mortal Wkly Rep 68(35):762–765. https://doi.org/10.15585/mmwr.mm6835a3

Phan HT, Blizzard CL, Reeves MJ, Thrift AG, Cadilhac DA, Sturm J, Heeley E, Otahal P, Rothwell P, Anderson CS, Parmar P, Krishnamurthi R, Barker-Collo S, Feigin V, Gall S (2019) Sex differences in long-term quality of life among survivors after stroke in the INSTRUCT. Stroke 50(9):2299–2306. https://doi.org/10.1161/STROKEAHA.118.024437

Phan HT, Reeves MJ, Gall S, Morgenstern LB, Xu Y, Lisabeth LD (2022) Factors contributing to sex differences in health-related quality of life after ischemic stroke: BASIC (Brain Attack Surveillance in Corpus Christi) project. J Am Heart Assoc 11(17):e026123. https://doi.org/10.1161/JAHA.122.026123

Poorthuis MH, Algra AM, Algra A, Kappelle LJ, Klijn CJ (2017) Female- and male-specific risk factors for stroke: a systematic review and meta-analysis. JAMA Neurol 74(1):75–81. https://doi.org/10.1001/jamaneurol.2016.3482

PRB (2000) Older women: living longer, living alone. https://www.prb.org/resources/older-women-living-longer-living-alone/. Accessed 28 Mar 2023

Rawlley B, Marchina S, Cappucci SP, Gogia B, Wang JY, Stillman A, Kumar S (2023) Investigation on gender differences in leadership of stroke-related clinical trials. Stroke 54(2):295–303. https://doi.org/10.1161/STROKEAHA.122.039173

Rexrode KM, Madsen TE, Yu AYX, Carcel C, Lichtman JH, Miller EC (2022) The impact of sex and gender on stroke. Circ Res 130(4):512–528. https://doi.org/10.1161/CIRCRESAHA.121.319915

Ridker PM, Cook NR, Lee IM, Gordon D, Gaziano JM, Manson JE, Hennekens CH, Buring JE (2005) A randomized trial of low-dose aspirin in the primary prevention of cardiovascular disease in women. N Engl J Med 352(13):1293–1304. https://doi.org/10.1056/NEJMoa050613

Rothwell PM, Goldstein LB (2004) Carotid endarterectomy for asymptomatic carotid stenosis: asymptomatic carotid surgery trial. Stroke 35(10):2425–2427. https://doi.org/10.1161/01.STR.0000141706.50170.a7

Rothwell PM, Eliasziw M, Gutnikov SA, Warlow CP, Barnett HJ, Carotid Endarterectomy Trialists Collaboration (2004) Endarterectomy for symptomatic carotid stenosis in relation to clinical subgroups and timing of surgery. Lancet 363(9413):915–924. https://doi.org/10.1016/S0140-6736(04)15785-1

Sabetta A, Lombardi L, Stefanini L (2022) Sex differences at the platelet-vascular interface. Intern Emerg Med 17(5):1267–1276. https://doi.org/10.1007/s11739-022-02994-y

Sacco RL, Diener HC, Yusuf S, Cotton D, Ounpuu S, Lawton WA, Palesch Y, Martin RH, Albers GW, Bath P, Bornstein N, Chan BP, Chen ST, Cunha L, Dahlöf B, De Keyser J, Donnan GA, Estol C, Gorelick P, Gu V, Hermansson K, Hilbrich L, Kaste M, Lu C, Machnig T, Pais P, Roberts R, Skvortsova V, Teal P, Toni D, Vandermaelen C, Voigt T, Weber M, Yoon BW, PRoFESS Study Group (2008) Aspirin and extended-release dipyridamole versus clopidogrel for recurrent stroke. N Engl J Med 359(12):1238–1251. https://doi.org/10.1056/NEJMoa0805002

Saiz LC, Gorricho J, Garjón J, Celaya MC, Erviti J, Leache L (2022) Blood pressure targets for the treatment of people with hypertension and cardiovascular disease. Cochrane Database Syst Rev 11(11):CD010315. https://doi.org/10.1002/14651858.CD010315.pub5

Sandset EC, Wang X, Carcel C, Sato S, Delcourt C, Arima H, Stapf C, Robinson T, Lavados P, Chalmers J, Woodward M, Anderson CS (2020) Sex differences in treatment, radiological features and outcome after intracerebral haemorrhage: pooled analysis of intensive blood pressure reduction in acute cerebral haemorrhage trials 1 and 2. Eur Stroke J 5(4):345–350. https://doi.org/10.1177/2396987320957513

Seshadri S, Beiser A, Kelly-Hayes M, Kase CS, Au R, Kannel WB, Wolf PA (2006) The lifetime risk of stroke: estimates from the Framingham study. Stroke 37(2):345–350. https://doi.org/10.1161/01.STR.0000199613.38911.b2

Shajahan S, Sun L, Harris K, Wang X, Sandset EC, Yu AY, Woodward M, Peters SA, Carcel C (2023) Sex differences in the symptom presentation of stroke: a systematic review and meta-analysis. Int J Stroke 18(2):144–153. https://doi.org/10.1177/17474930221090133

Sheikh HU, Pavlovic J, Loder E, Burch R (2018) Risk of stroke associated with use of estrogen containing contraceptives in women with migraine: a systematic review. Headache 58(1):5–21. https://doi.org/10.1111/head.13229

Sheth SA, Lee S, Warach SJ, Gralla J, Jahan R, Goyal M, Nogueira RG, Zaidat OO, Pereira VM, Siddiqui A, Lutsep H, Liebeskind DS, McCullough LD, Saver JL (2019) Sex differences in outcome after endovascular stroke therapy for acute ischemic stroke. Stroke 50(9):2420–2427. https://doi.org/10.1161/STROKEAHA.118.023867

Shinohara Y, Huang Y (2012) Abstract 2455: cilostazol for men, but aspirin for women in stroke prevention for patients with cerebral infarction – pooled analysis of CSPS 2 and CASISP. Stroke 43(suppl_1)

SPRINT Research Group, Wright JT Jr, Williamson JD, Whelton PK, Snyder JK, Sink KM, Rocco MV, Reboussin DM, Rahman M, Oparil S, Lewis CE, Kimmel PL, Johnson KC, Goff DC Jr, Fine LJ, Cutler JA, Cushman WC, Cheung AK, Ambrosius WT (2015) A randomized trial of intensive versus standard blood-pressure control. N Engl J Med 373(22):2103–2116. https://doi.org/10.1056/NEJMoa1511939. Erratum in: N Engl J Med. 2017 Dec 21;377(25):2506

SPS3 Investigators, Benavente OR, Hart RG, LA MC, Szychowski JM, Coffey CS, Pearce LA (2012) Effects of clopidogrel added to aspirin in patients with recent lacunar stroke. N Engl J Med 367(9):817–825. https://doi.org/10.1056/NEJMoa1204133

Strong B, Lisabeth LD, Reeves M (2020) Sex differences in IV thrombolysis treatment for acute ischemic stroke: a systematic review and meta-analysis. Neurology 95(1):e11–e22. https://doi.org/10.1212/WNL.0000000000009733

Sun D, Raynald HX, Jia B, Tong X, Ma G, Wang A, Ma N, Gao F, Mo D, Nguyen TN, Miao Z, ANGEL-ACT Study Group (2023) Sex-related differences in outcomes of endovascular treatment for anterior circulation large vessel occlusion. Stroke 54(2):327–336. https://doi.org/10.1161/STROKEAHA.122.041195

Swartz RH, Cayley ML, Foley N, Ladhani NNN, Leffert L, Bushnell C, McClure JA, Lindsay MP (2017) The incidence of pregnancy-related stroke: a systematic review and meta-analysis. Int J Stroke 12(7):687–697. https://doi.org/10.1177/1747493017723271

Tsao CW, Aday AW, Almarzooq ZI, Alonso A, Beaton AZ, Bittencourt MS, Boehme AK, Buxton AE, Carson AP, Commodore-Mensah Y, MSV E, Evenson KR, Eze-Nliam C, Ferguson JF, Generoso G, Ho JE, Kalani R, Khan SS, Kissela BM, Knutson KL, Levine DA, Lewis TT, Liu J, Loop MS, Ma J, Mussolino ME, Navaneethan SD, Perak AM, Poudel R, Rezk-Hanna M, Roth GA, Schroeder EB, Shah SH, Thacker EL, LB VW, Virani SS, Voecks JH, Wang NY, Yaffe K, Martin SS (2022) Heart disease and stroke statistics-2022 update: a report from the American Heart Association. Circulation 145(8):e153–e639. https://doi.org/10.1161/CIR.0000000000001052. Erratum in: Circulation. 2022 Sep 6;146(10):e141

Volz M, Ladwig S, Werheid K (2021) Gender differences in post-stroke depression: a longitudinal analysis of prevalence, persistence and predictive value of known risk factors. Neuropsychol Rehabil 31(1):1–17. https://doi.org/10.1080/09602011.2019.1648301

Vyas MV, Silver FL, Austin PC, Yu AYX, Pequeno P, Fang J, Laupacis A, Kapral MK (2021) Stroke incidence by sex across the lifespan. Stroke 52(2):447–451. https://doi.org/10.1161/STROKEAHA.120.032898

Wenger NK, Ferdinand KC, Bairey Merz CN, Walsh MN, Gulati M, Pepine CJ, American College of Cardiology Cardiovascular Disease in Women Committee (2016) Women, hypertension, and the systolic blood pressure intervention trial. Am J Med 129(10):1030–1036. https://doi.org/10.1016/j.amjmed.2016.06.022

Wouters A, Scheldeman L, Liessens H, Dupont P, Boutitie F, Cheng B, Ebinger M, Endres M, Fiebach JB, Gerloff C, Muir KW, Nighoghossian N, Pedraza S, Simonsen CZ, Thijs V, Thomalla G, Lemmens R (2023) Sex differences in imaging and clinical characteristics of patients from the WAKE-UP trial. Eur J Neurol 30(3):641–647. https://doi.org/10.1111/ene.15629

Yong CM, Tremmel JA, Lansberg MG, Fan J, Askari M, Turakhia MP (2020) Sex differences in oral anticoagulation and outcomes of stroke and intracranial bleeding in newly diagnosed atrial fibrillation. J Am Heart Assoc 9(10):e015689. https://doi.org/10.1161/JAHA.120.015689

Yu AYX, Penn AM, Lesperance ML, Croteau NS, Balshaw RF, Votova K, Bibok MB, Penn M, Saly V, Hegedus J, Zerna C, Klourfeld E, Bilston L, Hong ZM, Coutts SB, SpecTRA Study Group (2019) Sex differences in presentation and outcome after an acute transient or minor neurologic event. JAMA Neurol 76(8):962–968. https://doi.org/10.1001/jamaneurol.2019.1305

Yu AYX, Hill MD, Asdaghi N, Boulanger JM, Camden MC, Campbell BCV, Demchuk AM, Field TS, Goyal M, Krause M, Mandzia J, Menon BK, Mikulik R, Moreau F, Penn AM, Swartz RH, Coutts SB, Diagnosis of Uncertain-Origin Benign Transient Neurological Symptoms (DOUBT) Study Group (2021) Sex differences in diagnosis and diagnostic revision of suspected minor cerebral ischemic events. Neurology 96(5):e732–e739. https://doi.org/10.1212/WNL.0000000000011212

Yu AYX, Austin PC, Rashid M, Fang J, Porter J, Vyas MV, Smith EE, Joundi RA, Edwards JD, Reeves MJ, Kapral MK (2023) Sex differences in intensity of care and outcomes after acute ischemic stroke across the age continuum. Neurology 100(2):e163–e171. https://doi.org/10.1212/WNL.0000000000201372

Zeitler EP, Kearing S, Coylewright M, Nair D, Hsu JC, Darden D, O'Malley AJ, Russo AM, Al-Khatib SM (2023) Comparative effectiveness of left atrial appendage occlusion versus oral anticoagulation by sex. Circulation 147(7):586–596. https://doi.org/10.1161/CIRCULATIONAHA.122.062765

Sex Differences in Pain and Its Treatment

Kevin L. Zacharoff

Contents

Abstract

Pain is a highly personal experience. Pain is often considered to be a purely neurologic phenomenon, but in actuality, it is a combination of both sensory and emotional experiences. This has sometimes been translated clinically toward a more mechanistic approach to the assessment and treatment of pain instead of one that does not discount pain mechanisms, but also is more inclusive of the need for humanism – considering the individual. In today's medical environment, more than ever before there is a significant amount of attention being paid to educating clinicians to better understand that several physiological, neurophysiological, and psychosocial factors can significantly impact responses to pain. The composition of these factors will be unique to that individual's life narrative, context, sex, and prior life experiences. Thus, the concept that a templated approach to pain

K. L. Zacharoff (✉)
Department of Family, Population, and Preventive Medicine, Renaissance School of Medicine at Stony Brook University, Stony Brook, NY, USA

Anesthetic and Analgesic Drug Products Advisory Committee to the U.S. Food and Drug Administration, Silver Spring, MD, USA
e-mail: Kevin.Zacharoff@stonybrookmedicine.edu

S. E. Tsirka, M. Acosta-Martinez (eds.), *Sex and Gender Effects in Pharmacology*, Handbook of Experimental Pharmacology 282,
https://doi.org/10.1007/164_2023_686

assessment and pharmacotherapeutic treatment planning should not be expected to provide optimal patient satisfaction and treatment outcomes in the majority. The hypotheses that there may be sex-based differences in the pain experience in a variety of ways including pain sensitivity, tolerance to pain, threshold at which something becomes painful, and the effectiveness of endogenous pain modulation systems are not new and have been well represented in the literature. This chapter reviews important key findings in the scientific literature with respect to sex-based differences in pain and pain responses to experimentally induced painful stimuli, pain experienced in commonly occurring painful medical conditions, and variations in responses to pain treatments. Possible explanations to account for observed differences or similarities will also be discussed.

Keywords

Analgesia · Bias · Difference · Disparities · Nociception · Pain · Pain research · Sex · Sex-based differences · Sex-specific · Special patient population · Stereotype

1 Introduction

Today's medical environment is filled with controversy about pain and its management. Much of this controversy often surrounds the use of opioid analgesics in treating pain and their relationship to the overdose crisis our nation continues to face. But there is also significant controversy which involves other important aspects of how people with pain are assessed, treated, stigmatized, and in some cases, victims of bias, stereotyping, and undertreatment. In 2000, pain was designated as the "fifth vital sign" (Scher et al. 2018) and one intention of this action was to improve the frequency, accuracy, and overall quality of pain care in the USA, after recognizing that pain care was deficient in many regards with either patients with pain being left undertreated or untreated. After this designation, it became commonplace to ask patients about the presence or absence of pain during virtually every clinical encounter, followed by having the patient subjectively rate their pain if any was reported. What *did not* accompany this sea change in recognizing pain as a significant medical condition which needed to be paid more attention was the incorporation of pain education in healthcare professional training programs about how to proceed once pain was identified. Clinicians were in many cases left underprepared for what was to become the significant prevalence of pain in the general patient population, estimated today to be more than 50 million adults with chronic pain (Rikard et al. 2023) (pain persisting over a 3-month period or longer), which does not include those suffering from acute or subacute pain. Many have argued that this lack of preparedness in some ways has contributed to the overdose crisis the USA faces today (Scher et al. 2018), as opioid analgesics were often utilized or overutilized as part of a pain treatment plan to address the pain rating and improve patient satisfaction. But these educational deficits may have also amplified disparate pain assessment and treatment for certain patient populations at risk of being treated inequitably, in many cases with those patients being undertreated for their pain or left completely untreated. Clinicians unarmed with a substantial foundation of knowledge about pain and its treatment may have often sought to categorize all people with pain as being similar to each other, physically *and* physiologically when, in fact, they may be quite different in many ways which potentially could make not only their pain but their responses to pain treatment different as well.

Pain is a unique medical phenomenon in many ways. The experience of "feeling" pain not only involves the function of inherent neurologic sequences common to all humans regardless of sex consisting of transduction, transmission, modulation, and perception, but also involves the emotional experience of pain which can be impacted by a variety of factors and significantly affect the relationship between pain, suffering, functional impact, and quality of life. In many ways, as part of the pain assessment process, clinicians must not only consider the pain itself, but also the unique aspects of someone's life as the basis for the context for their pain, and how best to plan to treat it. Additionally, this relationship between the neurological, physiological, and emotional experience of pain can be bidirectional, meaning that someone's emotional state has the potential to impact their neurologic responses to pain, and vice versa. This can be an important contributor to substantiate the idea that people of a different sex could have identifiably different painful experiences, neurologically, physiologically, and psychologically. This variation can include different sensitivity to pain, different modulation of pain, and even different perceptions of pain. A person's sex, not unlike other demographics, such as age, cultural backgrounds, and belief systems, may even affect the likelihood of reporting pain in the first place. Particularly with respect to the pain experience, every person is a unique individual; it follows that exactly how pain may or may not be perceived or impact that person's life can vary and how it is addressed needs to be individualized as well.

Regardless of sex, pain most commonly serves as a protective mechanism to alert an individual about impending harm and can be *adaptive*, or it can continue past that point long after its protective role in avoiding tissue damage or healing has taken place, becoming *maladaptive*. Unlike objective serum glucose levels or hemoglobin A1c measures in patients with diabetes or systolic and diastolic blood pressure measurements in patients with hypertension, pain is one of the few medical conditions in which *the patient plays a significant role in determining whether the treatment outcome is successful or not*. The patient also plays an integral role in helping to identify the goals and expectations of pain treatment, and in assessing whether progress is being made or not toward those mutually defined goals. Additionally, pain rating is a subjective phenomenon, with its severity, duration, and location frequently identified solely by the person experiencing it. Pain is sometimes considered by clinicians to be a symptom, often when presenting in an acute situation such as accompanying an injury, and other times pain is considered to be a syndrome or a medical condition, such as when it persists sub-acutely (generally longer than 1 month), or chronically (generally 3 months or longer).

Pain is frequently "quantified" in clinical terms with respect to associated suffering, often designated by a subjective pain rating (e.g., numerical pain rating scale 0–10) with clinical goals and expectations often focused on the negotiation between pain and the rated degree of suffering or discomfort (Fernández-Salazar 2014). When formulating a treatment plan for people with pain, it is important to consider not only the neurophysiological, physical processes that are responsible for someone's pain and related suffering but also to consider the neuropsychological, mental processes that will play a role in helping to mitigate pain and suffering. Most clinicians are trained to apply biomedical modeling to pain treatment planning, which is often appropriate for relieving suffering associated with most acute types of pain (e.g., pain related to injury or postoperative pain). This approach emphasizes the peripheral nociceptive or neurological aspect of pain, focusing on specific pain mechanisms, using a reductionistic approach to decreasing a person's pain rating, and using that as a metric for success. Pharmacologic therapy is typically the hallmark of this biomedical pain treatment model and is rarely individualized to the patient (or to the sex of the patient) in a substantial way beyond adjustment in dosage based on variables such as weight, age, estimated volume of distribution, hepatic or renal function, etc.

However, when subacute or chronic pain exists, this conventional biomedical approach typically may ignore other factors which may often be involved with influencing the amount of suffering involved with pain. These factors include that central pain mechanisms are likely involved in the pain experience and that culture, past experience(s) with pain, individual character traits and beliefs, socioeconomic conditions, information processing, reasoning, decision-making, and emotional state likely all play a significant role in the pain experience as well. It is well established that a biopsychosocial model of pain treatment is more effective for persistent pain, such as subacute or chronic pain. This model incorporates the need for clinicians to identify these important neuropsychological factors, and to consider what role they might potentially play as part of the pain assessment process to best determine a treatment plan to help negotiate the intimate relationship between pain and suffering. For example, identifying whether or not a person is likely to participate in self-management pain treatment strategies substantially impacts the likelihood of satisfaction in chronic pain treatment. If females with chronic pain are more likely to participate in self-management strategies than men, then this needs to be taken into consideration in the treatment planning process. If females are more likely to experience chronic pain than men, it makes sense that the application of the biopsychosocial model may need to be tailored accordingly. This also underscores the need for clinicians to consider that despite the fact there are commonalities between virtually all humans which will play a role in the painful experience, there are also many more neurological *and* psychological processes which are unique to the individual, despite similarities in the anatomy, pathology, or the adaptive or maladaptive nature of pain.

This chapter explores the fact that from both a neurophysiological, neuropsychological, and emotional perspective, there is scientific evidence which supports that there are sex-based differences in the pain experience and that differences based on sex may potentially affect response to pain treatments as well. Other possible contributors to these differences will also be discussed including societal conditioning, cultural factors, potential for researcher bias, and knowledge deficits. Although the concept of sex differences in pain is not new, with much of the existing literature dating back several years, the idea that there are sex-based differences in pain may be either relatively new to many, completely unknown, or not considered to be clinically significant. The clinical consequences may often be insufficient assessment, misapplication of treatment, or undertreatment of pain. In the context of pain and its management, women are a disparate patient population. This translates to the idea that there is some degree of inequity in the assessment and treatment of pain in women, which may result from the fact that pain and response to its treatment can be significantly different in women compared to men, and this may not often be taken into consideration in clinical practice.

2 Sex Differences in Pain

In order to make a decision about sex-based differences in pain and its treatment, it is important to first have consensus with respect to *how* pain is defined. Unfortunately, many still consider pain to be defined solely based on its numerical rating by an individual on a subjective scale of 0–10, with 0 being no pain at all, and 10 being pain as "bad" or severe as it could possibly be. In 2020, after 2 years of deliberations, the International Association for the Study of Pain (IASP) published a revised definition of pain (Raja et al. 2020) with the intention of helping provide better consensus about what pain is. The last time that pain had been defined by the IASP was 41 years prior, in 1979. The major thrust of this revised definition was not only to reinforce the notion that pain is both "an unpleasant sensory *and* emotional experience" but to also offer guidance with six qualifying "notes" to build on that premise and ultimately help improve how clinicians and patients come to a better level of understanding about the personal nature of pain and how this may also contribute to variable responses to its management. These notes included addressing the need to consider the individualized nature of pain from person to person, emphasizing the fact that pain and nociception (the peripheral and central nervous system's processing of painful stimuli) are two *distinctly different* phenomena and that people likely "learn" the concept of pain and how to respond to it through past experiences in their lives. While the IASP is to be applauded for its work on taxonomy and helping clinicians to better understand the individuality in how people experience pain, and that pain-related complaints need to be respected despite the often-subjective nature of pain and its symptomatology, little to no attention was paid to previously identified sex differences which may contribute to the pain experience and impact response to treatment put forth by the IASP years earlier. In fact, in 2008, the IASP focused its entire global annual campaign to attract attention to this with its "*Real Women, Real Pain*" campaign, aiming to "empower women and raise awareness of pain issues in women worldwide." Other intended outcomes were to increase advocacy for women with pain, increase the focus of research in this area, and potentially develop different treatment strategies specific to females.

Research has been consistent for many years in showing that all things are not equal when it comes to chronic pain in women relative to men (Bartley and Fillingim 2013). In fact, numerous studies (Fillingim et al. 2009; Mogil 2012) have shown that not only is pain reported more frequently by women than by men, but that the prevalence of chronic pain conditions in women is higher than men, including certain common chronic pain syndromes like fibromyalgia, chronic recurring daily headache, and irritable bowel syndrome. While many might consider that these to be indicators that pain is likely to be more severe in women than in men, research does not necessarily bear that out for a number of reasons, with the most likely being the subjective nature of self-reported pain rating, difficulty in controlling for biases related to observers, and underrepresentation of study subjects with lower pain severity ratings who might be arbitrarily excluded from research investigation. It is also important to note that because pain is such a personalized experience, and because it is so very much influenced by the individual characteristics which define someone's personality, it can be difficult to make accurate comparisons. If one considers that the perception of pain is potentially influenced by some combination of the constellation of social, cultural, genetic, molecular, cellular, physiologic, hormonal, and psychosocial factors, along with prior life experiences, it is not difficult to imagine that differences in pain among the sexes exist.

A review of the literature reveals that the majority of scientific exploration surrounding sex differences in pain has involved one of two main strategies (Fillingim et al. 2009). The first has been to explore sex differences in response to experimentally induced painful stimuli, with the hypothesis that if the pain stimulus is standardized, observed variations in responses are valid to the greatest degree possible. The second approach has been to examine clinical conditions which are known to include pain as a primary or secondary symptom with the intention of making a comparison of both subjective and, if possible, objective markers which may differ between males and females.

3 Sex Differences in Response to Experimental Pain

As mentioned previously, one way that research has attempted to identify and answer some of the questions about sex differences in pain sensitivity has been by attempting to measure differences in response to the delivery of reproducible, controlled, experimentally induced painful stimuli, including thermal, electrical, chemical, ischemic, and pressure-based stimuli in volunteer subjects (Fillingim et al. 2009). Sensitivity to these painful stimuli has been assessed in these experiments by a variety of methods including first report of pain, pain intensity ratings, and ratings of unpleasantness associated with the stimulus. The rationale behind these studies seems logical and has been that if the painful stimulus is controlled, observed differences in response may be variable, and when evaluating subjects of different sex, this could be at least partially explained on the basis of sex-based differences in the subjects and their pain responses. These kinds of studies typically evaluate specific markers of pain responses to experimentally induced pain, including potential differences in temporal summation of pain (defined as the perception of increasing pain sensation or sensitivity in response to localized repetitive nociceptive stimuli (Cheng et al. 2015)), spatial summation of pain (defined as increasing pain sensation or sensitivity to multiple simultaneous repetitive nociceptive stimuli (Nie et al. 2009)), pro-nociceptive pain modulatory imbalance (defined as enhanced facilitation or diminished inhibition in endogenous pain modulation processes) (Overstreet et al. 2021; Owens et al. 2019), or behavioral indices of pain threshold perception (generally defined by criteria such as time to first painful sensation, tolerance to painful stimulus, or self-reported level of unpleasant nature of a painful stimulus).

Fillingim et al. (2009) performed one of the most comprehensive reviews of the literature looking at self-reported sex differences in pain response to experimental pain stimuli. This meta-analysis reported that a review of the literature supported that women are more sensitive to experimental pain than men. Interestingly, in some cases, the results have been dependent on the particular type of experimental pain stimulus, with some stimuli demonstrating increased sensitivity in women, and others showing no difference between the responses of women and men. For example, research investigating pain sensitivity to pressure-type painful stimuli has demonstrated that females *are* more sensitive to pressure-based pain stimuli than males (Sarlani et al. 2004). Females exposed to pressure-based painful stimuli have also displayed a lower pain threshold and lower likelihood of development of pain tolerance than males. Fillingim's review of scientific data regarding sensitivity of pain in women in response to electrical-based painful stimulus similarly reinforced a significantly lower pain threshold and pain tolerance in women, but mildly supported the hypothesis that women are more likely sensitive to pain than men. Analysis of available data with respect to response to thermal (heat or cold) painful stimuli also corroborated sex differences in sensitivity to pain, with increased sensitivity in females, along with mildly supportive results with respect to lower pain thresholds and pain tolerance compared to males. Transient receptor potential vanilloid 1 (TRPV1) is a calcium-permeable ion channel known for its response to stimuli like the red chili pepper, capsaicin, and other pain-inducing chemicals or noxious heat. Analysis of data with respect to the hypothesis of chemically induced pain through exposure to capsaicin suggested higher pain sensitivity in females, but these results varied with respect to a number of other factors, such as the female subject's phase in their menstrual cycle, or the use of oral contraceptives, etc. The overall conclusion of Fillingim's analysis was that capsaicin-induced experimental pain responses did not likely differ significantly between males and females. These results contrast with respect to data regarding chemically induced pain with intramuscular injections of glutamate or hypertonic saline, which have found that more females reported pain and pain sensitivity to these stimuli than males.

The limitations of these kinds of studies evaluating self-reported pain responses to experimental pain can be numerous. The use of a variety of different pain assessment measures and inventories by researchers alone may be responsible for being a confounder, along with the fact that these tools are often largely subjective in nature, subject to interpretation by the study subject, making standardizing the study subjects' responses difficult to control for across different clinical trials. Additionally, with all of the possible mechanisms which may influence response even to a standardized painful stimulus, it may be nearly impossible to create inclusion or exclusion criteria which control for the multitude of possibilities which may impact the pain response, even within subjects of the same sex. These include the subject's mood, affect, comorbid medical and psychological conditions, past experience (s) with pain, adverse events of childhood, genetics, hormone levels, cultural background, etc. It may not necessarily be a given that clinical studies of this type performed in populations in various parts of the world can be extrapolated to other geographically different populations with significantly different cultures. Another important limitation may also be subjectivity of estimation of pain severity or other data by the observer in terms of interpretation of the pain report itself, application of pain assessment rating measures, etc. which could potentially influence the responses recorded.

It has been suggested that all forms of conveyance of pain response be considered as part of a standardized experimental pain research protocol, including not only written responses, as many pain assessment tools often use, but also verbal responses, nonverbal responses, visual responses, wearable technology, and imaging (Berger and Baria 2022). However, it is important to remember that as mentioned earlier, how pain is defined is a critical piece of the puzzle, and even if there is a way to more objectively measure differences in the "biomarkers" of pain, these may not encapsulate the complex essence of the pain experience (Berger and Baria 2022). The oversimplification of pain along with observer sex-based biases, precognitive and cognitive sex-based stereotypical thinking, and clinically related sex-based expectations of the researcher may potentially influence both the administration of self-reported queries and the interpretation of the study subjects' responses as well, especially if the researcher is a clinician with predisposed expectations based on clinical experiences with male and female patients with pain.

There have been several studies which have attempted to address some of these limitations by examining more objective, reflexive physiologic responses to pain, such as pupillary dilation, muscle twitching, endogenous pain modulation activity measurements, and cerebral activation (France and Suchowiecki 1999; Serrao et al. 2004). Results of these types of research have been mixed with respect to sex differences in pain response, *suggestive* of differences, but in some cases not necessarily conclusive. Further research of this kind is warranted, but the general consensus overall by experts in the field is that research studies of this kind have reinforced that women have a greater sensitivity to an experimentally controlled painful stimulus compared to men, with many theories attempting to explain them. One often-mentioned theoretical explanation for this consensus about increased sensitivity to pain is that inherent sex-based differences in the nervous system may be at least in part responsible, particularly with respect to observed differences in the male and female temporal summation of pain, spatial summation of pain, and pain modulation capacity (Bartley and Fillingim 2013).

Similar to other types of clinical research measuring responses to experimental stimulus application, the clinical value proposition of these and other types of experimentally induced pain research may also suffer to a certain degree because they are taking place outside of the patient care setting. The output of these kinds of laboratory-based pain research projects may not be clinically applicable from an ethical or practical perspective. It has been suggested that purely quantitative data may be limited in its ability to significantly inform changes in clinical practice of pain and its management (Berger and Baria 2022). Additionally, measuring pain responses in healthy human subjects may not necessarily yield similar results compared to subjects with preexisting acute, subacute, or chronic pain, both from a neurological, hormonal, and psychosocial perspective.

4 Sex Differences in Pain: A Clinical Perspective

There has been abundant research attempting to complement the above-mentioned research exploring sex differences in pain related to controlled experimental stimuli. Other analyses of people with chronic pain have looked at sex differences in greater depth based on specific pain-related diagnoses. These types of studies have attempted to explore whether sex differences may be explained by examining the prevalence of certain acute or chronic painful conditions, and to identify whether or not there is consistency in pain differences with male and females within sufferers of those conditions. Common conditions studied include orofacial pain, post-surgical pain, cancer-related pain, neuropathic pain, musculoskeletal pain (including back pain, osteoarthritis, "widespread" pain, fibromyalgia), abdominal pain, and headache pain.

From a clinical perspective, a foundational understanding of the prevalence of pain is important. The prevalence of chronic pain alone (not including acute or subacute pain) is estimated to be more than 50 million adults in the USA at any given time (Rikard et al. 2023) moderately affecting females more frequently in the general population than males (22.0% vs. 19.7%). However, recently published data analyses from the Centers for Disease Control and Prevention (Rikard et al. 2023) from data supplied by the National Center for Health Statistics found that the incidence of high-impact pain, which was defined as "chronic pain that also limited daily life or work activities on most days or every day during the previous 3 months," was significantly higher in females compared to males.

It is well known that there is a higher incidence of chronic pain in children, adolescents, and adults with a history of adverse childhood experiences or mistreatment (Beal et al. 2020; Groenewald et al. 2020). Research has shown that females are at significantly greater risk of experiencing such adverse childhood experiences as physical, emotional, or sexual abuse than males (Jones et al. 2020). Additionally, females who experience adverse events of childhood are at increased risk for developing chronic pain compared to males, and are also more likely to report a higher sensitivity to pain as well as a greater number of simultaneous painful locations (widespread pain) as well. Similar research findings have indicated that post-traumatic stress resulting from adverse childhood experiences may also increase the risk of the development of persistent pain with an increased likelihood of females transitioning from acute to chronic pain compared to males (Burns et al. 2020).

It is recognized that hormonal sex differences likely play a key role as a risk factor for the incidence of pain in females and may also play an important role in increased pain sensitivity in females compared to males. For example, the early onset of menarche has been described in females as a risk factor for developing many types of chronic pain including abdominal pain, neck pain, upper extremity pain, and chronic widespread pain as well. This is hypothesized to be possibly due to differences in lifetime levels of hormone exposure (e.g., estrogen) (Lund et al. 2022). Similarly, menopause has been shown to play a role in differences in pain sensitivity in females compared to males with similar types of painful medical conditions, and is thought to be associated with decreasing levels of sex hormones such as estrogen (Meriggiola et al. 2012).

The prevalence of chronic orofacial pain in adults is between 10 and 15% and is regarded as one of the more common causes of chronic pain (Häggman-Henrikson et al. 2020). Unlike acute orofacial pain, which is most often tooth and dental in nature, chronic orofacial pain is most commonly related to temporomandibular dysfunction. Factors which are known to increase the likelihood of developing temporomandibular dysfunction include anxiety, depression, and catastrophizing behavior. The prevalence of orofacial pain increases from early adolescence with a preponderance in girls compared to boys (LeResche et al. 2007; Nilsson et al. 2005). This increases to a twofold prevalence of chronic orofacial pain in adulthood in females compared to males (Lovgren et al. 2016). The majority of evidence in the literature reveals a higher prevalence in women with orofacial-related pain than men for all ages, additionally with increased relative pain ratings by women with orofacial pain between the ages of 45 and 65. Research has shown that the presence of chronic orofacial pain may increase the likelihood of developing other types of musculoskeletal pain, along with increased sensitivity to pain (Häggman-Henrikson et al. 2020).

Post-surgical pain has historically served as a good proxy for evaluating responses to acute pain. Generally, there can be a reasonably high level of confidence with regard to the standardization of the surgically induced noxious stimulus, and if controlling for other possible influencing factors (such as age and body mass), most people will experience a similar level of severity of pain severity, etc. after a given surgical procedure. Several analyses which have looked at sex differences in pain severity in acute post-surgical pain models have yielded mixed or less consistent and compelling results with respect to sex differences in pain compared to studies evaluating responses to most types of experimentally induced pain (Munk et al. 2023; Rosseland and Stubhaug 2004; Craft 2007; Taenzer et al. 2000). It is also possible that some of these study results may have been confounded or limited by other factors, such as variability in response to acute pain treatments which almost invariably include pharmacologic modalities, or the absence of request for the treatment of post-surgical pain by some subjects. These studies may also not have been able to adequately control for potential differences in response to those medication-based treatment interventions based on physiologic, psychologic, hormonal variation between subjects of different sex, which could have played a potential role in response to those treatments, or the severity of reported pain.

Fillingim et al. (2009) included in their large-scale literature review an examination of sex differences in people with cancer-related pain. This analysis concluded that in patients with cancer-related pain (which typically occurs in 30–85% of patients with cancer, depending on the diagnosis and stage of the disease) overall, there was little scientific evidence showing significant differences between pain in men or women with cancer pain. It was also acknowledged, however, that not unlike women with temporomandibular pain, there have been reports of increased incidence of depression in women with cancer compared to men, which could potentially lead to increased likelihood in frequency of reporting pain, impressions of or rating of pain severity, and significant functional impact or disability in women compared to men. Another factor which needs to be considered is that it has been reported that women with cancer-related pain may be more likely to suffer from other types of comorbid noncancer-related pain in addition to their cancer pain (Valeberg et al. 2008), potentially increasing the likelihood of experiencing more severe cancer-related pain than men.

Epidemiologically, chronic neuropathic pain is estimated to occur more frequently (8% vs. ~5.7%) in adult women than in men in the general population (Colloca et al. 2017). Fillingim and colleagues (2009) also reported that their review of the literature revealed that with respect to people with chronic neuropathic pain, which is commonly defined as "pain caused by a lesion or disease of the somatosensory nervous system" (Murnion 2018), women are more both more likely to experience neuropathic pain and are at increased risk of developing chronic neuropathic pain compared to men.

A review of differences in pain in people with chronic musculoskeletal pain, one of the most common types of chronic pain, was performed by Rollman and Lautenbacher (2001) and found that women have a greater incidence (45% vs. 31%) of musculoskeletal pain than men at any single specific body location related to musculoskeletal pain (e.g., shoulder, hip, knee, and back). Fillingim's review (Fillingim et al. 2009) also looked at chronic musculoskeletal pain based on more stratified types of musculoskeletal pain, including back pain, fibromyalgia, osteoarthritis, and orofacial pain, abdominal pain, and headache pain. This review found that the evidence leaned toward a higher prevalence of back pain in women with a greater likelihood of reporting back-related pain, a higher prevalence of fibromyalgia pain in women, and a higher level of pain severity related to osteoarthritis in women than men. Overall, Fillingim's conclusions were that irrespective of the specific origin or type of musculoskeletal pain, women with musculoskeletal pain were more likely to report the fact that they were experiencing pain than men.

Abdominal pain in females includes not only gastrointestinal conditions such as irritable bowel syndrome (IBS) but pelvic and gynecologic pain as well. It has been consistently reported that there is a higher prevalence of abdominal pain in women compared to men (Unruh 1996). IBS occurs more frequently in females than in males (Kim and Kim 2018), with women more likely to report increased pain severity and pain perception compared to men as well. Once again, it has been postulated that at least part of the responsibility for these differences may be related to increased sex-based differences in comorbid incidences of anxiety, depression, and other psychosocial behaviors. Interestingly, women with IBS more often complain of abdominal pain and constipation symptoms, while men with IBS more often complain of abdominal pain and diarrhea symptoms (Kim and Kim 2018). Research comparing visceral perception in women without a diagnosis of IBS to women with a diagnosis of IBS has shown no difference between the two groups (Chang et al. 2006).

With respect to headache-related pain, there is a preponderance of evidence which has shown that the prevalence of primary chronic daily recurring headaches (e.g., tension-type headaches and cluster headaches) and migraines to be higher in women compared to men; 1–16% in men vs. 3–33% in women (Lipton et al. 2001, 2004). The prevalence of chronic headache pain is sex-specific, and is known to change not only in frequency but also in severity with aging, being nearly identical in frequency in boys and girls in childhood, increasing in adolescent pubescent females, and continuing to increase comparatively up until menopause (Delaruelle et al. 2018). Along with suspected relationship to changes in sex hormones corresponding to these shifts in prevalence, some investigators have also postulated whether or not specific differences in the brains of males and females with chronic headache or other types of chronic pain, both functionally and morphologically, might play a role in differences in pain sensitivity, development of tolerance, and perception as well (Fauchon et al. 2021).

5 Possible Explanations for Sex Differences in People with Pain

When thinking about the sex differences in pain, it is important to reiterate something that the IASP's 2020 revised definition of pain emphasized (Raja et al. 2020): "*pain is always a personal experience that is influenced to varying degrees by biological, psychological, and social factors*." When attempting to explain the possible reasons for sex differences in pain and response to pain treatment, it is likely that some of the answers for these differences can be explained on the basis of these variables. Pain is a highly personalized experience, and it may be that people of one sex may share commonalities in their life experiences which then have the potential to influence the pain experience and certainly the negotiation between pain, suffering, and impact on quality of life. If one considers that pain is indeed in part a learned experience, then it makes sense that people of different sex may "learn" about pain as well.

From a purely biological perspective, both endogenous and exogenous hormonal influences may be contributing factors to sex differences in pain sensitivity, tolerance, modulation, and threshold and should always be considered. One of the first things to consider is the possible influence that sex hormones may have on the pain experience and that this impact can be neurological, psychological, or both. It is possible that estradiol, progesterone, and testosterone may have different and complex effects on pain transmission (Craft et al. 2004; Smith et al. 2006; Mogil 2000), nociception, pain perception, and brain activation. It is also possible that sex hormones affect both mu-opioid receptor binding and the effectiveness of the body's own endogenous "opioid" systems which play a significant role in reflexively mediating pain. Genetics may play a role as well in terms of pain sensitivity (Mogil 2000), with some researchers also suggesting that there may be sex-related physiologic differences in pain responses resulting from variations all the way down to the chromosomal level (Mogil 2012). Differences in pain transduction, transmission, and modulation may also exist due to sex differences related to serotonergic, dopamine, and NMDA receptor functioning (Fillingim et al. 2009), all with the potential of impacting pain sensitivity and perception.

From a psychosocial perspective, a number of other factors may contribute to sex differences in pain and its management. It has been well established in the research literature that catastrophizing increases pain sensitivity and may contribute to diminished functional capacity and alter one's ability to perform activities of daily living (Sullivan et al. 2001; Forsythe et al. 2011). Simply defined, catastrophizing is a type of cognitive aberrant behavior where the person exaggerates the impact of their pain, expect the worst possible outcome with respect to its treatment, and become fearfully disengaged, unmotivated, in many cases physically deconditioned as a result. Catastrophizing has also been shown to have physiologic effects as well, including altered inherent central nervous system pain inhibition (Quartana et al. 2009). There is evidence in the literature to show that women may be more likely to engage in catastrophizing behavior(s) than men (Forsythe et al. 2011), potentially leading to differences between men and women with respect to pain sensitivity. It is well known that higher levels of anxiety or predisposition to anxiety may be typically associated with increased pain sensitivity (Robin et al. 1987). Anxiety tends to be more likely in women than men, with women being at increased risk for developing anxiety disorders compared to men (Bekker and van Mens-Verhulst 2007). Similarly, the relationship between comorbid pain and depression is well known, with depression being more prevalent in women than men (Munce and Stewart 2007). Women with diagnosed clinical depression are more likely to complain of pain compared to men with a similar diagnosis (Marcus et al. 2008).

More significantly with respect to subacute or chronic pain conditions, self-efficacy is often considered to be a key component of a pain treatment plan, with self-efficacy defined by the American Psychological Association as an individual's belief in their capacity to execute behaviors necessary to produce specific results. There is a lower likelihood of a successful pain treatment outcome in people with chronic pain with purely passive and paternalistic approaches in the absence of patient involvement, motivation, and some degree of self-efficacy. A decreased level of self-efficacy has been associated with increased pain ratings and pain-related symptoms (Somers et al. 2012). Women may be more likely to participate in self-efficacy-based treatment strategies compared to men (Fisher et al. 2023).

Cultural norms involving gender roles among men and women may also impact how and whether or not pain is reported. As mentioned earlier regarding the IASP's revised definition of pain in 2020, people learn the concept of pain through experiences in their lives, and it is not common across many cultures to consider that reports of pain are more "acceptable" and more expected from women than men. Fowler et al. referred to this as social priming (Fowler et al. 2011) and reported that this phenomenon may be in part responsible for sex differences in pain reporting based on pain reports in response to experimental cold pressor stimulus.

Differences in pain coping strategies in men and women have been reported as possibly contributing to differences in pain response (Jackson et al. 2005). These include differences in support-seeking, problem-focused coping, internalization, and distraction-based strategies. As cultural norms shift, not unlike with other medical conditions, in the context of pain and its management it is equally important to consider that sex and gender are distinctly different terms, with sex referring to biological distinctions and gender referring to sex-related social roles and all of the potential contributors of social and psychological intricacies which may be involved (Wizemann and Pardue 2001).

It is also important to consider that other factors may play a role in sex differences in pain, and in some ways, research *and* clinical data may be deficient in providing some needed explanations for those differences. In an editorial about sex differences in pain and pain inhibition, Mogil (2012) proposed that there are a number of factors which may contribute to this deficiency, including: it is possible that women are more likely to seek medical attention for a pain-related problem than men, or more willing to report pain in medical intake surveys, it is possible that women may have a different level of susceptibility to pain because of the difference of incidence of pain-causing medical conditions in women (e.g., chronic headache and fibromyalgia), and it is also possible that women have a greater level of sensitivity and/or lower tolerance to pain compared to men.

6 Sex Differences in Pain Treatment

An omnipresent factor which has important clinical implications for pain treatment has to do with the possibility that clinicians providing pain care may assess patients with pain differently based on the patient's sex, which could then potentially impact treatment planning, especially when pharmacotherapeutic analgesic agents are employed. On one hand, this could potentially be beneficial, especially if the goal is individualized care based on an awareness of the sex differences in pain sensitivity, modulation, and perception described earlier in this chapter. Alternatively, this could also possibly result in treatment planning founded on precognitively or cognitively biased or stereotypical beliefs of the treating clinician, which could result in disparate assessment and treatment if the clinician's biased thinking leads them to believe that a female's pain rating is higher because they are more likely to complain about their pain more or to report a higher degree of impact on quality of life than a male would (Leresche 2011). There is also some research to support the possibility that sex of the clinician may impact their behavior, judgment, assessment, and treatment planning of female patients with pain compared to men (Feleus et al. 2009). For example, some research when presented utilizing standardized pain patient cases (Feleus et al. 2009) has shown that female physicians being more likely to inquire about the potentially contributing psychosocial history with female patients than male physicians would, or male physicians being more likely to prescribe analgesics or psychoactive medications to female patients compared to male patients. This has also been found to be the case when prescribing opioid analgesics, with women with noncancer pain more likely to be prescribed an opioid analgesic by their healthcare professional on a long-term basis compared to men (Campbell et al. 2010). Biases on the part of the clinician which may result in differences in how women with pain are treated are real and significant. This may be due to differences in communication between women and men and their healthcare providers about their pain, or differences in the way healthcare providers respond to them. In some cases, the higher sensitivity to pain in women may be falsely interpreted as exaggerating or complaining, which could potentially lead to a woman's complaint of pain being taken less seriously than the same complaint from a man, resulting in less aggressive pain treatment approaches (Hoffmann and Tarzian 2001). Clinicians may also empirically consider that women may typically be better able to cope with pain compared to men and that they therefore do not require the same level of aggressiveness with respect to pain treatment compared to men. Additionally, women may be more likely to report a pain-related complaint than men, leading to those reports being minimized by their assessing clinician or labeled as catastrophizing behavior.

Research has been mixed with respect to sex-specific differences in analgesic treatment responses in both clinical and experimentally induced pain, particularly with respect to the use of analgesic medication treatments, including both opioid and non-opioid analgesics, in addition to adjunctive pharmacologic treatments such as antidepressants and antileptic drugs. For example, many studies have shown decreased opioid consumption by women compared to men with post-surgical pain when administered via patient-controlled analgesia modalities (Miaskowski and Levine 1999). However, there is also a significant body of literature which shows mixed results or little differences with respect to sex-based opioid consumption with respect to cancer pain treatment, acute pain treatment in the emergency department setting, or in post-oral surgery patients (Fillingim et al. 2009). There is not a preponderance of research providing an evidence basis for sex differences with respect to multimodal and multidisciplinary pain treatments. However, it is important to note that goals and expectations of pain treatment outcomes on the basis of sex may vary significantly because of all the possible previously mentioned biological, psychological, and social variables involved. This means that one could potentially be better prepared to consider that the sex of the patient with pain might influence earlier consideration of potential benefits of employment of adjunctive medication therapy (e.g., an antidepressant) given different incidences of certain comorbid conditions such as clinical depression, which may significantly enhance pain treatment outcomes.

7 Implications for Pain Treatment

The goals of pain treatment always involve several considerations: primarily, the formulation of a treatment plan is mutually determined and individualized to *each and every patient*, taking into consideration the patient's unique narrative, context, and needs. While one should not assume that this will likely be the same across all members of the same sex, it requires an understanding of the above-mentioned differences in pain based on sex which may potentially exist, from both a mechanistic *and* humanistic perspective.

As has been discussed throughout this chapter, sometimes the experimental science affirms the clinical or observational science, and sometimes it does not. Real-world pain treatment based on sex differences may or may not coincide with research findings. Pain is such a complex phenomenon that it can often be difficult to separate differences based on the multitude of factors which may contribute or alter its expression. Differences in the prevalence of pain conditions based on sex alone are *not* a sufficient proxy for clinical pain treatment planning decision-making.

The employment of pharmacotherapeutic agents as a component of a pain treatment plan is virtually universal. Clinicians expect to use them, and patients expect to have them prescribed. Understanding sex-based differences in pain including likelihood of pain reporting, estimation of pain severity, pain modulation, pain threshold, and pain perception should be routinely considered to help clinicians develop the most intelligent and effective decisions about the role of pharmacotherapy to deliver the most tailored pain care possible.

Most importantly, if one considers that women are indeed a "special patient population," (Grimsrud et al. 2015), then it is critical from the perspective of pain assessment and treatment to consider them as such. A person's sex may place them at significant risk of undertreatment or being left untreated entirely. This requires reflection and understanding on the part of the clinician, particularly with respect to potential for bias and stereotyping. The IASP redefined pain in 2020 (Raja et al. 2020) with the intention of promoting a better understanding of the complex nature of pain, and how to best help people with pain negotiate pain and suffering with the right combination of biomedical *and* biopsychosocial approaches. If one considers that effective pain treatment must take into account potential patient differences in disease severity, nociception, inflammation, brain function, mood, affect, likelihood of catastrophizing, stressors, coping skills, cultural and social environment, and social support mechanisms, then it is not difficult to comprehend how much of a pivotal role the sex of an individual with pain should play in this process.

References

Bartley EJ, Fillingim RB (2013) Sex differences in pain: a brief review of clinical and experimental findings. Br J Anaesth 111(1):52–58

Beal SJ, Kashikar-Zuck S, King C, Black W, Barnes J, Noll JG (2020) Heightened risk of pain in young adult women with a history of childhood maltreatment: a prospective longitudinal study. Pain 161(1):156–165

Bekker MH, van Mens-Verhulst J (2007) Anxiety disorders: sex differences in prevalence, degree, and background, but gender-neutral treatment. Gend Med 4(Suppl B):S178–S193

Berger SE, Baria AT (2022) Assessing pain research: a narrative review of emerging pain methods, their technosocial implications, and opportunities for multidisciplinary approaches. Front Pain Res 3:896276

Burns JW, Janssen I, Lillis T, Mulcahy M, Purim-Shem-Tov YA, Bruehl S, Burgess HJ, Fischer A, Rim K, Aranda F, Pinkerton L, Hobfoll S (2020) The transition from acute to persistent pain: the identification of distinct trajectories among women presenting to an emergency department. Pain 161(11):2511–2519

Campbell CI, Weisner C, Leresche L, Ray GT, Saunders K, Sullivan MD, Banta-Green CJ, Merrill JO, Silverberg MJ, Boudreau D, Satre DD, Von Korff M (2010) Age and gender trends in long-term opioid analgesic use for noncancer pain. Am J Public Health 100(12):2541–2547

Chang L, Mayer EA, Labus JS et al (2006) Effect of sex on perception of rectosigmoid stimuli in irritable bowel syndrome. Am J Physiol Regul Integr Comp Physiol 291:R277–R284

Cheng JC, Erpelding N, Kucyi A, DeSouza DD, Davis KD (2015) Individual differences in temporal summation of pain reflect pronociceptive and antinociceptive brain structure and function. J Neurosci 35(26):9689–9700

Colloca L, Ludman T, Bouhassira D, Baron R, Dickenson AH, Yarnitsky D, Freeman R, Truini A, Attal N, Finnerup NB, Eccleston C, Kalso E, Bennett DL, Dworkin RH, Raja SN (2017) Neuropathic pain. Nat Rev Dis Primers 3:17002

Craft RM (2007) Modulation of pain by estrogens. Pain 132:S3–S12

Craft RM, Mogil JS, Aloisi AM (2004) Sex differences in pain and analgesia: the role of gonadal hormones. Eur J Pain 8:397

Delaruelle Z, Ivanova TA, Khan S et al (2018) Male and female sex hormones in primary headaches. J Headache Pain 19:117

Fauchon C, Meunier D, Rogachov A, Hemington KS, Cheng JC, Bosma RL, Osborne NR, Kim JA, Hung PS-P, Inman RD, Davis KD (2021) Sex differences in brain modular organization in chronic pain. Pain 162(4):1188–1200

Feleus A, Bierma-Zeinstra SM, Bernsen RM, Miedema HS, Verhaar JA, Koes BW (2009) Management decisions in nontraumatic complaints of arm, neck, and shoulder in general practice. Ann Fam Med 7:446–454

Fernández-Salazar M (2014) Cortical plasticity related to chronic pain in a continuous interaction of neuronal and mental processes

Fillingim RB, King CD, Ribeiro-Dasilva MC, Rahim-Williams B, Riley JL III (2009) Sex, gender, and pain: a review of recent clinical and experimental findings. J Pain 10(5):447–485. https://doi.org/10.1016/j.jpain.2008.12.001

Fisher HM, Stalls J, Winger JG, Miller SN, Plumb Vilardaga JC, Majestic C, Kelleher SA, Somers TJ (2023) Role of self-efficacy for pain management and pain catastrophizing in the relationship between pain severity and depressive symptoms in women with breast cancer and pain. J Psychosoc Oncol 41(1):87–103

Forsythe LP, Thorn B, Day M, Shelby G (2011) Race and sex differences in primary appraisals, catastrophizing, and experimental pain outcomes. J Pain 12:563–572

Fowler SL, Rasinski HM, Geers AL, Helfer SG, France CR (2011) Concept priming and pain: an experimental approach to understanding gender roles in sex-related pain differences. J Behav Med

France CR, Suchowiecki S (1999) A comparison of diffuse noxious inhibitory controls in men and women. Pain 81:77–84

Grimsrud KN, Sherwin CM, Constance JE, Tak C, Zuppa AF, Spigarelli MG, Mihalopoulos NL (2015) Special population considerations and regulatory affairs for clinical research. Clin Res Regul Aff 32(2):47–56

Groenewald CB, Murray CB, Palermo TM (2020) Adverse childhood experiences and chronic pain among children and adolescents in the United States. Pain Rep 5(5):e839

Häggman-Henrikson B, Liv P, Ilgunas A, Visscher CM, Lobbezoo F, Durham J, Lövgren A (2020) Increasing gender differences in the prevalence and chronification of orofacial pain in the population. Pain 161(8):1768–1775

Hoffmann DE, Tarzian AJ (2001) The girl who cried pain: a bias against women in the treatment of pain. Fac Scholar:145

Jackson T, Iezzi T, Chen H, Ebnet S, Eglitis K (2005) Gender, interpersonal transactions, and the perception of pain: an experimental analysis. J Pain 6:228–236

Jones CM, Merrick MT, Houry DE (2020) Identifying and preventing adverse childhood experiences: implications for clinical practice. JAMA 323(1):25–26

Kim YS, Kim N (2018) Sex-gender differences in irritable bowel syndrome. J Neurogastroenterol Motil 24(4):544–558

Leresche L (2011 Jul) Defining gender disparities in pain management. Clin Orthop Relat Res 469(7):1871–1877

LeResche L, Mancl LA, Drangsholt MT, Huang G, Von Korff M (2007) Predictors of onset of facial pain and temporomandibular disorders in early adolescence. Pain 129:269–278

Lipton RB, Stewart WF, Diamond S, Diamond ML, Reed M (2001) Prevalence and burden of migraine in the United States: data from the American Migraine Study II. Headache 41:646–657

Lipton RB, Bigal ME, Steiner TJ, Silberstein SD, Olesen J (2004) Classification of primary headaches. Neurology 63:427–435

Lovgren A, Haggman-Henrikson B, Visscher CM, Lobbezoo F, Marklund S, W¨anman A. (2016) Temporomandibular pain and jaw dysfunction at different ages covering the lifespan – a population based study. Eur J Pain 20:532–540

Lund CI, Engdahl B, Rosseland LA, Stubhaug A, Grimnes G, Furberg A-S, Steingrímsdóttir ÓA, Nielsen CS (2022) The association between age at menarche and chronic pain outcomes in women: the Tromsø Study, 2007 to 2016. Pain 163(9):1790–1799

Marcus SM, Kerber KB, Rush AJ, Wisniewski SR, Nierenberg A, Balasubramani GK, Ritz L, Kornstein S, Young EA, Trivedi MH (2008) Sex differences in depression symptoms in treatment-seeking adults: confirmatory analyses from the Sequenced Treatment Alternatives to Relieve Depression study. Compr Psychiatry 49:238–246

Meriggiola MC, Nanni M, Bachiocco V, Vodo S, Aloisi AM (2012) Menopause affects pain depending on pain type and characteristics. Menopause 19(5):517–523

Miaskowski C, Levine JD (1999) Does opioid analgesia show a gender preference for females? Pain Forum 8:34–44

Mogil JS (2000) Interactions between sex and genotype in the mediation and modulation of nociception in rodents. In: Fillingim RB (ed) Sex, gender, and pain (progress in pain research and management), vol 17. IASP Press, Seattle, pp 25–40

Mogil JS (2012) Sex differences in pain and pain inhibition: multiple explanations of a controversial phenomenon. Nat Rev Neurosci 13(12):859–866. https://doi.org/10.1038/nrn3360

Munce SE, Stewart DE (2007) Gender differences in depression and chronic pain conditions in a national epidemiologic survey. Psychosomatics 48:394–399

Munk A, Jacobsen HB, Schnur J, Montgomery G, Reme SE (2023) Acute and subacute postsurgical pain in women with breast cancer: incidence and associations with biopsychosocial predictors – a secondary analysis of a randomized controlled trial. Pain Rep 8(1):e1058

Murnion BP (2018) Neuropathic pain: current definition and review of drug treatment. Aust Prescr 41(3):60–63

Nie H, Graven-Nielsen T, Arendt-Nielsen L (2009) Spatial and temporal summation of pain evoked by mechanical pressure stimulation. Eur J Pain 13(6):592–599

Nilsson IM, List T, Drangsholt M (2005) Prevalence of temporomandibular pain and subsequent dental treatment in Swedish adolescents. J Orofac Pain 19:144–150

Overstreet DS, Michl AN, Penn TM et al (2021) Temporal summation of mechanical pain prospectively predicts movement-evoked pain severity in adults with chronic low back pain. BMC Musculoskelet Disord 22:429

Owens MA, Parker R, Rainey RL, Gonzalez CE, White DM, Ata AE, Okunbor JI, Heath SL, Merlin JS, Goodin BR (2019) Enhanced facilitation and diminished inhibition characterizes the pronociceptive endogenous pain modulatory balance of persons living with HIV and chronic pain. J Neurovirol 25(1):57–71

Quartana PJ, Campbell CM, Edwards RR (2009) Pain catastrophizing: a critical review. Expert Rev Neurother 9(5):745–758. https://doi.org/10.1586/ern.09.34

Raja SN, Carr DB, Cohen M, Finnerup NB, Flor H, Gibson S, Keefe FJ, Mogil JS, Ringkamp M, Sluka KA, Song XJ, Stevens B, Sullivan MD, Tutelman PR, Ushida T, Vader K (2020) The revised International Association for the Study of Pain definition of pain: concepts, challenges, and compromises. Pain 161(9):1976–1982

Rikard SM, Strahan AE, Schmit KM, Guy GP Jr (2023) Chronic pain among adults – United States, 2019–2021. MMWR Morb Mortal Wkly Rep 72:379–385

Robin O, Vinard H, Vernet Maury E, Saumet JL (1987) Influence of sex and anxiety on pain threshold and tolerance. Funct Neurol 2:173–179

Rollman GB, Lautenbacher S (2001) Sex differences in musculoskeletal pain. Clin J Pain 17:20–24

Rosseland LA, Stubhaug A (2004) Gender is a confounding factor in pain trials: women report more pain than men after arthroscopic surgery. Pain 112:248–253

Sarlani E, Grace EG, Reynolds MA, Greenspan JD (2004) Sex differences in temporal summation of pain and aftersensations following repetitive noxious mechanical stimulation. Pain 109(1–2): 115–123

Scher C, Meador L, Van Cleave JH, Reid MC (2018) Moving beyond pain as the fifth vital sign and patient satisfaction scores to improve pain care in the 21st century. Pain Manag Nurs 19(2): 125–129. https://doi.org/10.1016/j.pmn.2017.10.010

Serrao M, Rossi P, Sandrini G, Parisi L, Amabile GA, Nappi G, Pierelli F (2004) Effects of diffuse noxious inhibitory controls on temporal summation of the RIII reflex in humans. Pain 112:353–360

Smith YR, Stohler CS, Nichols TE, Bueller JA, Koeppe RA, Zubieta JK (2006) Pronociceptive and antinociceptive effects of estradiol through endogenous opioid neurotransmission in women. J Neurosci 26:5777–5785

Somers TJ, Kurakula PC, Criscione-Schreiber L, Keefe FJ, Clowse MEB (2012) Self-efficacy and pain catastrophizing in systemic lupus erythematosus: relationship to pain, stiffness, fatigue, and psychological distress. Arthritis Care Res 64:1334–1340

Sullivan MJ, Thorn B, Haythornthwaite JA et al (2001) Theoretical perspectives on the relation between catastrophizing and pain. Clin J Pain 17:52–64

Taenzer AH, Clark C, Curry CS (2000) Gender affects report of pain and function after arthroscopic anterior cruciate ligament reconstruction. Anesthesiology 93:670–675

Unruh AM (1996) Gender variations in clinical pain experience. Pain 65:123–167

Valeberg BT, Rustoen T, Bjordal K, Hanestad BR, Paul S, Miaskowski C (2008) Self-reported prevalence, etiology, and characteristics of pain in oncology outpatients. Eur J Pain 12:582–590

Wizemann TM, Pardue ML (2001) Exploring the biological contributions to human health: does sex matter? National Academy Press, Washington

Therapeutics for Substance-Using Women: The Need to Elucidate Sex-Specific Targets for Better-Tailored Treatments

Helen C. Fox, Verica Milivojevic, and Rajita Sinha

Contents

Abstract

In the last decade, alcohol consumption in the US has risen by 84% in women compared with 35% in men. Furthermore, research has shown that sex- and gender-related differences may disadvantage women in terms of developing a

H. C. Fox (✉)
Department of Psychiatry and Behavioral Health, Renaissance School of Medicine, Stony Brook University, Stony Brook, NY, USA
e-mail: Helen.Fox@stonybrookmedicine.edu

V. Milivojevic · R. Sinha
The Yale Stress Center, Department of Psychiatry, Yale University School of Medicine, New Haven, CT, USA

S. E. Tsirka, M. Acosta-Martinez (eds.), *Sex and Gender Effects in Pharmacology*, Handbook of Experimental Pharmacology 282,
https://doi.org/10.1007/164_2023_687

range of psychological, cognitive, and medical problems considerably earlier in their drinking history than men, and despite consuming a similar quantity of substances. While this "telescoping" process has been acknowledged in the literature, a concomitant understanding of the underlying biobehavioral mechanisms, and an increase in the development of specific treatments tailored to women, has not occurred. In the current chapter we focus on understanding why the need for personalized, sex-specific medications is imperative, and highlight some of the potential sex-specific gonadal and stress-related adaptations underpinning the accelerated progress from controlled to compulsive drug and alcohol seeking in women. We additionally discuss the efficacy of these mechanisms as novel targets for medications development, using exogenous progesterone and guanfacine as examples. Finally, we assess some of the challenges faced and progress made in terms of developing innovative medications in women. We suggest that agents such as exogenous progesterone and adrenergic medications, such as guanfacine, may provide some efficacy in terms of attenuating stress-induced craving for several substances, as well as improving the ability to emotionally regulate in the face of stress, preferentially in women. However, to fully leverage the potential of these therapeutics in substance-using women, greater focus needs to the placed on reducing barriers to treatment and research by encouraging women into clinical trials.

Keywords

Alcohol use · Substance use · Women · Sex-differences · Gender · Medication development · Progesterone · Guanfacine

1 Introduction

Until the middle of the last century, alcohol and substance use was viewed as a largely marginal issue for women and portrayed predominantly as a male problem. Today, however, extensive epidemiology data indicate that the well-established and universal gender gap in alcohol and substance use, along with its negative consequences, has been gradually narrowing since the 1960s, affecting all ages and socio-economic groups (White et al. 2015; Slade et al. 2016; McKetta and Keyes 2020; Dawson et al. 2015). In the last 10 years, alcohol consumption in the USA has risen by 84% in women compared to 35% in men (Peltier et al. 2019; Grant et al. 2017). Furthermore, adolescent females between the ages of 12 and 20 have higher rates of underage and binge drinking compared with males of the same age (Substance Abuse and Mental Health Services Administration U.S. Department of Health and Human Services 2020), and while the complex psycho-socio-cultural reasons for this converging pattern of alcohol and substance use still need to be fully clarified (White et al. 2015), there is an overwhelming research consensus regarding its health-related ramifications for women. For example, extensive research has shown that sex- and gender-related differences may disadvantage women in terms of developing psychological, cognitive, and medical problems considerably earlier in their drinking history than men, and despite consuming a similar quantity of substances to men, and in some cases less (Fama et al. 2020; Fox and Sinha 2009; Hernandez-Avila et al. 2004; Becker 2016). This accelerated progression through landmark symptoms pertaining to the addiction cycle in women (Brady and Randall 1999; Mann et al. 2005) has been labeled "telescoping" (Marks and Clark 2018; Piazza et al. 1989). However, while telescoping is generally acknowledged in the literature, *a concomitant understanding of the mechanisms underpinning the telescoping process, as well as an increase in the development of specific treatments tailored to women, has not occurred.*

Experimental studies elucidating mechanisms and possible therapeutic targets underpinning craving and relapse behaviors have either been conducted in predominantly male samples or have not incorporated sex-based analyses, leading to sex-bias in interpretations (Peltier et al. 2019; Fox 2007). For example, in the alcohol literature, stress-induced suppression of cortisol has been deemed a biomarker of risk for alcohol craving, relapse, and dependence (Breese et al. 2005). However, many of the formative studies characterizing this dampening of Hypothalamic-Pituitary-Adrenal (HPA)-axis systems during stress have been conducted in either all male or predominantly male samples (Wand and Dobs 1991; Lovallo et al. 2000; Errico et al. 1993; Junghanns et al. 2003; Adinoff et al. 2005a; Vescovi et al. 1997). Indeed, our own research has shown that while alcohol-using men demonstrate a dampened cortisol and ACTH response to stress, a *sensitized* response is observed in women alongside a marked dysregulation of sympathetic systems (Fox et al. 2009). This may have important sex-related ramifications for the effects of FDA-approved drugs like naltrexone, which target hypothalamic tone. This is borne out by the fact that *only one* of the seven studies assessing sex differences in the effectiveness of naltrexone has reported a significant improvement in drinking outcomes for women (Canidate et al. 2017). While an increase in federal initiatives over the last four decades has focused on mitigating some of these issues by implementing policies from requiring the inclusion of women in research (1993) (Clayton and Collins 2014), to its current policy on Sex as a Biological Variable (SABV; Jan 2016), women remain highly challenging to recruit into clinical trials. This is due, in most part, to feeling stigmatized, to transportation constraints, and family or caregiving commitments (Schamp et al. 2021; Greenfield et al. 2010a).

When considered together, the steady increase in alcohol and substance use in women, alongside accelerated mental health sequelae and lack of personalized FDA-approved medications, reflects a growing public health crisis unique to women. In the current chapter, we focus on several pertinent aspects of this issue. First, we determine *why* the development of personalized, sex-specific medications is required to improve prognosis in alcohol- and substance-using women, particularly given the wide variation in bio-psycho-social and cultural differences that set women at a disadvantage for telescoping and poor treatment outcome. Second, focus is given to some of the possible sex-specific gonadal and stress-related factors underpinning the accelerated progress from controlled to compulsive drug- and alcohol-seeking in women. Third, we discuss the efficacy of these mechanisms as novel targets for medications development, using exogenous progesterone and guanfacine as examples. Fourth, we discuss some of the challenges faced and progress made in terms of developing innovative medications for alcohol and substance-using women.

2 Differences Between Men and Women Regarding Initiation of Drug Use and Maintenance-Related Behaviors: Why We Need Sex-Specific Medications

One of the most comprehensive heuristic models of addiction uses evidence-based research to support a three-stage cycle, comprising binge/intoxication, withdrawal/negative affect, and preoccupation/anticipation. Each stage reflects corresponding functional dysregulations including the development of incentive salience, negative mood sensitivity, and dysexecutive function, respectively, and these biobehavioral processes are mediated by changes in three major neurocircuitry systems (basal ganglia, extended amygdala, and prefrontal cortex) (Koob and Le Moal 2008; Koob and Le Moal 2001; Koob 2021). In view of this model, how men and women use drugs and hence, where men and women enter this addiction cycle maybe very different and dependent upon complex psychosocial and cultural experiences, including body image, family roles, and caregiving commitments, in addition to biological differences. For example, studies indicate that while peer pressure and the role of deviant peers play a more significant role in drug initiation in adolescent boys compared with girls, the influence of a romantic partner, early childhood trauma, and societal pressures impact initiation of drug and alcohol use to a greater extent in both adolescent girls and women compared to their male counterparts (Haas and Peters 2000; Kuntsche and Müller 2012; Fonseca et al. 2021). From a broad perspective then, sex and gender may impact the neural adaptations underpinning both the hedonic and dysphoric reinforcing effects of addictive substances during initiation of drug use, which in turn could culminate in very different paths to addiction.

This is further demonstrated by cultural norms and expectations regarding women's roles which have been shown to affect how substance-using women are perceived by not only society in general, but also by health care practitioners (Becker 2016). Historically, substance-using women have been vilified for acting contrary to their internalized gender stereotypes (Auvinen et al. 2021). Campbell (2000) states that they are often constructed as *"willfully wayward women, who are morally corrupt and "deviant" in socially inacceptable ways."* Hence, they are likely to experience greater epistemic injustice (Ettorre 2015), be perceived as more pathological than men, and prescribed psychotropic drugs to a far greater extent than men (Riaz 2019). This is supported by epidemiological data indicating that women with addictive behaviors tend to exhibit higher comorbid neuropsychiatric disorders than men, including anxiety, depression, phobias, and stress-related disorders (Fonseca et al. 2021).

In particular, sociocultural expectations around caregiving and maternal roles serve to further increase barriers to treatment and research (Fiddian-Green et al.

2022; Campbell and Ettorre 2011; Choi et al. 2015). Many women face higher risks regarding sexual and reproductive health, and those who are mothers additionally risk losing custody of their children (Fonseca et al. 2021; Holbrook 2015) potentially accounting for elevated feelings of shame, self-accusation, depreciating thoughts, and depression (Auvinen et al. 2021). Multifaceted societal issues relating to weight control (especially in relation to tobacco use (Kuo et al. 2022)) alongside potential menstrual cycle effects (Fattore et al. 2008; Fox et al. 2008a) additionally place women at a greater disadvantage of addiction facilitators such as fatigue, sleep disorders, and co-occurring anxiety and panic disorder (Ek et al. 2021; Just-Østergaard et al. 2018; Martin et al. 2022; Perkins et al. 1995; Evans et al. 2020).

Hence, as addiction is a chronic stress disorder (Fox and Sinha 2009; Sinha 2008), extensive social and cultural norms may play an intricate and marked role in amplifying biological and psychological correlates of alcohol and substance use in women. In particular, negative reinforcement behaviors (a prominent process in the addiction cycle) may be exacerbated in women compared to men. The pertinence of the self-medication/tension reduction theory of addiction in women is also supported by extensive public health data showing that substance-using women are more likely than men to have a lower Socio-Economic Status (SES), violent partners, history of sexual violence, fractured relationships, and less social support (Fonseca et al. 2021; Devries et al. 2014).

Given the wide gender-specific social and cultural differences pertaining to the etiology of substance use in men and women, it is not surprising that marked differences are also observed with regard to *how* men and women progress from controlled to compulsive alcohol and substance use, and most importantly *how* biological stress and reward systems integral to motivation for substance use and relapse are sex-specific and impacted by gonadal hormones.

3 Women Progress to Dependence Faster than Men: The Role of Stress and Gonadal Hormones in (a) Underpinning Telescoping, and (b) as Targets for Treatment Development

In both animal and human research, maintenance of drug use and the movement from controlled to compulsive drug and alcohol seeking have been characterized by allostatic decreases in the function of reward neurocircuitry (via development of processes such as incentive salience) alongside elevations in the upregulation and sensitivity of core Hypothalamic-Pituitary-Adrenal and Sympathetic-Adrenal-Medullary (HPA-SAM) system markers (via negative mood sensitivity) (Holbrook 2015), potentiating a shift from positive to negative reinforcing behaviors (George et al. 2014; Koob 2010). This has been demonstrated extensively in the clinical and preclinical literature by a wealth of studies linking elevations in tonic levels of stress system markers such as Corticotropin-Releasing Factor (CRF), cortisol, Adrenocorticotropic Hormone (ACTH), and Norepinephrine (NE), to increased intake of cocaine, opioids, alcohol, tobacco, and marijuana in both current and abstinent substance users (Koob and Kreek 2007; Goeders 2002). Phasic dysregulation of these markers in response to a range of psychological stressors has also been shown to predict relapse factors in psychostimulant, alcohol, opioid, and nicotine using individuals (Sinha et al. 2006; Adinoff et al. 2005b; Milivojevic and Sinha 2018; Jensen and Sofuoglu 2016; Wemm and Sinha 2019). Most importantly, extensive research has shown that dysregulation of these stress mechanisms underlying craving and relapse *is both sex-specific and affected by gonadal hormones and menstrual cycle (MC) phase in women.*

For example, substantial preclinical evidence indicates that female rats demonstrate a more robust behavioral and stress response to acute cocaine administration compared to male rats (Festa et al. 2010), even without stress provocation. This is demonstrated by the fact that female rats show greater HPA axis response to alcohol (Ogilvie and Rivier 1997) and greater locomotor activity following cocaine exposure compared to male rats (Carroll et al. 2007). Female rats also show significantly increased locomotor activity, orofacial activity, and ACTH and cortisol levels, as well as a decrease in D3 dopamine transporters, in response to nicotine compared to male rats (Harrod et al. 2005; Harrod et al. 2004; Faraday et al. 2005). Preclinical murine models have also shown that female rats and mice self-administer more cocaine (Templeton et al. 2023) and alcohol (Cozzoli et al. 2014) following exposure to a range of stressors (tail suspension, isolation, predator odor), compared with males. They are additionally more sensitive to the anxiolytic effects of nicotine and cannabis than male rats (Cheeta et al. 2001; Fabris et al. 2022; Salviato et al. 2021) and more sensitive to the biological and behavioral effects of stress during withdrawal to nicotine (Torres et al. 2013), cocaine, and cannabis.

3.1 Menstrual Cycle (MC) Processes Underlying Motivation for Drugs and Alcohol: Progesterone as a Target Mechanism

The literature has been far more ambiguous in humans, although many studies have shown that both substance-using and non-using women have demonstrated sensitized subjective (anxious/nervous/feeling good) and cardiovascular responses to the acute administration of both cocaine (Kosten et al. 1996; Singha et al. 2000; Lukas et al. 1996) and nicotine (Netter et al. 1994; Acheson et al. 2006). Importantly, however, findings have been dependent upon type of drug and stage of Menstrual Cycle (MC), compounding further the potential for vulnerability and consumption acceleration in women. For example, with regard to psychostimulants, studies in healthy women have shown that the positive subjective effects of d-amphetamine such as "High," "Euphoria," and "Like Drug" were potentiated during the follicular phase (when estradiol levels were high), compared to the mid-luteal phase (when progesterone levels were elevated) (Justice and de Wit 1999). Similar subjective effects of cocaine were also potentiated in follicular compared with mid-luteal phase women following smoked cocaine, although ratings were dependent upon dose (Evans et al. 2002). Other studies indicated that the subjective response to smoked cocaine, specifically, was greater in the follicular phase than the luteal phase and that sex differences were more likely to be observed when men were compared to women in the luteal phase, again emphasizing the possible role of progesterone in attenuating the rewarding effects of cocaine (Evans et al. 2002; Sofuoglu et al. 1999; Evans and Foltin 2010; Evans and Foltin 2006). Follow-up research comparing women in both the early (low estradiol) and late (high estradiol) follicular phase of their MC found no significant differences in the subjective effects of d-amphetamine, again suggesting less of a role for estradiol in potentiating the effects of amphetamines and a potentially greater role for progesterone in masking the acute effects (Justice and De Wit 2000; Evans 2007). In support of this, studies examining the role of exogenous administration of estradiol were not shown to enhance either the subjective or pharmacokinetic effects of d-amphetamine in either normal cycling (Justice and De Wit 2000) or postmenopausal (Schleifer et al. 2002) women.

Findings from our own laboratory have also lent some support to the theory that progesterone may have a buffering effect on certain stress-related processes in women that are known to be associated with compulsive drug seeking. In one study, we compared daily salivary cortisol and progesterone levels across the menstrual cycle (MC) in $N = 12$ cocaine-dependent women during 4 weeks of inpatient abstinence vs $N = 10$ healthy control women (Fox et al. 2008a). Cocaine-dependent women demonstrated significantly higher levels of both daily salivary cortisol (Fig. 1a) and daily salivary progesterone (Fig. 1b) across the entire menstrual cycle, compared with healthy control women (Fox et al. 2008a), highlighting two pertinent points with regard to sex-specific factors relating to drug maintenance. First, an upregulation of cortisol across the entire MC in the substance-using women may represent stress system sensitivity known to underpin higher levels of anxiety, negative affect, and drug craving; all of which are associated with relapse (Koob 2010; Fox et al. 2008b; Sinha et al. 2006). To support this, negative mood was also significantly higher across the MC in the cocaine women compared with the healthy women [$F\ (1,20) = 5.43, p < 0.03$]. Second, an upregulation of progesterone in the cocaine-dependent women could potentially reflect a compensatory adaptation to an enhanced distressed state, characterized in the current sample, by increased levels of cortisol and enhanced negative mood. Cocaine-dependent females also demonstrated significantly lower estradiol/progesterone (E2/P) ratios across their MC compared with healthy controls, reflecting the significantly increased progesterone levels particularly during the follicular and ovulation phases.

Although little is known regarding the specific pathophysiological consequences of upregulated progesterone levels and low E2/P ratios, one possibility is that it may eventually culminate in progesterone deficiency and adrenal exhaustion (Studd 2006). While stress-related increases in neurosteroids such as progesterone and allopregnanolone may be adaptive at first, the longer-term consequences of these agents may have opposing effects resulting in increased anxiety (Gulinello and Smith 2003). Repeated biological adaptations to stress have also culminated in depleted basal levels of allopregnanolone as well as blunted response to stress in depressive disorders and premenstrual dysphoric disorder (PMDD) (Girdler and Klatzkin 2007; Romeo et al. 1998). Importantly therefore, persistently high

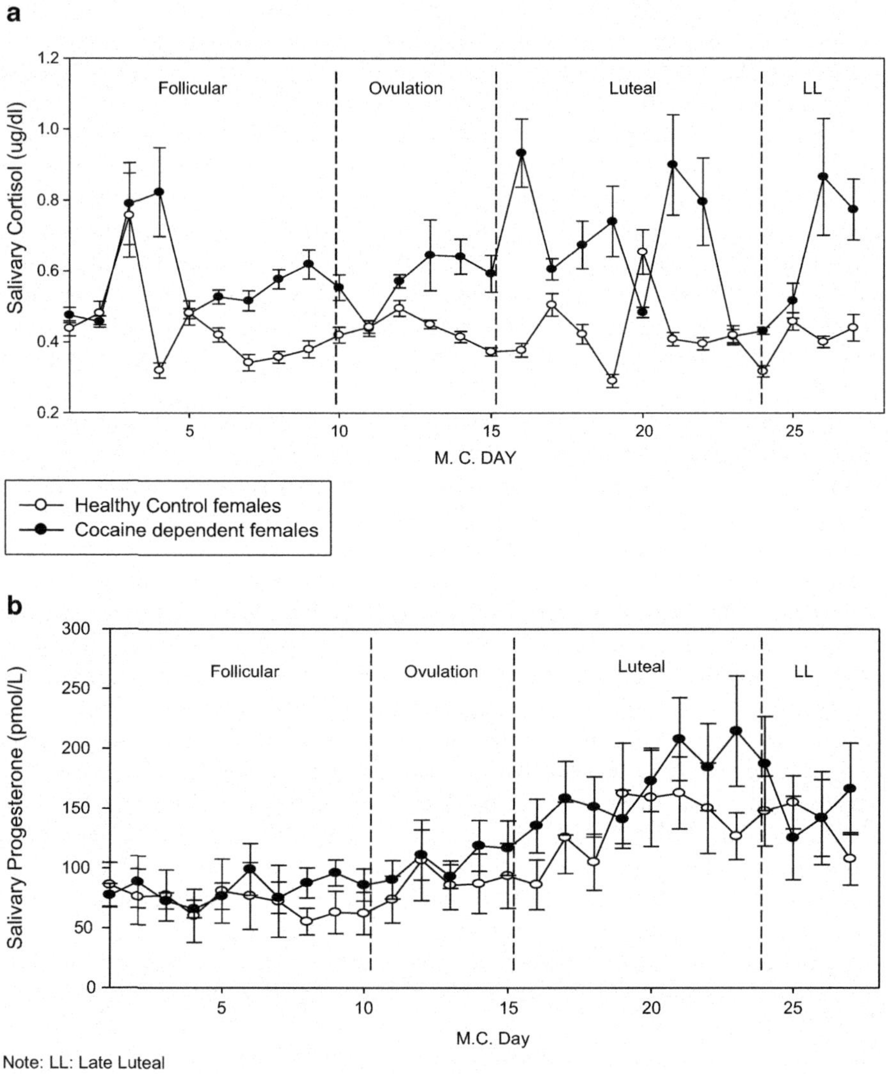

Fig. 1 (**a**) Daily salivary cortisol levels for cocaine-dependent women vs. healthy women at each stage of the menstrual cycle. (**b**) Daily salivary progesterone levels for cocaine-dependent women vs. healthy women at each stage of the menstrual cycle

progesterone levels and low E2/P ratios may eventually predispose females to increased anxiety, reduced tolerance for stress, mood swings, and agitated depression (Fiad et al. 1996; Kaplan and Manuck 2004). As these stress-related behaviors are associated with abstinence symptoms and relapse susceptibility in recently abstinent cocaine-dependent patients (Kampman et al. 2004; Sinha et al. 2006), these hormonal neuroadaptations may have important implications for relapse susceptibility in women.

Another study from our laboratory has highlighted the importance of MC phase with regard to emotional management during stress (Milivojevic et al. 2014), which again can be linked to a set of regulatory goal-oriented behaviors associated with relapse vulnerability and treatment outcome, including decision-making, self-monitoring, and impulse control (Loree et al. 2015; Blume and Marlatt 2009). We administered an online version of the Mayer, Salovey, and Caruso Emotional Intelligence Test (MSCEIT) to $N = 98$ comorbid chronic cocaine and alcohol users (55M/43F) and $N = 56$ healthy controls (28M/28F) and categorized the women into two groups dependent on their MC phase. These comprised a High Progesterone group (luteal phase of the menstrual cycle, DAYS 20–25) and a Low Progesterone group (follicular phase, DAYS 1–19, and premenstrual (late luteal) phase of the menstrual cycle (DAYS 26–32)) at the time of MSCEIT administration. Findings highlighted first the potential vulnerability of substance-using women with regard to being able to regulate emotions during distress compared with their male counterparts, and second, the role of endogenous progesterone in possibly mitigating these issues. Specifically, we found that in the healthy group, females were significantly better at managing emotions compared with males ($p = 0.004$), while in the substance and alcohol-using group, this discrepancy was not observed due to the fact that the substance-using females performed significantly *worse* than the healthy females ($p < 0.001$; Fig. 2a). In a follow-up analyses, we examined the effects of progesterone level as characterized by MC on MSCEIT performance in both the healthy and substance/alcohol-using women. Findings indicated that women in the high endogenous progesterone group performed better with regard to managing emotions, particularly in terms of interpersonal relations (Fig. 2b). As such, these findings potentially highlight the fact that emotion regulation and the ability to manage emotions during protracted withdrawal from cocaine and alcohol may represent an important relapse-related biobehavioral target in women that may be improved by progesterone levels.

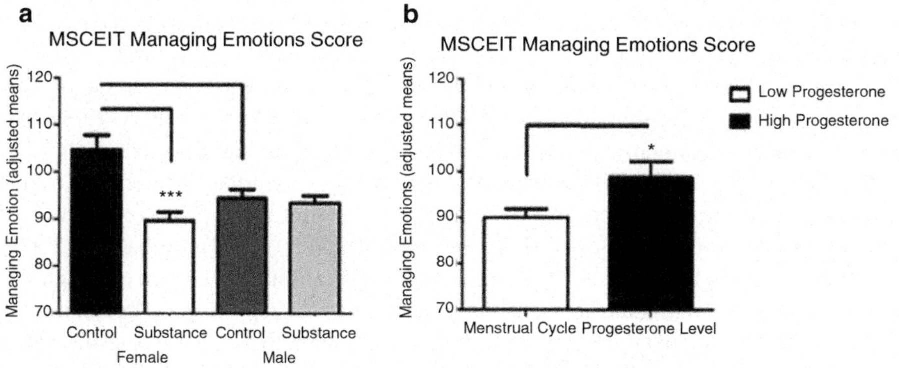

Fig. 2 (**a**) MSCEIT Managing Emotions Score. (**b**) MSCEIT Managing Emotions Score

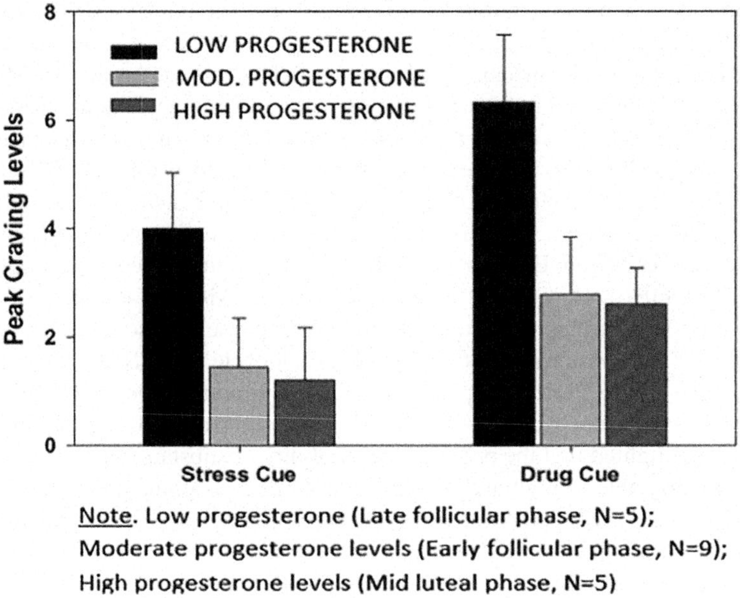

Fig. 3 Cocaine craving response to stress and drug cue imagery

Taken together, these studies serve to highlight the impact of endogenous progesterone levels and MC phase on addictive and relapse-related behaviors. Findings point to the fact that substance-using women may be vulnerable to chronic progesterone deficiency due to persistent stress system sensitization from drug use, as well as natural hormonal fluctuations such as the late luteal phase of their MC (characterized by a progesterone "crash"). For example, it is notable that in the previous study, attenuated E2/P ratios in the late luteal phase were also associated with increased cocaine craving (Fox et al. 2008a). Further support is provided by studies that have shown premenstrual (late luteal) syndrome complaints to contribute to higher levels of craving in women seeking treatment for alcohol, cocaine, and cannabis (Qurishi et al. 2022), as well as studies that have demonstrated elevated craving during the follicular MC phase (low progesterone) in social drinkers (Warren et al. 2021). Again, in our laboratory we have shown that during exposure to personalized psychological stress imagery and drug cue imagery (a variant stressor), early abstinent cocaine-dependent women in the later follicular phase of their cycle (characterized by low progesterone levels) reported significantly higher ratings of cocaine craving compared to women in the mid-luteal phase (characterized by high progesterone levels; $p < 0.05$, in both conditions. Fig. 3) (Sinha et al. 2007).

Findings such as these also have important implications for women experiencing dynamic hormonal flux during transitional periods of the reproductive cycle, including menarche, pregnancy, postpartum, and menopause, where progesterone levels may be vulnerable to either age-related or metabolic-related dysregulation (Stefaniak et al. 2023). This is borne out by the fact that adolescence reflects both a pivotal time for alcohol and substance misuse and peak onset of depression and anxiety-related disorders, with a female preponderance of both (Altemus et al. 2014; Gater et al. 1998). Recent studies have also highlighted the increase in both alcohol and prescription opioids in women over 50 in the USA (Kuerbis et al. 2014). Moreover, while menopause in women may indirectly lead to greater severity of substance and alcohol use in an attempt to cope with accompanying affective menopausal transition symptoms (Milic et al. 2018; Faravelli et al. 2013), researchers should also consider the direct role of gonadal hormones, and specifically fluctuations in endogenous progesterone, in potentially exacerbating the addiction process (Epstein et al. 2007).

In summary, these studies show that female gonadal hormones, such as progesterone, may play a pivotal role in influencing stress/reward system engagement in response to acute drug administration and acute psychological stress, as well as impact ability to emotionally regulate in the face of stress. All of these behaviors are integral to craving and relapse vulnerability in women, via positive and negative reinforcement processes. Notably, these studies also show that substance-using women may be particularly vulnerable to progesterone deficiencies due to both persistent and chronic stress system upregulation, as well as normal transitional changes in the MC, including late luteal phase decreases, adolescence, and menopause. Such progesterone fluctuations may therefore reflect a promising new target for medications development in women, and exogenous progesterone a potentially efficacious medication.

3.2 Stress System Processes Underlying Motivation for Drugs and Alcohol: The Sympathetic System as a Target Mechanism

In addition to hormonal fluctuations setting women at a possible disadvantage in terms of telescoping and exacerbating motivational behaviors, aberrations within sympathetic stress systems may similarly provide another sex-specific target pertinent to substance-using women. For example, growing evidence suggests that greater emotional sensitivity to stress in women alongside higher autonomic disruption may represent unique risk factors for substance use in women, compared with men (Fox et al. 2009; Chaplin et al. 2008; Nolen-Hoeksema et al. 2008; Heinsbroek et al. 1991; Waldrop et al. 2010). In view of this, stress-induced craving has been seen to be both a quantitatively and qualitatively different motivational biobehavioral experience in men compared with women. Several studies have indicated higher stress-related increases in craving and drinking in females (Bertholomey et al. 2016; Vengeliene et al. 2005). Furthermore, while the stress-induced craving state in both male and female alcohol and substance users is characterized by sensitized anxiety, arousal, and negative mood compared with control groups (Fox et al. 2007), this response is generally exacerbated in females (Chaplin et al. 2008; Fox et al. 2009; Gilmore et al. 2019; Back et al. 2008). These findings are also compatible with extensive clinical surveys and longitudinal studies which have shown that internalizing emotions such as negative mood and anxiety are predictive of binge drinking, problem use, and dependence to a greater extent in both adolescent (Johannessen et al. 2017) and adult females compared with males (Anker et al. 2017; Anker et al. 2018). Other studies have shown that while females may demonstrate less withdrawal symptoms from alcohol and opioids, they do demonstrate greater negative affect (Becker and Koob 2016). Notably, the clinical importance of this sensitized mood response to stress is illustrated by experimental research highlighting the robust link between stress-provoked negative affect and relapse factors in chronic drinkers, smokers, stimulant users, and opioid users (Shiffman et al. 2020; Cooney et al. 1997; Litt et al. 2000; Preston and Epstein 2011).

In addition, the craving state during early abstinence from alcohol in men and women is also qualitatively different, in terms of both sympathetic tone and phasic response to stress. This is important in terms of motivational behaviors, as high levels of central NE induce sympathomimetic states associated with withdrawal and elevated craving as well as negative motivational states robustly associated with relapse risk (Becker 2012; Weinshenker and Schroeder 2007; Sofuoglu and Sewell 2009) including sensitized anxiety and inhibitory control. For example, high central NE and sympathetic overdrive impacts medial prefrontal (mPFC) circuits (Smith and Aston-Jones 2008) inducing α1 receptor stimulation and desensitizing of α2 receptors in the prefrontal cortex, commonly documented following repeated cocaine and alcohol exposure (Derlet and Albertson 1990; Drouin et al. 2002; Baumann et al. 2004; Porrino et al. 2004; Porrino et al. 2007; Beveridge et al. 2005). Most importantly, these processes are critical to effective cognitive flexibility (Arnsten and Li 2005; Sawaguchi and Goldman-Rakic 1994; Zahrt et al. 1997) and allocation of attention (Weinshenker and Schroeder 2007), by attenuating salient "signals" and increasing irrelevant "noise." In support of this, high tonic and low phasic activity of Locus Coeruleus (LC-NE) innervations within cortical control regions (Aron 2007; Aron and Poldrack 2005) are key to the stopping and monitoring components of inhibitory control, a key aspect of cognitive flexibility (Aston-Jones and Cohen 2005; Aston-Jones and Gold 2009). Moreover, the ability to successfully cognitively inhibit in the fact of stress is known to underpin multiple goal-oriented behaviors associated with good treatment outcome in substance-using individuals.

In view of this, it is important to consider that high basal heart rate and NE levels, as well as sympathetic dysregulation during stress, have been shown to be specific to substance use disordered women (Fox and Sinha 2014), *suggesting that the noradrenergic upregulation may be sex-specific* (McRae-Clark et al. 2017). These findings again corroborate the extensive preclinical work showing that female animals show higher reactivity to early life stress and greater sensitivity to stress-related increases in cocaine acquisition (Kosten et al. 2005; Kosten et al. 2004; Anker and Carroll 2010; Buffalari et al. 2012; Curtis et al. 2006; Bangasser et al. 2010), and greater responses to acquisition and escalation of cocaine use than males (Lynch et al. 2002; Lynch and Taylor 2004; Lynch et al. 2005; Lynch et al. 2007). In addition, sexual dimorphism of LC-NE activation, dendritic morphology, feedforward regulation of the HPA axis (Curtis et al. 2006; Bangasser et al. 2010; Bangasser 2013; Bangasser et al. 2011), and expression of adrenergic receptors in the mPFC (Ferris et al. 2007) suggest that chronic drug abuse may manifest as vulnerability to autonomic and sympathetic hyperarousal along with high drug craving and poor cognitive flexibility during early abstinence, specifically in substance-using women.

For example, studies in female rats have shown that NE signaling potentiates stress-induced reinstatement of alcohol to a greater extent than in male rats (Haass-Koffler et al. 2018). In particular, several research studies using the alpha2 antagonist, yohimbine, have emphasized a potential sex-specific role played by alpha2 receptors in manipulating NE-LC stress circuitry. Female rats are more sensitive to alcohol seeking than male rats following the administration of yohimbine (Bertholomey et al. 2016). Furthermore, this has also been corroborated in both substance-using and healthy women compared with men, where pre-treatment with yohimbine is associated with higher ratings of cue-related craving and anxiety (Moran-Santa Maria et al. 2014), and elevated amygdala and decreased prefrontal activity following fearful faces, respectively (Schwabe et al. 2013). Findings from our own studies have additionally shown that compared with men, 4-week abstinent women demonstrate elevated basal levels of autonomic markers including heart rate and norepinephrine (Fox et al. 2009; Fox and Sinha 2009) alongside phasic elevations in alcohol craving and blunted autonomic and norepinephrine response to stress (Fox et al. 2009; Fox and Sinha 2009). This may reflect a risk-related inability to mount a typical arousal response to stress due to the elevated levels of sympathetic tone. Given that a similar pattern of tonic and phasic dysregulation in cortisol and ACTH has been linked to alcohol craving and relapse factors (Adinoff et al. 2005b; Breese et al. 2005; Sinha et al. 2011) in predominantly male samples (Fox 2007), *sympathetic overdrive and subsequent dampening during stress provocation in women may provide a sex-sensitive pathway that is related to relapse and qualitatively different to that observed in men* (Fox et al. 2009).

As LC-NE anxiety and arousal systems may be more sensitized in women, this may also have implications for sex-specific differences in associated regulatory systems underpinning affect regulation. For example, upregulation of LC-NE during stress is known to impinge upon medial prefrontal circuits (Kawahara et al. 2000) leading to α1 receptor stimulation and a2 receptor desensitization (Marek and Aghajanian 1999; Birnbaum et al. 1999; Arnsten et al. 1999a). This, in turn, may serve to impair attentional and regulatory processes by decreasing salient "signals" and increasing irrelevant "noise" (Birnbaum et al. 1999; Arnsten et al. 1999b) *to a greater extent in women*.

In line with this, preliminary findings from our own laboratory have shown that comorbid alcohol and cocaine-using women performed significantly worse on cognitive control performance during psychological stress and cue-related stress compared with their male counterparts and healthy women. In this study we exposed N=107 treatment-seeking alcohol and cocaine using individuals, and N=74 social drinkers, to three personalized imagery conditions (stress, drug-cue, neutral/relaxing), in a randomized and counterbalanced manner, using identical procedures to those conducted in our prior work (Fox et al. 2007, 2008b; Sinha et al. 2009, 2011). The Stroop Color/Word Test was presented both prior to and following each imagery condition, and change from baseline findings showed that the

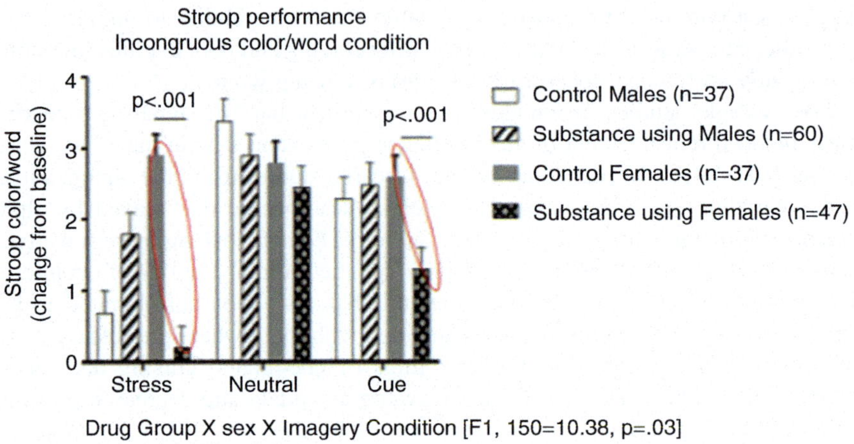

Fig. 4 Stroop performance, incongruous color/word condition

substance using women performed significantly worse on the incongruous color/word condition compared with the control women. This discrepancy was not observed between the substance using men and control men (Fig. 4). Given that cognitive flexibility in the face of stress may underpin a host of goal-oriented behaviors (D'Esposito 2007) linked to treatment outcome in alcohol and substance-using populations and has additionally been linked to a fewer number of days to relapse in our own prior research, the control process of affect regulation may reflect another salient sex-specific pathway to relapse in women.

Other pilot data from our lab showing poor management of emotions during distress in 4-week abstinent comorbid alcohol and cocaine-using women compared with both healthy female controls and substance-using males (Milivojevic et al. 2014) again corroborate this (Fig. 2a) and emphasize the possible utility of emotion regulation as a therapeutic target for women. *Taken together, these studies highlight the fact that possible sympathetic and adrenergic stress system dysregulation underlying stress-related craving and ability to successfully cognitively and emotionally regulate in the face of stress seem to be particularly specific to substance-using women.*

In sum, evidence-based research indicates that stress system adaptations (including negative mood severity during withdrawal and response to stress) underpin the movement from controlled to compulsive drug seeking (Koob 2010; Koob and Kreek 2007; Koob 2013). As complex sex-specific biological and hormonal as well as psychosocial and cultural factors impact these core stress pathways, with potentially greater severity in women, hormonal and sympathetic markers may play a role in underpinning the telescoping processes in substance-using women, *and hence provide innovative markers for therapeutics development in women.*

4 Medications

The body of work presented in the current chapter serves to highlight the robust role stress and gonadal hormones on sex-specific motivation for drug and alcohol seeking. As such, we postulate that hormonal and adrenergic agents which can target both stress-induced anxiety and negative mood, as well as improve the ability to cognitively and emotionally regulate in the face of stress, might preferentially attenuate craving and relapse factors in alcohol and substance-using women.

4.1 Exogenous Progesterone

In view of this, previous studies highlighting some of the non-reproductive functions of progesterone on stress and reward behaviors suggest that progesterone may represent a potential therapeutic for attenuating craving and relapse-related behaviors in substance-using women. For example, progesterone is known to have potent anxiolytic and anti-stress effects due to the actions of its metabolite allopregnanolone on the allosteric modulation of GABAA receptors (Bitran et al. 1995; Wenzel et al. 2021; Sundström-Poromaa et al. 2020; Rupprecht 2003). Moreover, the potential "masking effects" of progesterone on sensitized reward and stress-related drug reinforcement behaviors (discussed in Sect. 3.1) are consistent with the fact that luteal phase deficiency has been most commonly associated with premenstrual dysphoric disorders (Stefaniak et al. 2023; Patel et al. 2017). This has led to the recent FDA approval of allopregnanolone in the treatment of postpartum depression (Meltzer-Brody et al. 2018). Functional MRI studies have also indicated that progesterone-related increases in amygdala reactivity may play a role in mediating levels of anxiety and negative mood (van Wingen et al. 2008) known to underlie elevations in craving and relapse. In addition, recent research has shown that low to moderate concentrations of progesterone and allopregnanolone elevate amygdala activity in women to the same degree as that observed during anxiety responses (Bäckström et al. 2014).

While evidence for the effects of progesterone in improving other non-reproductive processes, such as cognitive regulation and neuroprotection, are relatively modest, certain studies have found progesterone and allopregnanolone to be protective against schizophrenia-related cognitive dysfunction (Cai et al. 2018; Cao et al. 2021). Exogenous progesterone treatment, 200 mg/day, has also been shown to significantly improve cognitive inhibitory performance in the Stroop and the Digit Symbol Substitution Test in a group of male and female smokers (Sofuoglu et al. 2011). In addition, psychological stress has been shown to influence menstrual cycle effects on activity in emotion regulation circuitry, such that higher levels of allopregnanolone were associated with smaller amygdala and medial prefrontal cortex responses to stress during the late luteal phase (Ossewaarde et al. 2010) (characterized by a progesterone "crash"). Similarly, in corroboration with our own findings suggesting progesterone to have a buffering effect on stress and cortisol levels (Fig. 1a), studies have also shown that progesterone levels increase alongside decreasing levels of HPA axis hormones (Stephens et al. 2016), providing further parsimonious support for its effects on emotion regulation. Hence, with regard to the stress/regulation model of addiction, progesterone's anti-stress properties alongside an impact on neuroregulatory processes may underpin potential therapeutic properties that may be more efficacious in women. This is corroborated by several studies highlighting the ability of both endogenous and exogenous progesterone to attenuate nicotine craving and relapse, preferentially in a range of female smokers (Sofuoglu et al. 2001; Allen et al. 2016; Tosun et al. 2019; Allen et al. 2008; Forray et al. 2017). Notably, a recent study has shown that endogenous basal levels of progesterone were significantly negatively associated with craving ratings during withdrawal in postmenopausal women, but not men (Weinland et al. 2021). Intriguingly, another study has found progesterone to have deleterious effects on motivational behaviors in men, showing endogenous levels to be *positively* associated with alcohol craving during early abstinence (Ho et al. 2019).

These findings also concur broadly with a study from our own laboratory, where 200 mg (b.i.d.) of micronized progesterone was administered to early abstinent men and women with cocaine use disorder, across 7 days. Results showed attenuations in the overall stress-induced craving state, slightly more in early abstinent cocaine-using women compared with men, as well as demonstrating a generalized improvement in inhibitory control in both cocaine-using men and women (Fox et al. 2013). Following approximately 4 weeks of abstinence from cocaine, $N = 41$ individuals receiving treatment for cocaine use disorder were randomized to either exogenous progesterone (12M/9F) or placebo (12M/9F). After 7 days, they were then exposed to three personalized 5-min imagery scenarios: (1) stress, (2) cocaine cue (a variant stressor), and (3) relaxing (intra-individual control); one imagery per day, across three consecutive days, in a randomized and counterbalanced order. Measures of reported cocaine craving, negative mood, and anxiety were collected, as well as inhibitory "Stroop" performance, and levels of cortisol and ACTH, at baseline, immediately following exposure to the imagery conditions, and at various recovery time-points. Findings indicated that progesterone compared with placebo significantly reduced ratings of cocaine craving following exposure to the cocaine cue condition in both men and women ($p < 0.05$). With regard to negative affective response to stress, however, placebo women demonstrated a significantly sensitized response to stress compared with the placebo men ($p < 0.0001$), in corroboration with extensive human literature. Moreover, progesterone was able to significantly reduce negative mood in women to a significantly greater extent than placebo women ($p = 0.04$; Fig. 5). Exogenous progesterone was also observed to have a broad effect on improving cognitive control across all three imagery conditions compared with the placebo group ($p < 0.01$; Fig. 6). A recent 10-week treatment trial in $N = 21$ (11 progesterone; 10 placebo) women with cocaine use disorder also showed that, while progesterone had no effect on relapse, it was found to be safe and well-tolerated, supporting the possibility of a larger study to fully test efficacy (Oliva et al. 2022).

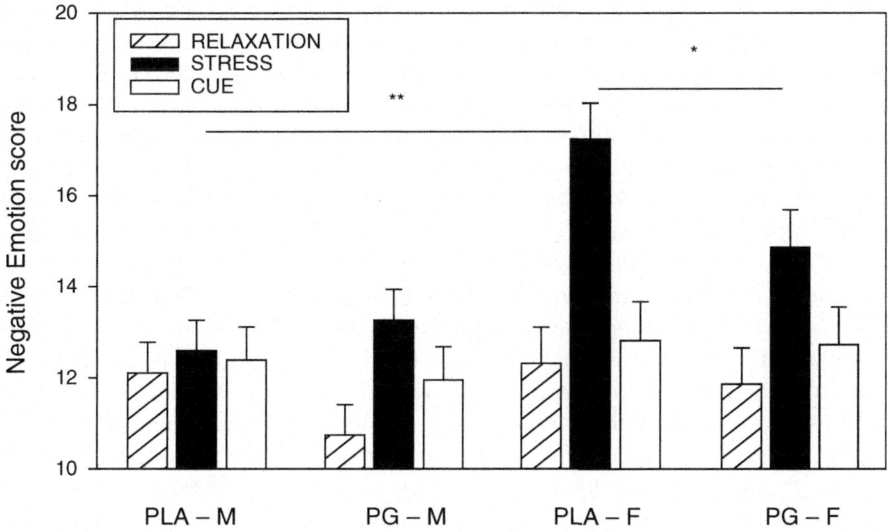

Fig. 5 Negative emotion response to stress, cue & relaxing imagery in progesterone vs. placebo men and women

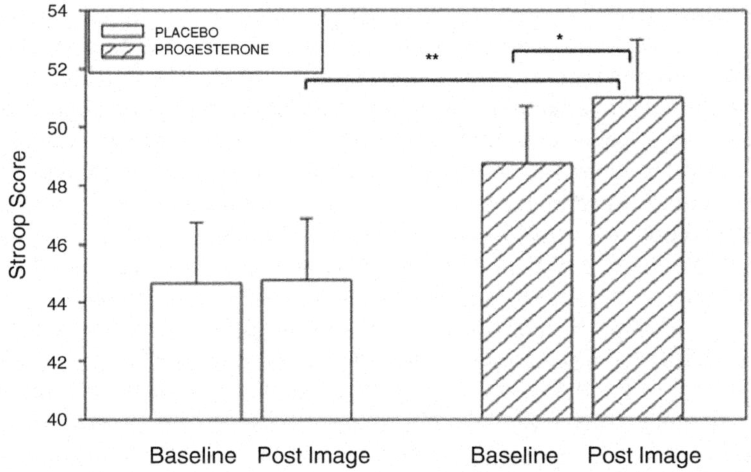

Fig. 6 Stroop color/word "interference" score at baseline and following exposure to all three imagery conditions

4.2 Guanfacine

Another medication that has recently been assessed in the context of reducing stress-related craving and improving inhibitory control, preferentially in women is the alpha-2 agonist, guanfacine. We postulated that as an alpha2-adrenergic agonist, guanfacine might be particularly effective in targeting sympathetic overdrive, specific to craving and emotion dysregulation in alcohol and substance-using women, by inhibiting norepinephrine (NE) centrally (Ramos and Arnsten 2007) via feedback inhibition of its release through stimulation of presynaptic α2 receptors (Ramos and Arnsten 2007; Arnsten 2007). We additionally postulated that guanfacine might decrease the emotional dysregulation observed in substance-using women (Fig. 2a) by mimicking the effects of NE at postsynaptic α(2A)-receptors in the prefrontal cortex (PFC) and decreasing excitatory postsynaptic transmission in the medial prefrontal cortex (Ji et al. 2008; Lê et al. 2011). In addition, as previous research had shown substance-using women to be more sensitive to the alpha2 manipulation of LC-NE systems (Bangasser et al. 2016; McRae-Clark et al. 2017) we also postulated that guanfacine might be effective in both attenuating the sensitized negative mood, arousal and anxiety experienced during stress-induced craving, as well as improve the ability to reappraise and regulate these enhanced emotions during stress, preferentially in women. In support of this, guanfacine has been shown to attenuate smoking lapse, cigarette smoking, and tobacco craving to a greater extent in women compared with men (Verplaetse et al. 2015), and Glassman and colleagues (Glassman et al. 1993) also showed that another alpha2 agonist, clonidine, was able to reduce nicotine withdrawal and promote smoking cessation in women as compared to men.

In a post hoc analysis examining the effects of sex on guanfacine's efficacy in reducing stress-related craving, we compared $N = 29$ men with $N = 13$ women all of whom were 4-week abstinent co-users of cocaine, alcohol, and tobacco (Fox et al. 2014). We assessed their response to 3 types of personalized stress imagery (stress, drug cue-related stress, and combined stress and drug cue) after titration to 3 mg guanfacine vs placebo (Fox et al. 2014). The three stress imagery scenarios were presented over headphones, one imagery per day, across 3 days, in a randomized and counterbalanced order. Self-report measures of cocaine craving, alcohol craving, nicotine craving, negative mood, anxiety, and arousal, as well as cardiovascular output and Stroop Color/Word performance were collected at baseline, immediately following imagery exposure, and at various "recovery" time-points until 1-h post imagery. Following data analysis, a series of Treatment Group X Sex X Time-point interactions for cocaine craving [F5, 501 = 5.1, $p < 0.0001$; Fig. 7a], alcohol craving [F5, 492 = 3.4, $p = 0.005$; Fig. 7b], nicotine craving (Main effect of Medication: [F1,37 = 9.9, $p = 0.003$]; Fig. 7c), and anxiety [F5, 520 = 7.0, $p < 0.0001$; Fig. 8a] were observed, indicating that guanfacine was able to successfully attenuate craving and anxiety compared with placebo, but only in the women. The positive effects of guanfacine were not seen in the men, possibly due to the fact that in all cases, placebo women reported significantly higher craving and anxiety compared with placebo men, again in support of extensive previous literature (Fox and Sinha 2009). Similarly, a Treatment Group X Sex interaction for negative mood [F1, 84 = 4.0, $p < 0.05$; Fig. 8b], also showed a decrease in negative affect following all three imagery conditions and all time-points in the guanfacine women only. Regarding assessment of executive control in the face of stress, a similar pattern was observed on Stroop performance where the placebo women performed significantly worse

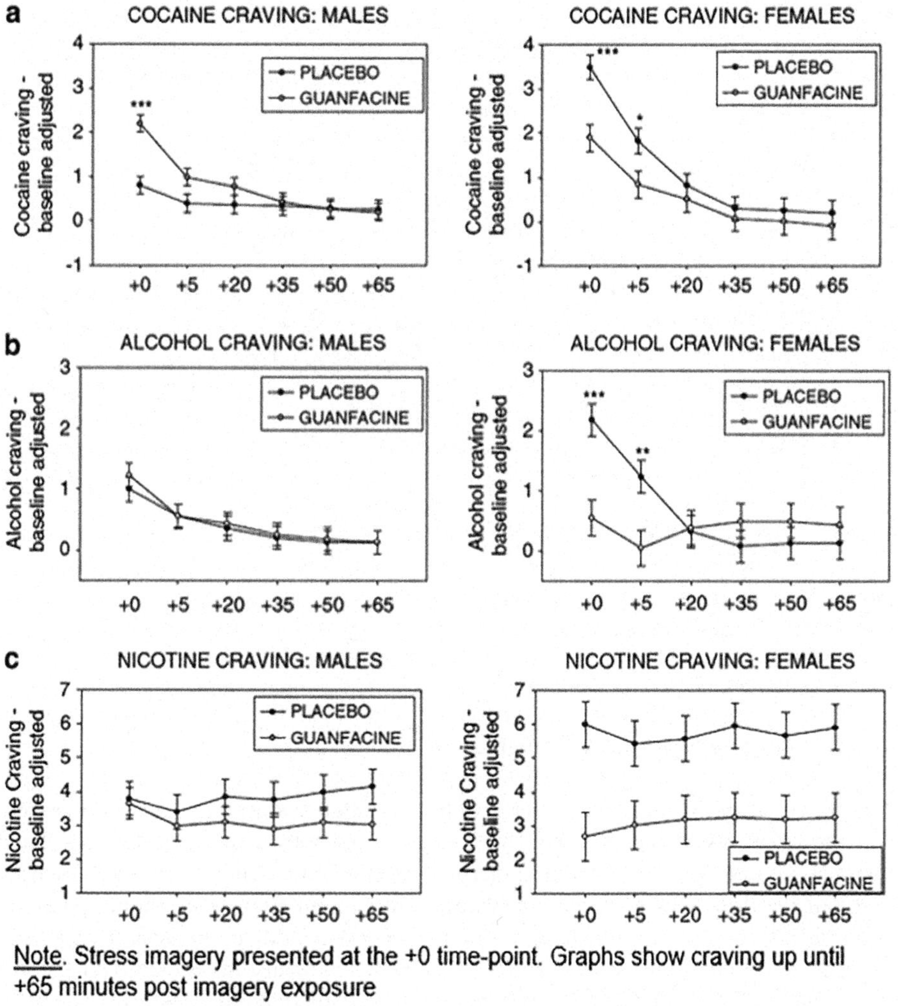

Fig. 7 Sex effects of guanfacine vs. placebo on (**a**) cocaine craving, (**b**) alcohol craving, (**c**) nicotine craving, during exposure to 10 min of stressful imagery

than the placebo men, and guanfacine women demonstrated a significant improvement compared with placebo women (Fox et al. 2014). Overall findings support the literature showing an enhanced craving, anxiety, arousal, and cognitive dysregulation "threshold" during stress in women compared with men during early abstinence from poly substances including alcohol. Importantly, findings indicate that guanfacine can attenuate this negatively reinforcing state preferentially in women.

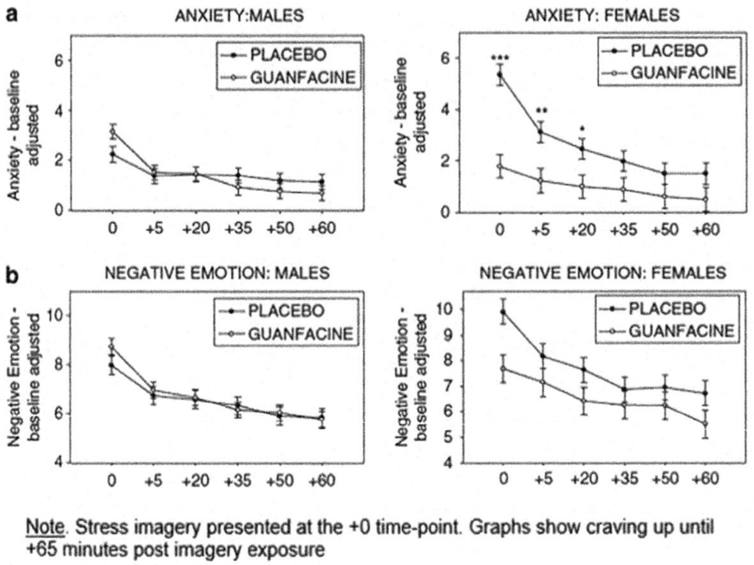

Fig. 8 Sex effects of guanfacine vs. placebo on (**a**) anxiety and (**b**) negative emotion, during exposure to 10 min of stressful imagery

5 Challenges and Progress

As presented in the current chapter, extensive evidence suggests that chronic stress and gonadal system adaptations (including sympathetic and progesterone-related processes) may play a role in underpinning the movement from controlled to compulsive drug seeking more substantially in women. Hence, providing potential *sex-specific targets for medications development* in addiction. Despite this, and despite the gradual increases in drinking and substance use in women over the last few decades in the context of telescoping, there still remains a pressing need for well-tailored sex-specific therapeutics. There may be several factors that contribute to this situation.

First, the need for better sex-specific medications within the addiction field is also exacerbated by broader systemic issues pertaining to addiction in general. For example, despite the enormous potential benefits gained from addiction therapeutics, treatment medications are still relatively rare compared with other chronic and clinical disorders, including cardiovascular disease, diabetes, and asthma. There are still only three FDA-approved medications for alcohol, including disulfiram, naltrexone (oral and long-acting injectable), and acamprosate, all of which have demonstrated only moderate efficacy (Jonas et al. 2014; Kranzler and Soyka 2018), possibly due to the heterogeneity of addictive disorders. Most notably, none of these medications have been thoroughly developed in women. In addition to this, there are currently no FDA-approved medications for cocaine and other psychostimulants, and this is compared to >70 new FDA-approved agents for hypertension in the last decade (Davis and Oparil 2018). As such, there is a need not only to develop new and better-tailored medications for female alcohol and substance users, but also to elucidate novel medications and medication targets, in general, for both men and women. This is likely due to both social stigma and the fact that barriers to treatment have meant that many substance users are not treatment-seeking (Substance Abuse and Mental Health Services Administration 2017). In addition to this, systemic factors including typically slow adoption and implementation of novel therapies into medical practice (Grol and Wensing 2004) are likely to be exacerbated in the case of addiction therapies (Saxon and McCarty 2005). For instance, dissemination issues may be due, in part, to the frequent need for combined behavioral therapies, many of which may comprise total abstinence-based orientations opposed to pharmacotherapies, poor organization support, complex legislative issues, and insurance reimbursement (Butelman and Kreek 2017). In support of this, US National Survey on Drug Use and Health (NSDUH) data from 2015 indicated that only approximately 10% of substance-using individuals requiring treatment were receiving it (Center for Behavioral Health Statistics and Quality 2018), highlighting a wide social and systemic issue undermining the development of new treatments and new treatment targets for both men and women.

Although these issues represent a general problem, it is clear that female substance users experience more severe barriers to treatment compared with their male counterparts, for many of the psychosocial and cultural reasons mentioned in the earlier sections of the chapter, including stigmatization, greater psychological comorbidities, and caregiving commitments (Ait-Daoud et al. 2019; Altemus et al. 2014). In response to this, specific federal guidelines and policies were developed by NIH and the FDA over the last few decades to help ensure the inclusion of women in clinical trials as well as encourage gender-specific analyses on outcome measures. However, despite initiatives including the Clinical Equity Provision in the 1993 NIH Revitalization Act (Federal Register 1994), the lifting of FDA restrictions pertaining to the inclusion of women of childbearing potential in clinical trials (Weinberger et al. 2010) and the current NIH consideration of Sex as A Biological Variable (2016), women continue to remain markedly under-represented in clinical trials and there continues to be poor compliance with these guidelines (Bierer et al. 2022).

A second issue effecting the relatively slow development of medications for addiction in general has been related to a need to establish a new paradigm within which to elucidate biobehavioral targets underpinning the transition from controlled to compulsive alcohol and drug seeking. Until relatively recently, the most commonly adopted paradigms for medications development in alcohol and cocaine addiction were to examine an agent's potential for attenuating either reward or acute withdrawal symptoms (Gorelick et al. 2004). Broadly, this included but was not limited to potentiating dopamine transmission via agonist and partial agonist therapies, as well as targeting anxiolytic mechanisms via GABAergic and glutamatergic medications, many of which posed long-term issues relating to high abuse liability and sedation, attention, memory, and language (Diana 2011; Addolorato et al. 2012; Ijff and Aldenkamp 2013; Haney et al. 2010; Evans 2011;

Sommer et al. 2013). Furthermore, it has only been in the last two decades that the focus of medications development for addiction has shifted from reward attenuation to targeting longer-term relapse prevention strategies. As discussed in the current chapter, these have included the improvement of cognitive and executive performance and attenuation of provoked, stress-related craving states (Sinha 2008; Sofuoglu et al. 2016; Sofuoglu 2010; Fox and Verica 2018; Fox et al. 2007), both of which reflect biobehavioral adaptations associated with motivation for drugs during protracted abstinence, when the acute withdrawal symptoms have dissipated. This is also reflected by the fact that while maintenance assisted treatments for opioid use disorder (such as buprenorphine and methadone) are known to provide the essential receptor occupancy for safe and stable detoxification, there is little evidence to suggest that they are also able to engage core stress, reward or prefrontal circuitry adequately enough to strengthen emotion regulation, and mitigate craving in the face of provocation (i.e., stress/cue) (Kowalczyk et al. 2015; Leri et al. 2004; Biernacki et al. 2022). Moreover, despite the fact that myriad experimental and Ecological Momentary Assessment (EMA) research has shown craving, stress, cognitive flexibility, and negatively valanced mood states to robustly predict lapses to many drugs (Fatseas et al. 2018; Mayhugh et al. 2018; Kowalczyk et al. 2018; Pedersen et al. 2022), the development of anti-craving medications that specifically target provoked craving, via neurobehavioral adaptations in affective and regulatory circuitry, remains a relatively burgeoning field.

Despite such challenges, the current chapter serves to highlight some of the progress that has been made over the past decade with regard to the development of potential addiction medications for women. The main examples provided include exogenous progesterone and guanfacine, both of which have the potential to target sex-specific aspects of both craving and relapse as well as the executive control of emotion during stressful states. Moreover, recent studies are showing guanfacine, exogenous progesterone (and its metabolite, allopregnanolone) to be safe and well-tolerated in female alcohol and substance users (Fox and Sinha 2014; Oliva et al. 2022; Fox et al. 2015; Fox et al. 2012), encouraging the conduct of larger, outpatient clinical trials. In addition, multimodal research focusing on the moderating effects of sex on positive reinforcement processes as well as withdrawal-related negative reinforcement continues to expand (Slabbert et al. 2020; Bobzean et al. 2014).

As greater emphasis continues to be placed on the development of precision medicine it is also expected that better-tailored treatments will continue to emerge in the next 5–10 years for both women and other minority groups due to the elucidation of both genetic and epigenetic moderators of treatment response.

The ability to further advance research and treatment equity for under-served populations also means increasing treatment access by targeting some of the key systemic, structural, and personal-level barriers frequently encountered by women. As mentioned previously, these primarily include real and perceived stigma, child care resources, transportation, and economic hardship (Greenfield et al. 2010b; McCrady et al. 2020). In view of our own research, the *pandemic* enabled us to fast-track the implementation of telehealth procedures and utilize the benefits of a remote platform to assuage some of these issues while maintaining a solid flow of women into our clinical trials to test the effects of guanfacine in substance-using women with a promising adherence rate. Except for two safety checks, remote methods allowed women to take part in 12-week clinical trials with minimal in-person contact, by monitoring ongoing safety over Teams and compliance via encrypted FDA-approved video software showing participants consuming the medication daily. Packages mailed out to women taking part in the study included medication, urine cups, where the strips could be held up to the camera to monitor substance use, and UV lights to assess riboflavin content to ensure that urine samples had not been swapped out.

Regarding this research study, we also made a comparison of screening and recruitment rates of substance-using women between the initial 6 months at the start of the study, which was in-person and pre-pandemic (Sep 2019 to March 2020), to the initial 6 months following approval of our remote platform (Dec 2020 to June 2021). Marked increases in screening, enrollment, and randomization were observed, where the number of women screened increased from $N = 5$ (in-person) to $N = 22$ (remote), and the number of women consented increased from $N = 1$ during the initial 6 months of in-person to $N = 10$ during the initial 6 months of remote, with $N = 28$ women consented after 14 months of using our remote platform. By the final year of the project, we were randomizing approximately 1.5 women per month onto the study medication. Given the flexibility regarding time and travel afforded by using a remote platform, plus the relative anonymity of not physically having to attend a health facility, we suggest that such approaches should be used to encourage alcohol and substance-using women into clinical trials research. As such, further research is warranted to fully establish safe, effective, and standardized medication delivery and virtual data collection procedures for the development of future standardized protocols using a paradigm that has the potential to be uniquely beneficial to women with addictive disorders. In the long-term this will help address a range of major public health disparities not only in women, but also in other under-served populations.

6 Conclusions

Alcohol and substance use in women has increased dramatically over the last few decades compared with men. This reflects a public health crisis as women experience an accelerated progression through landmark symptoms pertaining to the addiction cycle known as "telescoping," and there are no FDA-approved medications currently tailored to the needs of substance-using women. This is primarily related to a number of systemic, structural, and personal-level barriers to treatment and research unique to women.

The movement from controlled to compulsive drug and alcohol seeking is associated with allostatic adaptations to the stress and reward circuits of the brain. Moreover, extensive research indicates that these chronic changes are sex-specific and influenced by gonadal hormones. As such, in the current chapter we explore the role of both endogenous progesterone fluctuations and sympathetic stress system dysregulation as potential therapeutic targets underlying relapse-related behaviors, such as provoked craving and emotional and cognitive regulation.

Findings to date indicate that exogenous progesterone and adrenergic medications, such as guanfacine, may provide some efficacy in terms of attenuating stress-induced craving for several substances, as well as improving the ability to emotionally regulate in the face of stress, preferentially in women. However, to fully leverage the potential of certain therapeutics in substance-using women, more focus needs to the placed on reducing barriers to treatment and research by encouraging women into clinical trials. Developing and refining a remote clinical trials platform may offer one potential solution.

References

Acheson A, Mahler SV, Chi H, de Wit H (2006) Differential effects of nicotine on alcohol consumption in men and women. Psychopharmacology (Berl) 186(1):54–63

Addolorato G, Leggio L, Hopf FW, Diana M, Bonci A (2012) Novel therapeutic strategies for alcohol and drug addiction: focus on GABA, ion channels and transcranial magnetic stimulation. Neuropsychopharmacology 37(1):163–177

Adinoff B, Krebaum SR, Chandler PA, Ye W, Brown MB, Williams MJ (2005a) Dissection of hypothalamic-pituitary-adrenal axis pathology in 1-month-abstinent alcohol-dependent men, part 2: response to ovine corticotropin-releasing factor and naloxone. Alcohol Clin Exp Res 29(4):528–537

Adinoff B, Junghanns K, Kiefer F, Krishnan-Sarin S (2005b) Suppression of the HPA Axis stress-response: implications for relapse. Alcohol Clin Exp Res 29(7):1351–1355

Ait-Daoud N, Blevins D, Khanna S, Sharma S, Holstege CP, Amin P (2019) Women and addiction: an update. Med Clin North Am 103(4):699–711

Allen SS, Bade T, Center B, Finstad D, Hatsukami D (2008) Menstrual phase effects on smoking relapse. Addiction 103(5):809–821

Allen SS, Allen AM, Lunos S, Tosun N (2016) Progesterone and postpartum smoking relapse: a pilot double-blind placebo-controlled randomized trial. Nicotine Tob Res 18(11):2145–2153

Altemus M, Sarvaiya N, Neill EC (2014) Sex differences in anxiety and depression clinical perspectives. Front Neuroendocrinol 35(3):320–330

Anker JJ, Carroll ME (2010) The role of progestins in the behavioral effects of cocaine and other drugs of abuse: human and animal research. Neurosci Biobehav Rev 35(2):315–333

Anker JJ, Forbes MK, Almquist ZW, Menk JS, Thuras P, Unruh AS, Kushner MG (2017) A network approach to modeling comorbid internalizing and alcohol use disorders. J Abnorm Psychol 126(3):325–339

Anker E, Bendiksen B, Heir T (2018) Comorbid psychiatric disorders in a clinical sample of adults with ADHD, and associations with education, work and social characteristics: a cross-sectional study. BMJ Open 8(3):e019700

Arnsten AFT (2007) Catecholamine and second messenger influences on prefrontal cortical networks of "representational knowledge": a rational bridge between genetics and the symptoms of mental illness. Cereb Cortex 17(Suppl 1):i6–i15

Arnsten AFT, Li BM (2005) Neurobiology of executive functions: catecholamine influences on prefrontal cortical functions. Biol Psychiatry 57(11):1377–1384

Arnsten AF, Mathew R, Ubriani R, Taylor JR, Li BM (1999a) Alpha-1 noradrenergic receptor stimulation impairs prefrontal cortical cognitive function. Biol Psychiatry 45(1):26–31

Arnsten AFT, Mathew R, Ubriani R, Taylor JR, Li BM (1999b) α-1 noradrenergic receptor stimulation impairs prefrontal cortical cognitive function. Biol Psychiatry 45(1):26–31

Aron AR (2007) The neural basis of inhibition in cognitive control. Neuroscientist 13(3):214–228

Aron AR, Poldrack RA (2005) The cognitive neuroscience of response inhibition: relevance for genetic research in attention-deficit/hyperactivity disorder. Biol Psychiatry 57(11):1285–1292

Aston-Jones G, Cohen JD (2005) Adaptive gain and the role of the locus coeruleus-norepinephrine system in optimal performance. J Comp Neurol 493(1):99–110

Aston-Jones G, Gold JI (2009) How we say no: norepinephrine, inferior frontal gyrus, and response inhibition. Biol Psychiatry 65(7):548–549

Auvinen P, Parviainen J, Lahikainen L, Palukka H (2021) Discussion protocol for alleviating epistemic injustice: the case of community rehabilitation interaction and female substance abusers. Soc Sci 10(2):45

Back SE, Waldrop AE, Saladin ME, Yeatts SD, Simpson A, McRae AL, Upadhyaya HP, Contini Sisson R, Spratt EG, Allen J, Kreek MJ, Brady KT (2008) Effects of gender and cigarette smoking on reactivity to psychological and pharmacological stress provocation. Psychoneuroendocrinology 33(5):560–568

Bäckström T, Bixo M, Johansson M, Nyberg S, Ossewaarde L, Ragagnin G, Savic I, Strömberg J, Timby E, van Broekhoven F, van Wingen G (2014) Allopregnanolone and mood disorders. Prog Neurobiol 113:88–94

Bangasser DA (2013) Sex differences in stress-related receptors: "micro" differences with "macro" implications for mood and anxiety disorders. Biol Sex Differ 4(1):2

Bangasser DA, Curtis A, Reyes BAS, Bethea TT, Parastatidis I, Ischiropoulos H, Van Bockstaele EJ, Valentino RJ (2010) Sex differences in corticotropin-releasing factor receptor signaling and trafficking: potential role in female vulnerability to stress-related psychopathology. Mol Psychiatry 15(9):877, 896–877, 904

Bangasser DA, Zhang X, Garachh V, Hanhauser E, Valentino RJ (2011) Sexual dimorphism in locus coeruleus dendritic morphology: a structural basis for sex differences in emotional arousal. Physiol Behav 103(3–4):342–351

Bangasser DA, Wiersielis KR, Khantsis S (2016) Sex differences in the locus coeruleus-norepinephrine system and its regulation by stress. Brain Res 1641(Pt B):177–188

Baumann MH, Milchanowski AB, Rothman RB (2004) Evidence for alterations in alpha2-adrenergic receptor sensitivity in rats exposed to repeated cocaine administration. Neuroscience 125(3):683–690

Becker HC (2012) Effects of alcohol dependence and withdrawal on stress responsiveness and alcohol consumption. Alcohol Res 34(4):448–458

Becker JB (2016) Sex differences in addiction. Dialogues Clin Neurosci 18(4):395–402

Becker JB, Koob GF (2016) Sex differences in animal models: focus on addiction. Pharmacol Rev 68(2):242–263

Bertholomey ML, Nagarajan V, Torregrossa MM (2016) Sex differences in reinstatement of alcohol seeking in response to cues and yohimbine in rats with and without a history of adolescent corticosterone exposure. Psychopharmacology (Berl) 233(12):2277–2287

Beveridge TJR, Smith HR, Nader MA, Porrino LJ (2005) Effects of chronic cocaine self-administration on norepinephrine transporters in the nonhuman primate brain. Psychopharmacology (Berl) 180(4):781–788

Bierer BE, Meloney LG, Ahmed HR, White SA (2022) Advancing the inclusion of underrepresented women in clinical research. Cell Rep Med 3(4):100553

Biernacki K, Lopez-Guzman S, Messinger JC, Banavar NV, Rotrosen J, Glimcher PW, Konova AB (2022) A neuroeconomic signature of opioid craving: how fluctuations in craving bias drug-related and nondrug-related value. Neuropsychopharmacology 47(8):1440–1448

Birnbaum S, Gobeske KT, Auerbach J, Taylor JR, Arnsten AF (1999) A role for norepinephrine in stress-induced cognitive deficits: alpha-1-adrenoceptor mediation in the prefrontal cortex. Biol Psychiatry 46(9):1266–1274

Bitran D, Shiekh M, McLeod M (1995) Anxiolytic effect of progesterone is mediated by the neurosteroid allopregnanolone at brain GABAA receptors. J Neuroendocrinol 7(3):171–177

Blume AW, Marlatt GA (2009) The role of executive cognitive functions in changing substance use: what we know and what we need to know. Ann Behav Med 37(2):117–125

Bobzean SAM, DeNobrega AK, Perrotti LI (2014) Sex differences in the neurobiology of drug addiction. Exp Neurol 259:64–74

Brady KT, Randall CL (1999) Gender differences in substance use disorders. Psychiatr Clin North Am 22(2):241–252

Breese GR, Chu K, Dayas CV, Funk D, Knapp DJ, Koob GF, Lê DA, O'Dell LE, Overstreet DH, Roberts AJ, Sinha R, Valdez GR, Weiss F (2005) Stress enhancement of craving during sobriety: a risk for relapse. Alcohol Clin Exp Res 29(2):185–195

Buffalari DM, Baldwin CK, See RE (2012) Treatment of cocaine withdrawal anxiety with guanfacine: relationships to cocaine intake and reinstatement of cocaine seeking in rats. Psychopharmacology (Berl) 223(2):179–190

Butelman ER, Kreek MJ (2017) Medications for substance use disorders (SUD): emerging approaches. Expert Opin Emerg Drugs 22(4):301–315

Cai H, Cao T, Zhou X, Yao JK (2018) Neurosteroids in schizophrenia: pathogenic and therapeutic implications. Front Psych 9:73

Campbell N (2000) Using women: gender, drug policy, and social justice. Routledge, New York

Campbell ND, Ettorre E (2011) Gendering addiction. Palgrave Macmillan, London

Canidate SS, Carnaby GD, Cook CL, Cook RL (2017) A systematic review of naltrexone for attenuating alcohol consumption in women with alcohol use disorders. Alcohol Clin Exp Res 41(3):466–472

Cao KX, Ma ML, Wang CZ, Iqbal J, Si JJ, Xue YX, Yang JL (2021) TMS-EEG: an emerging tool to study the neurophysiologic biomarkers of psychiatric disorders. Neuropharmacology 197: 108574

Carroll ME, Anderson MM, Morgan AD (2007) Higher locomotor response to cocaine in female (vs. male) rats selectively bred for high (HiS) and low (LoS) saccharin intake. Pharmacol Biochem Behav 88(1):94–104

Center for Behavioral Health Statistics and Quality (2018) 2017 National Survey on Drug Use and Health: Detailed Tables. Substance Abuse and Mental Health Services Administration, Rockville

Chaplin TM, Hong K, Bergquist K, Sinha R (2008) Gender differences in response to emotional stress: an assessment across subjective, behavioral, and physiological domains and relations to alcohol craving. Alcohol Clin Exp Res 32(7):1242–1250

Cheeta S, Irvine EE, Tucci S, Sandhu J, File SE (2001) In adolescence, female rats are more sensitive to the anxiolytic effect of nicotine than are male rats. Neuropsychopharmacology 25(4):601–607

Choi S, Adams SM, Morse SA, MacMaster S (2015) Gender differences in treatment retention among individuals with co-occurring substance abuse and mental health disorders. Subst Use Misuse 50(5):653–663

Clayton JA, Collins FS (2014) Policy: NIH to balance sex in cell and animal studies. Nature 509(7500):282–283

Cooney NL, Litt MD, Morse PA, Bauer LO, Gaupp L (1997) Alcohol cue reactivity, negative-mood reactivity, and relapse in treated alcoholic men. J Abnorm Psychol 106(2):243–250

Cozzoli DK, Tanchuck-Nipper MA, Kaufman MN, Horowitz CB, Finn DA (2014) Environmental stressors influence limited-access ethanol consumption by C57BL/6J mice in a sex-dependent manner. Alcohol 48(8):741–754

Curtis AL, Bethea T, Valentino RJ (2006) Sexually dimorphic responses of the brain norepinephrine system to stress and corticotropin-releasing factor. Neuropsychopharmacology 31(3): 544–554

D'Esposito M (2007) From cognitive to neural models of working memory. Philos Trans R Soc Lond B Biol Sci 362(1481):761–772

Davis J, Oparil S (2018) Novel medical treatments for hypertension and related comorbidities. Curr Hypertens Rep 20(10):90

Dawson DA, Goldstein RB, Saha TD, Grant BF (2015) Changes in alcohol consumption: United States, 2001-2002 to 2012-2013. Drug Alcohol Depend 148:56–61

Derlet RW, Albertson TE (1990) Acute cocaine toxicity: antagonism by agents interacting with adrenoceptors. Pharmacol Biochem Behav 36(2):225–231

Devries KM, Child JC, Bacchus LJ, Mak J, Falder G, Graham K, Watts C, Heise L (2014) Intimate partner violence victimization and alcohol consumption in women: a systematic review and meta-analysis. Addiction 109(3):379–391

Diana M (2011) The dopamine hypothesis of drug addiction and its potential therapeutic value. Front Psych 2:64

Drouin C, Blanc G, Villégier AS, Glowinski J, Tassin JP (2002) Critical role of alpha1-adrenergic receptors in acute and sensitized locomotor effects of D-amphetamine, cocaine, and GBR 12783: influence of preexposure conditions and pharmacological characteristics. Synapse 43(1):51–61

Ek J, Jacobs W, Kaylor B, McCall WV (2021) Addiction and sleep disorders. Adv Exp Med Biol 1297:163–171

Epstein EE, Fischer-Elber K, Al-Otaiba Z (2007) Women, aging, and alcohol use disorders. J Women Aging 19(1–2):31–48

Errico AL, Parsons OA, King AC, Lovallo WR (1993) Attenuated cortisol response to biobehavioral stressors in sober alcoholics. J Stud Alcohol 54(4):393–398

Ettorre E (2015) Embodied deviance, gender, and epistemologies of ignorance: re-visioning drugs use in a neurochemical. Unjust World Subst Use Misuse 50(6):794–805

Evans SM (2007) The role of estradiol and progesterone in modulating the subjective effects of stimulants in humans. Exp Clin Psychopharmacol 15(5):418–426

Evans A (2011) Dopamine agonist-induced substance addiction: the next piece of the puzzle. J Clin Neurosci 18(2):191–192

Evans SM, Foltin RW (2006) Exogenous progesterone attenuates the subjective effects of smoked cocaine in women, but not in men. Neuropsychopharmacology 31(3):659–674

Evans SM, Foltin RW (2010) Does the response to cocaine differ as a function of sex or hormonal status in human and non-human primates? Horm Behav 58(1):13–21

Evans SM, Haney M, Foltin RW (2002) The effects of smoked cocaine during the follicular and luteal phases of the menstrual cycle in women. Psychopharmacology (Berl) 159(4):397–406

Evans EA, Goff SL, Upchurch DM, Grella CE (2020) Childhood adversity and mental health comorbidity in men and women with opioid use disorders. Addict Behav 102:106149

Fabris D, Carvalho MC, Brandão ML, Prado WA, Zuardi AW, Crippa JA, de Oliveira AR, Lovick TA, Genaro K (2022) Sex-dependent differences in the anxiolytic-like effect of cannabidiol in the elevated plus-maze. J Psychopharmacol 36(12):1371–1383

Fama R, Le Berre AP, Sullivan EV (2020) Alcohol's unique effects on cognition in women: a 2020 (re)view to envision future research and treatment. Alcohol Res 40(2):03

Faraday MM, Blakeman KH, Grunberg NE (2005) Strain and sex alter effects of stress and nicotine on feeding, body weight, and HPA axis hormones. Pharmacol Biochem Behav 80(4):577–589

Faravelli C, Alessandra Scarpato M, Castellini G, Lo SC (2013) Gender differences in depression and anxiety: the role of age. Psychiatry Res 210(3):1301–1303

Fatseas M, Serre F, Swendsen J, Auriacombe M (2018) Effects of anxiety and mood disorders on craving and substance use among patients with substance use disorder: an ecological momentary assessment study. Drug Alcohol Depend 187:242–248

Fattore L, Altea S, Fratta W (2008) Sex differences in drug addiction: a review of animal and human studies. Womens Health 4(1):51–65

Ferris MJ, Mactutus CF, Silvers JM, Hasselrot U, Beaudin SA, Strupp BJ, Booze RM (2007) Sex mediates dopamine and adrenergic receptor expression in adult rats exposed prenatally to cocaine. Int J Dev Neurosci 25(7):445–454

Festa ED, Shivers KY, Jenab S, Quiñones-Jenab V (2010) Cocaine-induced sex differences in D1 dopamine receptor mRNA levels after acute cocaine administration. Ethn Dis 20(1 Suppl 1):S1-24-7

Fiad TM, Cunningham SK, McKenna TJ (1996) Role of progesterone deficiency in the development of luteinizing hormone and androgen abnormalities in polycystic ovary syndrome. Eur J Endocrinol 135(3):335–339

Fiddian-Green A, Gubrium A, Harrington C, Evans EA (2022) Women-reported barriers and facilitators of continued engagement with medications for opioid use disorder. Int J Environ Res Public Health 19(15):9346

Fonseca F, Robles-Martínez M, Tirado-Muñoz J, Alías-Ferri M, Mestre-Pintó JI, Coratu AM, Torrens M (2021) A gender perspective of addictive disorders. Curr Addict Rep 8(1):89–99

Forray A, Gilstad-Hayden K, Suppies C, Bogen D, Sofuoglu M, Yonkers KA (2017) Progesterone for smoking relapse prevention following delivery: a pilot, randomized, double-blind study. Psychoneuroendocrinology 86:96–103

Fox HC (2007) Gender differences in neurobiological response to stress and alcohol cues: implications for treatment and relapse. 30th Annual Research Society on Alcoholism Scientific Meeting, Chicago, IL, July 7–12, 2007

Fox HC, Sinha R (2009) Sex differences in drug-related stress-system changes: implications for treatment in substance-abusing women. Harv Rev Psychiatry 17(2):103–119

Fox H, Sinha R (2014) The role of guanfacine as a therapeutic agent to address stress-related pathophysiology in cocaine-dependent individuals. Adv Pharmacol 69:217–265

Fox HM, Verica BSK, SR (2018) Stress system sensitivity and emotion regulation in early abstinence from substance use disorders – targets for medications development. In: Foti DSS (ed) Emotion and motivated behaviors: integrating animal and human neurobiology research. Elsevier, pp 120–141

Fox HC, Bergquist KL, Hong KI, Sinha R (2007) Stress-induced and alcohol cue-induced craving in recently abstinent alcohol-dependent individuals. Alcohol Clin Exp Res 31(3):395–403

Fox HC, Hong KA, Paliwal P, Morgan PT, Sinha R (2008a) Altered levels of sex and stress steroid hormones assessed daily over a 28-day cycle in early abstinent cocaine-dependent females. Psychopharmacology (Berl) 195(4):527–536

Fox HC, Hong KIA, Siedlarz K, Sinha R (2008b) Enhanced sensitivity to stress and drug/alcohol craving in abstinent cocaine-dependent individuals compared to social drinkers. Neuropsychopharmacology 33(4):796–805

Fox HC, Hong KIA, Siedlarz KM, Bergquist K, Anderson G, Kreek MJ, Sinha R (2009) Sex-specific dissociations in autonomic and HPA responses to stress and cues in alcohol-dependent patients with cocaine abuse. Alcohol 44(6):575–585

Fox HC, Seo D, Tuit K, Hansen J, Kimmerling A, Morgan PT, Sinha R (2012) Guanfacine effects on stress, drug craving and prefrontal activation in cocaine dependent individuals: preliminary findings. J Psychopharmacol 26(7):958–972

Fox HC, Sofuoglu M, Morgan PT, Tuit KL, Sinha R (2013) The effects of exogenous progesterone on drug craving and stress arousal in cocaine dependence: impact of gender and cue type. Psychoneuroendocrinology 38(9):1532–1544

Fox HC, Morgan PT, Sinha R (2014) Sex differences in guanfacine effects on drug craving and stress arousal in cocaine-dependent individuals. Neuropsychopharmacology 39(6):1527–1537

Fox H, Sofuoglu M, Sinha R (2015) Guanfacine enhances inhibitory control and attentional shifting in early abstinent cocaine-dependent individuals. J Psychopharmacol 29(3):312–323

Fox HC, Hong KIA, Siedlarz KM, Bergquist K, Anderson G, Kreek MJ, Sinha R (2009) Sex-specific dissociations in autonomic and HPA responses to stress and cues in alcohol-dependent patients with cocaine abuse. Alcohol 44(6):575–585

Gater R, Tansella M, Korten A, Tiemens BG, Mavreas VG, Olatawura MO (1998) Sex differences in the prevalence and detection of depressive and anxiety disorders in general health care settings. Arch Gen Psychiatry 55(5):405

George O, Koob GF, Vendruscolo LF (2014) Negative reinforcement via motivational withdrawal is the driving force behind the transition to addiction. Psychopharmacology (Berl) 231(19): 3911–3917

Gilmore AK, Guille C, Baker NL, Brady KT, Hahn CK, Davis CM, McCauley JL, Back SE (2019) Gender differences in subjective stress and neuroendocrine response to a stress task among individuals with opioid dependence: a pilot study. Addict Behav 92:148–154

Girdler SS, Klatzkin R (2007) Neurosteroids in the context of stress: implications for depressive disorders. Pharmacol Ther 116(1):125–139

Glassman AH, Covey LS, Dalack GW, Stetner F, Rivelli SK, Fleiss J, Cooper TB (1993) Smoking cessation, clonidine, and vulnerability to nicotine among dependent smokers. Clin Pharmacol Ther 54(6):670–679

Goeders NE (2002) The HPA axis and cocaine reinforcement. Psychoneuroendocrinology 27(1–2): 13–33

Gorelick DA, Gardner EL, Xi ZX (2004) Agents in development for the management of cocaine abuse. Drugs 64(14):1547–1573

Grant BF, Chou SP, Saha TD, Pickering RP, Kerridge BT, Ruan WJ, Huang B, Jung J, Zhang H, Fan A, Hasin DS (2017) Prevalence of 12-month alcohol use, high-risk drinking, and DSM-IV alcohol use disorder in the United States, 2001-2002 to 2012-2013: results from the National Epidemiologic Survey on alcohol and related conditions. JAMA Psychiatry 74(9):911–923

Greenfield SF, Back SE, Lawson K, Brady KT (2010a) Substance abuse in women. Psychiatr Clin North Am 33(2):339–355

Greenfield SF, Back SE, Lawson K, Brady KT (2010b) Substance abuse in women. Psychiatr Clin N Am 33(2):339–355

Grol R, Wensing M (2004) What drives change? Barriers to and incentives for achieving evidence-based practice. Med J Aust 180(S6):S57–S60

Gulinello M, Smith SS (2003) Anxiogenic effects of neurosteroid exposure: sex differences and altered GABAA receptor pharmacology in adult rats. J Pharmacol Exp Ther 305(2):541–548

Haas AL, Peters RH (2000) Development of substance abuse problems among drug-involved offenders. Evidence for the telescoping effect. J Subst Abuse 12(3):241–253

Haass-Koffler CL, Swift RM, Leggio L (2018) Noradrenergic targets for the treatment of alcohol use disorder. Psychopharmacology (Berl) 235(6):1625–1634

Haney M, Hart CL, Vosburg SK, Comer SD, Reed SC, Cooper ZD, Foltin RW (2010) Effects of baclofen and mirtazapine on a laboratory model of marijuana withdrawal and relapse. Psychopharmacology (Berl) 211(2):233–244

Harrod SB, Mactutus CF, Bennett K, Hasselrot U, Wu G, Welch M, Booze RM (2004) Sex differences and repeated intravenous nicotine: behavioral sensitization and dopamine receptors. Pharmacol Biochem Behav 78(3):581–592

Harrod SB, Booze RM, Welch M, Browning CE, Mactutus CF (2005) Acute and repeated intravenous cocaine-induced locomotor activity is altered as a function of sex and gonadectomy. Pharmacol Biochem Behav 82(1):170–181

Heinsbroek RP, van Haaren F, Feenstra MG, Boon P, van de Poll NE (1991) Controllable and uncontrollable footshock and monoaminergic activity in the frontal cortex of male and female rats. Brain Res 551(1–2):247–255

Hernandez-Avila CA, Rounsaville BJ, Kranzler HR (2004) Opioid-, cannabis- and alcohol-dependent women show more rapid progression to substance abuse treatment. Drug Alcohol Depend 74(3):265–272

Ho AMC, Geske JR, Bakalkin G, Winham SJ, Karpyak VM (2019) Correlations between sex-related hormones, alcohol dependence and alcohol craving. Drug Alcohol Depend 197: 183–190

Holbrook AM (2015) Methadone versus buprenorphine for the treatment of opioid abuse in pregnancy: science and stigma. Am J Drug Alcohol Abuse 41(5):371–373

Ijff DM, Aldenkamp AP (2013) Cognitive side-effects of antiepileptic drugs in children. Handb Clin Neurol 111:707–718

Jensen KP, Sofuoglu M (2016) Stress response genes and the severity of nicotine withdrawal. Pharmacogenomics 17(1):1–3

Ji XH, Ji JZ, Zhang H, Li BM (2008) Stimulation of alpha2-adrenoceptors suppresses excitatory synaptic transmission in the medial prefrontal cortex of rat. Neuropsychopharmacology 33(9): 2263–2271

Johannessen EL, Andersson HW, Bjørngaard JH, Pape K (2017) Anxiety and depression symptoms and alcohol use among adolescents – a cross sectional study of Norwegian secondary school students. BMC Public Health 17(1):494

Jonas DE, Amick HR, Feltner C, Bobashev G, Thomas K, Wines R, Kim MM, Shanahan E, Gass CE, Rowe CJ, Garbutt JC (2014) Pharmacotherapy for adults with alcohol use disorders in outpatient settings. JAMA 311(18):1889

Junghanns K, Backhaus J, Tietz U, Lange W, Bernzen J, Wetterling T, Rink L, Driessen M (2003) Impaired serum cortisol stress response is a predictor of early relapse. Alcohol 38(2):189–193

Justice AJ, de Wit H (1999) Acute effects of d-amphetamine during the follicular and luteal phases of the menstrual cycle in women. Psychopharmacology (Berl) 145(1):67–75

Justice AJ, De Wit H (2000) Acute effects of d-amphetamine during the early and late follicular phases of the menstrual cycle in women. Pharmacol Biochem Behav 66(3):509–515

Just-Østergaard E, Mortensen EL, Tolstrup JS, Flensborg-Madsen T (2018) Vital exhaustion and risk of alcohol use disorders: a prospective cohort study. J Psychosom Res 114:25–30

Kampman KM, Pettinati HM, Volpicelli JR, Oslin DM, Lipkin C, Sparkman T, O'Brien CP (2004) Cocaine dependence severity predicts outcome in outpatient detoxification from cocaine and alcohol. Am J Addict 13(1):74–82

Kaplan JR, Manuck SB (2004) Ovarian dysfunction, stress, and disease: a primate continuum. ILAR J 45(2):89–115

Kawahara H, Kawahara Y, Westerink BHC (2000) The role of afferents to the locus coeruleus in the handling stress-induced increase in the release of noradrenaline in the medial prefrontal cortex: a dual-probe microdialysis study in the rat brain. Eur J Pharmacol 387(3):279–286

Koob GF (2010) The role of CRF and CRF-related peptides in the dark side of addiction. Brain Res 1314:3–14

Koob GF (2013) Negative reinforcement in drug addiction: the darkness within. Curr Opin Neurobiol 23(4):559–563

Koob GF (2021) Drug addiction: hyperkatifeia/negative reinforcement as a framework for medications development. Pharmacol Rev 73(1):163–201

Koob G, Kreek MJ (2007) Stress, dysregulation of drug reward pathways, and the transition to drug dependence. Am J Psychiatry 164(8):1149–1159

Koob GF, Le Moal M (2001) Drug addiction, dysregulation of reward, and allostasis. Neuropsychopharmacology 24(2):97–129

Koob GF, Le Moal M (2008) Review. Neurobiological mechanisms for opponent motivational processes in addiction. Philos Trans R Soc Lond B Biol Sci 363(1507):3113–3123

Kosten TR, Kosten TA, McDougle CJ, Hameedi FA, McCance EF, Rosen MI, Oliveto AH, Price LH (1996) Gender differences in response to intranasal cocaine administration to humans. Biol Psychiatry 39(2):147–148

Kosten TA, Sanchez H, Zhang XY, Kehoe P (2004) Neonatal isolation enhances acquisition of cocaine self-administration and food responding in female rats. Behav Brain Res 151(1–2): 137–149

Kosten TA, Miserendino MJD, Bombace JC, Lee HJ, Kim JJ (2005) Sex-selective effects of neonatal isolation on fear conditioning and foot shock sensitivity. Behav Brain Res 157(2): 235–244

Kowalczyk WJ, Phillips KA, Jobes ML, Kennedy AP, Ghitza UE, Agage DA, Schmittner JP, Epstein DH, Preston KL (2015) Clonidine maintenance prolongs opioid abstinence and decouples stress from craving in daily life: a randomized controlled trial with ecological momentary assessment. Am J Psychiatry 172(8):760–767

Kowalczyk WJ, Moran LM, Bertz JW, Phillips KA, Ghitza UE, Vahabzadeh M, Lin JL, Epstein DH, Preston KL (2018) Using ecological momentary assessment to examine the relationship between craving and affect with opioid use in a clinical trial of clonidine as an adjunct medication to buprenorphine treatment. Am J Drug Alcohol Abuse 44(5):502–511

Kranzler HR, Soyka M (2018) Diagnosis and pharmacotherapy of alcohol use disorder. JAMA 320(8):815

Kuerbis A, Sacco P, Blazer DG, Moore AA (2014) Substance abuse among older adults. Clin Geriatr Med 30(3):629–654

Kuntsche E, Müller S (2012) Why do young people start drinking? Motives for first-time alcohol consumption and links to risky drinking in early adolescence. Eur Addict Res 18(1):34–39

Kuo CW, Lin CF, Chen CY, Wang RH, Chou CY, Cheng HJ, Wu JS, Chen CW, Shieh CC, Yu T (2022) Body-weight gain in women during smoking cessation is a sex-specific predictor of 6-month abstinence: a retrospective cohort study. Front Public Health 10:872220

Lê AD, Funk D, Juzytsch W, Coen K, Navarre BM, Cifani C, Shaham Y (2011) Effect of prazosin and guanfacine on stress-induced reinstatement of alcohol and food seeking in rats. Psychopharmacology (Berl) 218(1):89–99

Leri F, Tremblay A, Sorge RE, Stewart J (2004) Methadone maintenance reduces heroin- and cocaine-induced relapse without affecting stress-induced relapse in a rodent model of poly-drug use. Neuropsychopharmacology 29(7):1312–1320

Litt MD, Cooney NL, Morse P (2000) Reactivity to alcohol-related stimuli in the laboratory and in the field: predictors of craving in treated alcoholics. Addiction 95(6):889–900

Loree AM, Lundahl LH, Ledgerwood DM (2015) Impulsivity as a predictor of treatment outcome in substance use disorders: review and synthesis. Drug Alcohol Rev 34(2):119–134

Lovallo WR, Dickensheets SL, Myers DA, Thomas TL, Nixon SJ (2000) Blunted stress cortisol response in abstinent alcoholic and polysubstance-abusing men. Alcohol Clin Exp Res 24(5): 651–658

Lukas SE, Sholar M, Lundahl LH, Lamas X, Kouri E, Wines JD, Kragie L, Mendelson JH (1996) Sex differences in plasma cocaine levels and subjective effects after acute cocaine administration in human volunteers. Psychopharmacology (Berl) 125(4):346–354

Lynch WJ, Taylor JR (2004) Sex differences in the behavioral effects of 24-h/day access to cocaine under a discrete trial procedure. Neuropsychopharmacology 29(5):943–951

Lynch WJ, Roth ME, Carroll ME (2002) Biological basis of sex differences in drug abuse: preclinical and clinical studies. Psychopharmacology (Berl) 164(2):121–137

Lynch WJ, Mangini LD, Taylor JR (2005) Neonatal isolation stress potentiates cocaine seeking behavior in adult male and female rats. Neuropsychopharmacology 30(2):322–329

Lynch WJ, Kiraly DD, Caldarone BJ, Picciotto MR, Taylor JR (2007) Effect of cocaine self-administration on striatal PKA-regulated signaling in male and female rats. Psychopharmacology (Berl) 191(2):263–271

Mann K, Ackermann K, Croissant B, Mundle G, Nakovics H, Diehl A (2005) Neuroimaging of gender differences in alcohol dependence: are women more vulnerable? Alcohol Clin Exp Res 29(5):896–901

Marek GJ, Aghajanian GK (1999) 5-HT2A receptor or alpha1-adrenoceptor activation induces excitatory postsynaptic currents in layer V pyramidal cells of the medial prefrontal cortex. Eur J Pharmacol 367(2–3):197–206

Marks KR, Clark CD (2018) The telescoping phenomenon: origins in gender bias and implications for contemporary scientific inquiry. Subst Use Misuse 53(6):901–909

Martin CE, Dzierzewski JM, Keyser-Marcus L, Donovan EK, Ramey T, Svikis DS, Moeller FG (2022) Sex specific sleep parameters among people with substance use disorder. Front Psych 13: 905332

Mayhugh RE, Rejeski WJ, Petrie MR, Laurienti PJ, Gauvin L (2018) Differing patterns of stress and craving across the day in moderate-heavy alcohol consumers during their typical drinking routine and an imposed period of alcohol abstinence. PloS One 13(4):e0195063

McCrady BS, Epstein EE, Fokas KF (2020) Treatment interventions for women with alcohol use disorder. Alcohol Res 40(2):8

McKetta SC, Keyes KM (2020) Trends in U.S. women's binge drinking in middle adulthood by socioeconomic status, 2006-2018. Drug Alcohol Depend 212:108026
McRae-Clark AL, Cason AM, Kohtz AS, Moran Santa-Maria M, Aston-Jones G, Brady KT (2017) Impact of gender on corticotropin-releasing factor and noradrenergic sensitivity in cocaine use disorder. J Neurosci Res 95(1–2):320–327
Meltzer-Brody S, Howard LM, Bergink V, Vigod S, Jones I, Munk-Olsen T, Honikman S, Milgrom J (2018) Postpartum psychiatric disorders. Nat Rev Dis Primers 4:18022
Milic J, Glisic M, Voortman T, Borba LP, Asllanaj E, Rojas LZ, Troup J, Kiefte-de Jong JC, van Beeck E, Muka T, Franco OH (2018) Menopause, ageing, and alcohol use disorders in women. Maturitas 111:100–109
Milivojevic V, Sinha R (2018) Central and peripheral biomarkers of stress response for addiction risk and relapse vulnerability. Trends Mol Med 24(2):173–186
Milivojevic V, Sinha R, Morgan PT, Sofuoglu M, Fox HC (2014) Effects of endogenous and exogenous progesterone on emotional intelligence in cocaine-dependent men and women who also abuse alcohol. Hum Psychopharmacol 29(6):589–598
Moran-Santa Maria MM, McRae-Clark A, Baker NL, Ramakrishnan V, Brady KT (2014) Yohimbine administration and cue-reactivity in cocaine-dependent individuals. Psychopharmacology (Berl) 231(21):4157–4165
Netter P, Müller MJ, Neumann A, Kamradik B (1994) The influence of nicotine on performance, mood, and physiological parameters as related to smoking habit, gender, and suggestibility. Clin Investig 72(7):512–518
Nolen-Hoeksema S, Wisco BE, Lyubomirsky S (2008) Rethinking rumination. Perspect Psychol Sci 3(5):400–424
Ogilvie KM, Rivier C (1997) Gender difference in hypothalamic-pituitary-adrenal axis response to alcohol in the rat: activational role of gonadal steroids. Brain Res 766(1–2):19–28
Oliva A, Reed SC, Brooks DJ, Levin FR, Evans SM (2022) Safety and tolerability of progesterone treatment for women with cocaine use disorder: a pilot treatment trial. Am J Drug Alcohol Abuse 48(5):586–595
Ossewaarde L, Hermans EJ, van Wingen GA, Kooijman SC, Johansson IM, Bäckström T, Fernández G (2010) Neural mechanisms underlying changes in stress-sensitivity across the menstrual cycle. Psychoneuroendocrinology 35(1):47–55
Patel BG, Rudnicki M, Yu J, Shu Y, Taylor RN (2017) Progesterone resistance in endometriosis: origins, consequences and interventions. Acta Obstet Gynecol Scand 96(6):623–632
Pedersen SL, Kennedy TM, Holmes J, Molina BSG (2022) Momentary associations between stress and alcohol craving in the naturalistic environment: differential associations for Black and White young adults. Addiction 117(5):1284–1294
Peltier MR, Verplaetse TL, Mineur YS, Petrakis IL, Cosgrove KP, Picciotto MR, McKee SA (2019) Sex differences in stress-related alcohol use. Neurobiol Stress 10:100149
Perkins KA, Sexton JE, DiMarco A, Grobe JE, Scierka A, Stiller RL (1995) Subjective and cardiovascular responses to nicotine combined with alcohol in male and female smokers. Psychopharmacology (Berl) 119(2):205–212
Piazza NJ, Vrbka JL, Yeager RD (1989) Telescoping of alcoholism in women alcoholics. Int J Addict 24(1):19–28
Porrino LJ, Lyons D, Smith HR, Daunais JB, Nader MA (2004) Cocaine self-administration produces a progressive involvement of limbic, association, and sensorimotor striatal domains. J Neurosci 24(14):3554–3562
Porrino LJ, Smith HR, Nader MA, Beveridge TJR (2007) The effects of cocaine: a shifting target over the course of addiction. Prog Neuropsychopharmacol Biol Psychiatry 31(8):1593–1600
Preston KL, Epstein DH (2011) Stress in the daily lives of cocaine and heroin users: relationship to mood, craving, relapse triggers, and cocaine use. Psychopharmacology (Berl) 218(1):29–37
Qurishi R, Drenth JPH, De Jong CAJ (2022) Premenstrual syndrome predicts alcohol craving in women with substance use disorders. Women Health 62(5):430–438

Ramos BP, Arnsten AFT (2007) Adrenergic pharmacology and cognition: focus on the prefrontal cortex. Pharmacol Ther 113(3):523–536

Riaz M (2019) Comparison of guilt and shame between men and women with drug addiction. J Forensic Sci Crim Investig 12(4):1–8

Romeo E, Ströhle A, Spalletta G, di Michele F, Hermann B, Holsboer F, Pasini A, Rupprecht R (1998) Effects of antidepressant treatment on neuroactive steroids in major depression. Am J Psychiatry 155(7):910–913

Rupprecht R (2003) Neuroactive steroids: mechanisms of action and neuropsychopharmacological properties. Psychoneuroendocrinology 28(2):139–168

Salviato BZ, Raymundi AM, Rodrigues da Silva T, Salemme BW, Batista Sohn JM, Araújo FS, Guimarães FS, Bertoglio LJ, Stern CA (2021) Female but not male rats show biphasic effects of low doses of Δ9-tetrahydrocannabinol on anxiety: can cannabidiol interfere with these effects? Neuropharmacology 196:108684

Sawaguchi T, Goldman-Rakic PS (1994) The role of D1-dopamine receptor in working memory: local injections of dopamine antagonists into the prefrontal cortex of rhesus monkeys performing an oculomotor delayed-response task. J Neurophysiol 71(2):515–528

Saxon AJ, McCarty D (2005) Challenges in the adoption of new pharmacotherapeutics for addiction to alcohol and other drugs. Pharmacol Ther 108(1):119–128

Schamp J, Simonis S, Roets G, Van Havere T, Gremeaux L, Vanderplasschen W (2021) Women's views on barriers and facilitators for seeking alcohol and drug treatment in Belgium. Nordisk Alkohol Nark 38(2):175–189

Schleifer LA, Justice AJH, de Wit H (2002) Lack of effects of acute estradiol on mood in postmenopausal women. Pharmacol Biochem Behav 71(1–2):71–77

Schwabe L, Höffken O, Tegenthoff M, Wolf OT (2013) Opposite effects of noradrenergic arousal on amygdala processing of fearful faces in men and women. Neuroimage 73:1–7

Shiffman S, Scholl SM, Mao J, Ferguson SG, Hedeker D, Tindle HA (2020) Ecological momentary assessment of temptations and lapses in non-daily smokers. Psychopharmacology (Berl) 237(8): 2353–2365

Singha AK, McCance-Katz EF, Petrakis I, Kosten TR, Oliveto A (2000) Sex differences in self-reported and physiological response to oral cocaine and placebo in humans. Am J Drug Alcohol Abuse 26(4):643–657

Sinha R (2008) Chronic stress, drug use, and vulnerability to addiction. Ann N Y Acad Sci 1141(1): 105–130

Sinha R, Garcia M, Paliwal P, Kreek MJ, Rounsaville BJ (2006) Stress-induced cocaine craving and hypothalamic-pituitary-adrenal responses are predictive of cocaine relapse outcomes. Arch Gen Psychiatry 63(3):324–331

Sinha R, Fox H, Hong KI, Sofuoglu M, Morgan PT, Bergquist KT (2007) Sex steroid hormones, stress response, and drug craving in cocaine-dependent women: implications for relapse susceptibility. Exp Clin Psychopharmacol 15(5):445–452

Sinha R, Fox HC, Hong KA, Bergquist K, Bhagwagar Z, Siedlarz KM (2009) Enhanced negative emotion and alcohol craving and altered physiological responses following stress and cue exposure in alcohol dependent individuals. Neuropsychopharmacology 34(5):1198–1208. https://doi.org/10.1038/npp.2008.78

Sinha R, Fox HC, Hong KIA, Hansen J, Tuit K, Kreek MJ (2011) Effects of adrenal sensitivity, stress- and cue-induced craving, and anxiety on subsequent alcohol relapse and treatment outcomes. Arch Gen Psychiatry 68(9):942–952

Slabbert I, Greene MC, Womersley JS, Olateju OI, Soboka M, Lemieux AM (2020) Women and substance use disorders in low- and middle-income countries: a call for advancing research equity in prevention and treatment. Subst Abus 41(1):6–10

Slade T, Chapman C, Swift W, Keyes K, Tonks Z, Teesson M (2016) Birth cohort trends in the global epidemiology of alcohol use and alcohol-related harms in men and women: systematic review and metaregression. BMJ Open 6(10):e011827

Smith RJ, Aston-Jones G (2008) Noradrenergic transmission in the extended amygdala: role in increased drug-seeking and relapse during protracted drug abstinence. Brain Struct Funct 213(1–2):43–61

Sofuoglu M (2010) Cognitive enhancement as a pharmacotherapy target for stimulant addiction. Addiction 105(1):38–48

Sofuoglu M, Sewell RA (2009) Norepinephrine and stimulant addiction. Addict Biol 14(2): 119–129

Sofuoglu M, Dudish-Poulsen S, Nelson D, Pentel PR, Hatsukami DK (1999) Sex and menstrual cycle differences in the subjective effects from smoked cocaine in humans. Exp Clin Psychopharmacol 7(3):274–283

Sofuoglu M, Babb DA, Hatsukami DK (2001) Progesterone treatment during the early follicular phase of the menstrual cycle: effects on smoking behavior in women. Pharmacol Biochem Behav 69(1–2):299–304

Sofuoglu M, Mouratidis M, Mooney M (2011) Progesterone improves cognitive performance and attenuates smoking urges in abstinent smokers. Psychoneuroendocrinology 36(1):123–132

Sofuoglu M, DeVito EE, Waters AJ, Carroll KM (2016) Cognitive function as a transdiagnostic treatment target in stimulant use disorders. J Dual Diagn 12(1):90–106

Sommer BR, Mitchell EL, Wroolie TE (2013) Topiramate: effects on cognition in patients with epilepsy, migraine headache and obesity. Ther Adv Neurol Disord 6(4):211–227

Stefaniak M, Dmoch-Gajzlerska E, Jankowska K, Rogowski A, Kajdy A, Maksym RB (2023) Progesterone and its metabolites play a beneficial role in affect regulation in the female brain. Pharmaceuticals (Basel) 16(4)

Stephens MAC, Mahon PB, McCaul ME, Wand GS (2016) Hypothalamic-pituitary-adrenal axis response to acute psychosocial stress: effects of biological sex and circulating sex hormones. Psychoneuroendocrinology 66:47–55

Studd J (2006) Ovariotomy for menstrual madness and premenstrual syndrome – 19th century history and lessons for current practice. Gynecol Endocrinol 22(8):411–415

Substance Abuse and Mental Health Services Administration (2017) Key substance use and mental health indicators in the United States: results from the 2016 National Survey on Drug Use and Health (HHS Publication No. SMA 17-5044, NSDUH Series H-52)

Substance Abuse and Mental Health Services Administration U.S. Department of Health and Human Services (2020) 2019 National Survey on Drug Use and Health: Women

Sundström-Poromaa I, Comasco E, Sumner R, Luders E (2020) Progesterone – friend or foe? Front Neuroendocrinol 59:100856

Templeton TJ, Diarra S, Gilpin NW (2023) Sex differences in cocaine self-administration by Wistar rats after predator odor exposure. bioRxiv

Torres OV, Gentil LG, Natividad LA, Carcoba LM, O'Dell LE (2013) Behavioral, biochemical, and molecular indices of stress are enhanced in female versus male rats experiencing nicotine withdrawal. Front Psych 4:38

Tosun NL, Fieberg AM, Eberly LE, Harrison KA, Tipp AR, Allen AM, Allen SS (2019) Exogenous progesterone for smoking cessation in men and women: a pilot double-blind, placebo-controlled randomized clinical trial. Addiction 114(10):1800–1813

van Wingen GA, van Broekhoven F, Verkes RJ, Petersson KM, Bäckström T, Buitelaar JK, Fernández G (2008) Progesterone selectively increases amygdala reactivity in women. Mol Psychiatry 13(3):325–333

Vengeliene V, Vollmayr B, Henn FA, Spanagel R (2005) Voluntary alcohol intake in two rat lines selectively bred for learned helpless and non-helpless behavior. Psychopharmacology (Berl) 178(2–3):125–132

Verplaetse TL, Weinberger AH, Smith PH, Cosgrove KP, Mineur YS, Picciotto MR, Mazure CM, McKee SA (2015) Targeting the noradrenergic system for gender-sensitive medication development for tobacco dependence. Nicotine Tob Res 17(4):486–495

Vescovi PP, DiGennaro C, Coiro V (1997) Hormonal (ACTH, cortisol, beta-endorphin, and met-enkephalin) and cardiovascular responses to hyperthermic stress in chronic alcoholics. Alcohol Clin Exp Res 21(7):1195–1198

Waldrop AE, Price KL, Desantis SM, Simpson AN, Back SE, McRae AL, Spratt EG, Kreek MJ, Brady KT (2010) Community-dwelling cocaine-dependent men and women respond differently to social stressors versus cocaine cues. Psychoneuroendocrinology 35(6):798–806

Wand GS, Dobs AS (1991) Alterations in the hypothalamic-pituitary-adrenal axis in actively drinking alcoholics. J Clin Endocrinol Metab 72(6):1290–1295

Warren JG, Fallon VM, Goodwin L, Gage SH, Rose AK (2021) Menstrual cycle phase, hormonal contraception, and alcohol consumption in premenopausal females: a systematic review. Front Glob Womens Health 2

Weinberger AH, McKee SA, Mazure CM (2010) Inclusion of women and gender-specific analyses in randomized clinical trials of treatments for depression. J Womens Health (Larchmt) 19(9): 1727–1732

Weinland C, Mühle C, Kornhuber J, Lenz B (2021) Progesterone serum levels correlate negatively with craving in female postmenopausal in-patients with alcohol use disorder: a sex- and menopausal status-separated study. Prog Neuropsychopharmacol Biol Psychiatry 110:110278

Weinshenker D, Schroeder JP (2007) There and back again: a tale of norepinephrine and drug addiction. Neuropsychopharmacology 32(7):1433–1451

Wemm SE, Sinha R (2019) Drug-induced stress responses and addiction risk and relapse. Neurobiol Stress 10:100148

Wenzel ES, Pinna G, Eisenlohr-Moul T, Bernabe BP, Tallon RR, Nagelli U, Davis J, Maki PM (2021) Neuroactive steroids and depression in early pregnancy. Psychoneuroendocrinology 134:105424

White A, Castle IJP, Chen CM, Shirley M, Roach D, Hingson R (2015) Converging patterns of alcohol use and related outcomes among females and males in the United States, 2002 to 2012. Alcohol Clin Exp Res 39(9):1712–1726

Zahrt J, Taylor JR, Mathew RG, Arnsten AF (1997) Supranormal stimulation of D1 dopamine receptors in the rodent prefrontal cortex impairs spatial working memory performance. J Neurosci 17(21):8528–8535

Intersection of Sex and Depression: Pathogenesis, Presentation, and Treatments

Dafni F. T. Frohman, Kimberly Nnah, and Stella E. Tsirka

Contents

Abstract

Major Depressive Disorder (MDD) is a highly prevalent, debilitating disorder. According to the World Health Organization, approximately 5% of adults suffer from depression worldwide and more women than men are affected. Yet, we have a very limited understanding of the pathogenesis of the disease, how sex and genetics influence the pathophenotype of MDD, and how they contribute to the responses to pharmacological treatment. This chapter addresses key theories about the etiology of depression, the variations in epidemiology and presentation,

D. F. T. Frohman
Renaissance School of Medicine at Stony Brook University, Stony Brook, NY, USA

K. Nnah · S. E. Tsirka (✉)
Renaissance School of Medicine at Stony Brook University, Stony Brook, NY, USA

Program in Neuroscience, Stony Brook, NY, USA

Department of Pharmacological Sciences, Stony Brook, NY, USA
e-mail: styliani-anna.tsirka@stonybrook.edu

S. E. Tsirka, M. Acosta-Martinez (eds.), *Sex and Gender Effects in Pharmacology*, Handbook of Experimental Pharmacology 282,
https://doi.org/10.1007/164_2023_670

and the treatment options with respect to sex and gender. Additionally, we discuss the emerging wave of treatment modalities, diagnosis, and research focusing on MDD.

Keywords

Animal models · Genetics · Hormones · Inflammation · Major depression disorder · Monoamine hypothesis · Sexual dimorphism

Depression is a chronic disease that affects approximately 280 million people worldwide, over 5.7% of people over 60 years old. The symptoms vary in severity and when they occur, they can cause significant disability in the affected people. In a systematic analysis for the Global Burden of Disease Study, it was reported that depressive disorders are the 13th leading cause of disability-adjusted life-years (DALYs) in 2019 (seventh among adult women, and sixth in the 25–49-year age group), a 61.1% increase from 1990 (Diseases and Injuries 2020). In its most severe form, depression can lead to suicide. Over 700,000 people die by suicide every year (Evaluation 2021).

1 Prevailing Theories on the Pathogenesis of Depression

An article was published recently outlining the current understanding of the pathogenesis of Major Depressive Disorder (MDD). The author used a tale of blind men who had never seen an elephant before but tried to describe the animal by each touching a part of its body, and using that limited experience as their definition, not comprehending its full size and shape (Nemeroff 2020). Similarly, our understanding of MDD is limited and tainted by the methodology we use to approach the disease.

Symptoms of the disease have been described extensively in the literature, starting from ancient years [from Hippocrates, Galen and Ishaq Ibn Imran (Nemeroff 2020)], and using a variety of phenotypes. Although several symptoms are documented in the manual of the American Psychiatric Association (2013), the diagnosis of MDD relies entirely on observation by the clinician and on self-reporting by the patient or a family member, which are inherently subjective data sources. As such, there are no objective diagnostic criteria to describe this heterogeneous disease. Currently, to be diagnosed with MDD, the patient must present with at least five of the following nine symptoms: (1) anhedonia, (2) depressed mood, (3) insomnia or hypersomnia, (4) changes in appetite or weight, (5) changes in psychomotor status, (6) fatigue or loss of energy, (7) worthlessness or guilt, (8) diminished concentration or indecisiveness, or (9) suicidal thoughts or behaviors. To evaluate for MDD, patients are given the Patient Health Questionnaire (PHQ-9), which scores each of the 9 DSM-IV criteria as "0" (not at all) to "3" (nearly every day) (Kroenke et al. 2001).

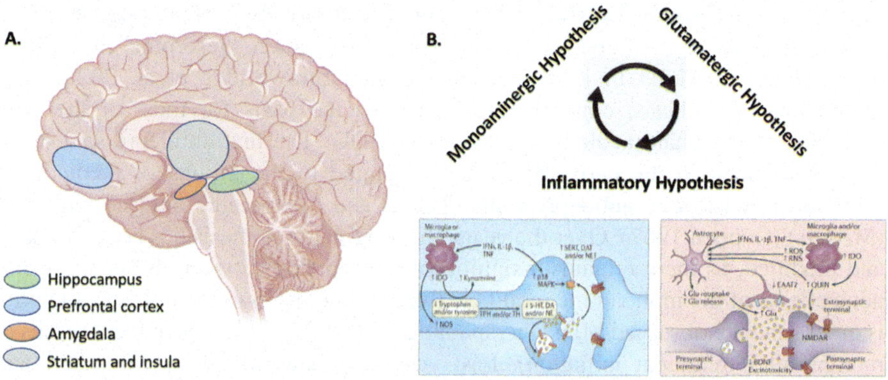

Fig. 1 Brain regions implicated in depression and current hypotheses for its etiology. (**a**) Structural differences have been reported in the prefrontal cortex, amygdala, hippocampus, insula and striatum in patients with depression. More recently imaging data were analyzed with a Canonical correlation analysis model to reveal components of cortical thickness and sub-cortical volumes relevant to four different clinical depression subgroups (Yu et al. 2021). (**b**) Inter-relation of the three current hypotheses leading to symptoms of depression, and main cellular and molecular effectors of the hypotheses. It is currently not clear what the initiating signals are. The bottom panels of **b** were adapted from Miller and Raison (2016)

A widely used, clinician-administered depression assessment scale is the Hamilton Depression Rating Scale (HDRS, also called Ham-D), which measures depression in patients before, during, and after treatment (Trajkovic et al. 2011). Other instruments include: the Beck Depression Inventory (BDI), which can be used for ages 13–80, and contains 21 self-report items (Osman et al. 2004); the Center for Epidemiologic Studies Depression Scale (CES-D) includes 20 self-report items and can be used for ages 6 and above (Radloff 1977); the EQ-5D is a tool to measure non-disease specific, health-related quality of life and exists in an adult and a child/adolescent version (Devlin and Brooks 2017); the Montgomery-Åsberg Depression Rating Scale (MADRS) quantifies depression in patients over 18 years and older (Davidson et al. 1986).

MDD also has a variety of subtypes, including MDD with atypical features, seasonal affective disorder (SAD), and dysthymia. MDD with atypical features is associated with increased appetite, hypersomnia, leaden paralysis, and mood reactivity. SAD is a subtype of MDD associated with specific seasonal patterns, commonly during fall or winter. Dysthymia is often viewed as a milder form of MDD but with a more chronic effect, lasting over 2 years. Regardless of the subtype, MDD is highly prevalent worldwide and constitutes a significant, long-term healthcare "burden" (Kessler 2012).

The etiology of MDD is not known. Over the years, various theories have been presented which account for some of the symptoms experienced by patients (Fig. 1). The predominant hypothesis is the *monoaminergic* hypothesis, which theorizes that the underlying pathophysiologic basis of depression is a deficiency or depletion in the levels of monoamines (serotonin, norepinephrine, and/or dopamine) in the central nervous system (Delgado 2000). This was discovered serendipitously in the 1950s, after the use of the anti-hypertensive medication "reserpine" led to the development of MDD in its respective patients (Strawbridge et al. 2022). The monoamine hypothesis, consequently, has been the basis for most of the drug discovery in the pharmacologic treatment of MDD. The first antidepressant drugs were introduced in the early 1950s and belonged to the groups of medications referred to as tricyclic antidepressants (TCAs) and monoamine oxidase inhibitors (MAOIs) (Coppen 1967). Over the years, this original hypothesis has been morphed and modified, as there remains a significant discrepancy between the pharmacokinetic effects of the monoamine modifiers (whose actions on monoamine availability is quick) and the observed MDD therapeutic effects (which become evident weeks or months after treatment initiation). Last year, a review article by Moncrieff and colleagues concluded that the evidence that decreased serotonin activity caused depression was not consistent (Moncrieff et al. 2022), but it has received a lot of pushback.

Another hypothesis for MDD is the *glutamatergic* hypothesis, which argues that extrasynaptic glutamate dysregulates glial amino acid (glutamate) transporters and results in aberrantly high levels of glutamate. This, in turn, activates extrasynaptic ionotropic N-methyl-D-aspartate (NMDA) receptors and presynaptic metabotropic glutamate receptors, both of which cause changes in synaptic receptor activation and in neurotransmission. Such circuit dysfunction results in dysregulation of the levels of neurotrophic factors, including brain-derived neurotrophic factor (BDNF), whose levels are decreased both in the central nervous system (CNS) and in the plasma of patients with MDD (Otte et al. 2016). Yet, some of the animal models commonly used to understand depression have not shown this associated modulation of BDNF, thus not supporting the glutamate hypothesis as a mono-etiology for MDD (Bjorkholm and Monteggia 2016).

An additional hypothesis that has been put forth for MDD is the *inflammatory* hypothesis. This has derived from reports that in the blood of patients with MDD, there is a positive association with neutrophils and $Ly6C^{hi}$ monocytes, as well as higher levels of the cytokines IL-6 (interleukin 6), IL-1β (interleukin 1-beta), CRP (C reactive protein), and TNF-α (tumor necrosis factor alpha). These markers are all classically used in assessing inflammation clinically. Population studies over time have revealed that elevated levels of CRP and IL-6 could be reliable prognostic markers for MDD diagnosis (Gimeno et al. 2011). In addition, elevated levels of cortisol and dysregulation of the Hypothalamic-Pituitary-Adrenal (HPA) axis have been described in MDD patients.

Though these theories present a variety of etiologies for MDD, none has shown to be superior, as treatment approaches focusing on only one of the hypotheses are not fully effective. In fact, approximately 30% of patients with MDD do not respond to any pharmacologic treatments, falling into the category of treatment-resistant patients (Conway et al. 2017). Basic and translational research findings conclude that all the hypotheses converge to contribute to the development of MDD and intersect with each other. For example, inflammatory cytokines decrease the levels of BDNF and hinder neuronal synaptic plasticity and neuronal circuits, just as noted in MDD.

2 Genetics and Sex in Depression

It has been extensively reported that women are more frequently diagnosed with MDD relative to men. In fact, many studies have described a 2:1 ratio for lifetime prevalence of MDD, respectively (Kuehner 2017). During the COVID-19 pandemic, data from 2020 showed an incidence of 53.2 million cases of patients with MDD, of whom 35.5 million were women and 17.7 million were men (Santomauro et al. 2021). This remains consistent in older adults (>65 years of age), of whom the incidence of reported depression is lower overall, but the percentage of women self-reporting MDD is still higher than that of men (Kuehner 2017). Do genetic differences account for this difference in disease occurrence? Broadly, there have not been any publications associating specific genes on the X chromosome with an increased risk of MDD (Hyde and Mezulis 2020). Instead, there is evidence that the rationale behind this is pleiotropic, including the contribution of sex hormones (ex. estradiol) during adolescence (Williams and Trainor 2018).

Twin studies strengthen the hypothesis that depression is affected by several genes, evident through analysis of Quantitative Trait Loci (QTL), which annotates genetic variants associated with a disease. The genes that have been correlated with depression include markers in the serotonin (5-HT) and dopamine (DA) systems (Zhao et al. 2020), which in turn change the availability of 5-HT or DA in the synapse. Within this category is 5-HT receptors, 5-HT transporters, monoamine oxidase A, Tryptophan hydroxylase 1, DA receptors, and catechol-*O*-methyltransferase. Recently, the 5-HT transporter gene-linked promoter region (5-HTTLPR) was also noted to correlate with increased susceptibility to depression (Iurescia et al. 2016). This promoter region was present in different individuals with variable number tandem repeats, however a consensus has yet to be reached on if aberrant concentrations of repeats increase or decrease MDD susceptibility [for a review, please see Zhao et al. (2020)].

Genome Wide Association Studies (GWAS) have identified single nucleotide polymorphisms (SNPs) in additional genes (14 in total) (Maul et al. 2020). Importantly, SNP rs6602398 has been associated with increased susceptibility to MDD in males. The SNP is present in the IL2RA gene (important for immune homeostasis). However, there is a lack of comprehensive GWAS that determine consistent specific susceptibility loci associated with MDD (Hyde and Mezulis 2020).

At the environmental level, there are several studies that link genetic factors, such as the length of the 5-HTTLPR tandem repeat, to a negative environment. Such correlations are more prevalent in females and link to a higher incidence of depression (Priess-Groben and Hyde 2013). Moreover, in addition to pubertal hormones, experiences of childhood sexual abuse (traditionally is more common in females than in males) may contribute to increased reported depression cases during adolescence in females (Kuehner 2017). These findings may also be corroborated in studying the connection between childhood sexual abuse (or other negative environments) and the incidence of MDD for people identifying as transgender or non-binary, who disproportionally suffer from mental health disorders (Tordoff et al. 2022).

3 Antidepressants Used in the Treatment of MDD

Depending on the severity of depressive symptoms, the treatment regimen can vary from predominantly psychotherapy to the addition of pharmacotherapy or electroconvulsive therapy (Table 1). A recent report noted that in the USA, among the 40.4 million adults aged 18–80, 16.7% were taking psychiatric medications, with 72% of those adults specifically taking antidepressants. The use of antidepressants was highest in White adults (15%), compared to Black (6.2%), Hispanic (5.7%), and Asian adults (3.1%) (Moore and Mattison 2017).

As previously mentioned, the first antidepressants used were TCAs (ex. imipramine, amitriptyline) and MAOIs (ex. iproniazid) (Lopez-Munoz and Alamo 2009). TCAs predominantly act as inhibitors of serotonin/norepinephrine reuptake. In addition, they exhibit anticholinergic, antiadrenergic, and antihistaminergic effects, which contribute to their large side effect profile. At higher concentrations, they may additionally block sodium channels. MAOIs primarily act by inhibiting the breakdown of monoamines. These were particularly used for the treatment of tuberculosis-exhibited antidepressant effects.

In the late 1980s and 1990s, fluoxetine was added to the arsenal against MDD. Fluoxetine is a selective serotonin reuptake inhibitor (SSRI) that began the wave of a new class of drugs used in MDD. Fluoxetine, along with other SSRIs (citalopram, sertraline) and selective norepinephrine reuptake inhibitors (SNRIs) (duloxetine, venlafaxine), was effective at countering depressive symptoms through inhibiting the reuptake of monoamines while minimizing the side effects associated with the

Table 1 Classes of antidepressants and the most frequently used medications

Major pharmacological options for treatment of MOD				
SSRIs	SNRIs	Atypicals	MAOIs	TCAs
Fluoxetine	Veniafaxine	Trazodone	Tranylcypromine	Nortriptyline
Paroxetine	Duloxetine	Nefazodone	Phenelzine	Desipramine
Sertraline	Desvenlafaxine	Mirtazipine	Selegiline	Protriptyline
Citalopram	Levomilnacipran	Bupropion	Isocarboxazid	Amoxapine
Escitalopram	Milnacipram	Vilazodone		Amitriptyline
Fluvoxamine		Vortioxetine		Clomipramine
		Buspirone		Doxepin
		Varenicline		Imipramine
		Ketamine		Trimipramine

SSRIs selective serotonin reuptake inhibitors, *SNRIs* serotonin-norepinephrine reuptake inhibitors, *MAOIs* monoamine oxidase inhibitors, *TCAs* tricyclic antidepressants older medications. Due to this major added benefit, SSRIs and SNRIs have become the first-line medication for initial pharmacologic treatment of MDD (Kendrick et al. 2019).

In the 1990s, atypical antidepressants such as bupropion and mirtazapine also became available for the treatment of MDD. While the medications in this subgroup vary in their mechanism of action, they all result indirectly or directly in increased monoamine levels. Bupropion, for example, does not affect serotonin levels, but causes increases in dopamine and norepinephrine. These treatment options provided important alternatives to the SSRIs and SNRIs, which still had notable side effects such as decreased libido and serotonin syndrome (Horst and Preskorn 1998).

One of the major drawbacks of traditional treatment options for MDD is the long delay to generate an effect once an individual starts taking the medication, i.e., about 4–6 weeks. A fast-acting antidepressant was recently approved (2019), namely ketamine, which produces long-lasting antidepressant effects within hours of administration. The duration of the therapeutic effect of a single dose of ketamine can last up to 2 weeks, even in patients typically resistant to treatment (Price et al. 2014; Zarate et al. 2006). How ketamine works as an antidepressant is not entirely understood. Traditionally, ketamine can bind and modulate NMDA receptors, acting as a non-competitive NMDA receptor antagonist. Ketamine has also been shown to modulate the responses of inflammatory microglia which then indirectly contribute to its anti-depressive effects (Yao et al. 2022). A very recent preclinical study showed that ketamine acted on a subset of adult immature EGR1+ granule cells in the dentate gyrus of the hippocampus, increasing their activity. Such changes along the pathway from the ventral hippocampus to the medial prefrontal cortex seem to underlie ketamine's acute antidepressant effects (Rawat et al. 2022). Despite its fast-acting effects, ketamine still needs to be studied for its long-term effects, as it has only recently become available for usage (Fig. 2).

Unfortunately, as alluded to in Sect. 1, the pharmacological treatments available are only partially effective for MDD patients, successfully treating less than 50% of patients (Conway et al. 2017). Moreover, we have yet to determine who would benefit best from one drug versus another, resulting in a random allocation on which medication to prescribe. Lastly, the medication efficacy seems to differ based on sex, which some studies postulate is based on differences in neuronal circuitry, hormone levels, or metabolism (LeGates et al. 2019).

4 Sex Differences in MDD Presentation of MDD and Prescription and Responses to Antidepressants

Women with depression report more atypical symptoms than do men, mainly increased appetite and hypersomnia (Kuehner 2017). They also report additional somatic symptoms such as low energy and fatigue, interpersonal sensitivity, gastrointestinal disturbances, and pain. In female patients, the symptoms are also more severe, present earlier, and occur in episodes that last longer than those in male patients (LeGates et al. 2019). Adolescent women are two to three times more likely

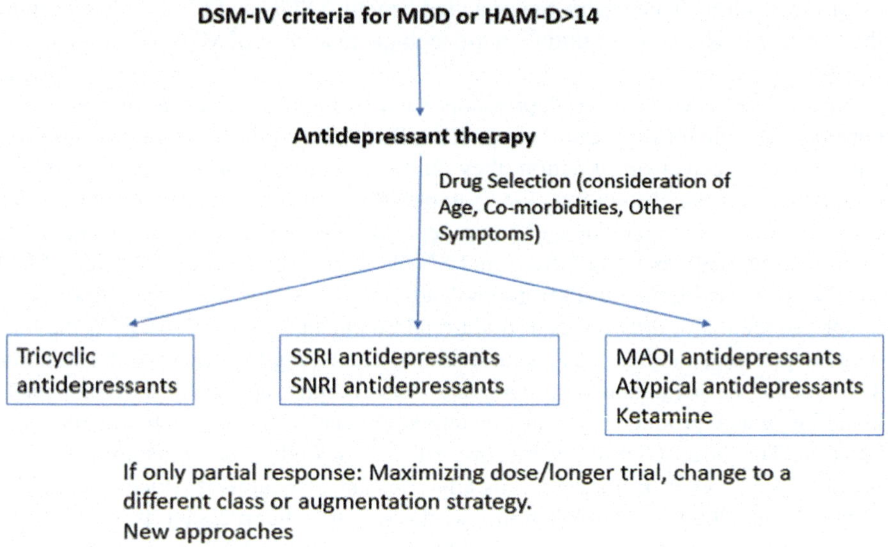

Fig. 2 Pharmacotherapy for MDD. Diagnostic criteria based on DSM- IV or the HAM-D Scale. Adapted from (Watkins et al. 2011)

to make suicide attempts than their counterparts, but these attempts are less likely to be lethal. The reproductive cycle additionally has effects on depressive symptoms. In the STAR*D trial, 66% of women reported premenstrual exacerbations in their symptoms (Haley et al. 2013). Men, meanwhile, more frequently report comorbid substance use disorder. Additionally, both sexes are equally likely to report irritability.

Translating this to prescription rates, an estimated 15.9% of adult women in the USA take antidepressants, compared to 7.7% of men, most likely reflecting the gender prevalence of the disease (Moore and Mattison 2017). While the mechanism is unclear, TCAs have shown to have more efficacy in males and SSRIs more in females (Khan et al. 2005). In the CRESCEND study, participants were given free choice of antidepressant medication and followed for 12 weeks after remission. Women in the study, who had chosen SSRIs or SNRIs, reported higher rates of response and remission (Kim et al. 2011). Even more, studies found that the efficacy of remission following SSRIs in women over age 50 was increased with the addition of hormone replacement therapy, thus suggesting an intersection between responsiveness to SSRIs and female hormones (Thase et al. 2005).

This increased therapeutic effectiveness of SSRIs for female patients in the presence of estradiol formed a basis for the exploration of other medications that could enhance the effectiveness of classic antidepressants. Through these efforts, folic acid was found to increase the efficacy of fluoxetine (De Long et al. 2014; Venkatasubramanian et al. 2013). Animal model studies, excitingly, corroborated the folic acid findings (Budni et al. 2021; Rosa et al. 2014). Similarly, triiodothyronine (T3) was reported to enhance the effects of TCAs in female patients (Altshuler et al. 2001; Giakoumatos and Osser 2019).

What could the underlying mechanisms be for these different, sex-specific responses to the anti-depressive drugs? The proposed mechanisms are speculative, but address potential differences in pharmacokinetics (Bigos et al. 2009), synaptic transmission (Bangasser and Cuarenta 2021), and compliance (that results from side effects).

4.1 Pharmacokinetics

A crucial physiological difference between males and females is the percentage of adipose tissue (higher in females), which may significantly increase the half-life of lipophilic drugs. Among the antidepressants, TCAs are the most lipophilic, have a long elimination half-life, and are associated with decreased gastrointestinal motility and delayed absorption (Marazziti et al. 2013).

Other characteristics noted to drive the difference in pharmacokinetics in men and women are the low acidity of the female gastric environment, the slower rate of gastric emptying, and the longer colonic transit times, all of which increase the rate of absorption and serum concentration of antidepressants (Bigos et al. 2009). Moreover, differences in the expression and activity of cytochrome P450 (CYP) enzymes may account for a different metabolic rate of these medications (Ferguson and Hill 2006). In tandem, the higher serum concentrations of SSRIs in women may also drive the increase in reported adverse effects (i.e., nausea, dry mouth, fatigue, and hyperhidrosis) (Ekhart et al. 2018).

Sex hormones such as estradiol affect the pharmacokinetics of antidepressants. This can be seen clinically as premenopausal women respond better to the medications than postmenopausal women (Pae et al. 2009). The use of oral contraceptives can also affect the efficacy of antidepressants, as they contain a combination of estrogen and progesterone. As with other drug–drug interactions, oral contraceptives can increase both the metabolism (through modifying CYPs) and the elimination of other medications (Damoiseaux et al. 2014). Along the same lines, pregnancy typically implies a decrease in medication use to minimize teratogenic risk. In the case of MDD, however, reports show that untreated MDD increases risk of preterm deliveries and of babies with low birth weight (Chan et al. 2014). As a result, women tend to stay on an antidepressant while pregnant, which has shown to be safe for most medications (Battle et al. 2013). Yet, the high levels of estrogen and progesterone during pregnancy may increase the pharmacokinetics of antidepressant metabolism, lowering their plasma concentration (Deligiannidis et al. 2014). Consequently, women may be prescribed a higher dose during pregnancy (Sit et al. 2008).

When women go through menopause, they are also at higher risk for depressive symptoms. This may be due to large fluctuations in hormone levels. At menopause, follicle-stimulating hormone (FSH) increases dramatically followed by a decrease in estradiol. Ryan et al. (2009) reported that the concentration change (but not the absolute plasma levels) of these hormones may contribute to depressive symptoms.

The authors also found that high levels of FSH may predict the response to antidepressant treatments in postmenopausal women (Ryan et al. 2009).

4.2 Synaptic Transmission

In MDD, excitatory synapse signals weaken, specifically in areas such as the prefrontal cortex (PFC), hippocampus, and nucleus accumbens (NAc). These findings have been supported in animal models used to mimic depressive-like behaviors (Cahill et al. 2021; LeGates et al. 2019). Decreased dendritic length and spine densities have been reported in the PFC and in the CA1, CA2 (the site assigned to social memory), and CA3 subregions of the hippocampus.

The use of SSRIs has restored neuronal activity in these areas, as well as increased the levels of BDNF. Similarly, increases in hippocampal and cortical expression of BDNF mRNA parallel the antidepressant-like response of SSRIs (Bjorkholm and Monteggia 2016).

One of the newly identified regulators of MDD is Sirtuin 1 (SIRT1), an NAD^+-dependent deacetylase. The deletion of SIRT1 selectively in excitatory neurons in the forebrain of male mice caused depression-like phenotypes, a result which was not replicated in female mice (Lei et al. 2020). Similar results were obtained in a model of lipopolysaccharide-induced depression which was associated with Estrogen Receptor-α/SIRT1 and the NFκB signaling pathway in old female mice but not in old male mice (Jiang et al. 2021), suggesting that age or sex-related depression may be associated with the different activation levels of this pathway. Specifically the administration of 17β-estradiol (E2) improved the LPS-induced behaviors and increased the levels of SIRT1, while downregulating NFκB and associated cytokines. This improvement was associated with ERα only, as inhibition of ERα reversed the E2 effects. ERβ had no effect (Jiang et al. 2021). In a recent study using single-cell RNA sequencing of the mouse ventromedial hypothalamus, genes associated with social behaviors were expressed at different concentrations in males and females, providing the first evidence of the existence of sex-specific neurons in the mammalian CNS (Kim et al. 2019), and further supporting these sex-specific behavioral differences.

In addition to genetic contributions affecting MDD, epigenetic target sites have been found to be modified in patients with MDD. Specifically, sex differences in the methylation of the promoter of *NR3C1* (Hill et al. 2019) and the regulatory region of the *FKBP5* locus (Wiechmann et al. 2019) have been observed, as well as methylation of the promoter of oxytocin gene (Sanwald et al. 2020), or the inflammation-specific gene Hepatocyte Growth Factor (HGF/c-MET) (Ciuculete et al. 2020). Such changes correlated with changes in the HDAC3 protein levels and H3K27me2 expression in relevant brain regions (Misztak et al. 2020). These epigenetic changes have also been shown to be consistent in patients with MDD and related animal models (Scarpa et al. 2020).

In the NAc, spine density remained consistent through its rostral/caudal extent in males but was increased in females. This difference was accompanied by increased frequency of miniature excitatory post-synaptic currents (mEPSCs), indicating differential dopaminergic modulation of these synapses (Wissman et al. 2012).

4.3 Compliance

Sex differences have also been reported by the patients in the side effects of the antidepressant treatment they receive. As above, women tolerate TCAs poorly and report dizziness, nausea, constipation, and somnolence while taking them (Ekhart et al. 2018; Greil et al. 2022). Men more frequently report sexual dysfunction and urinary complaints (Ekhart et al. 2018). Because of these side effects, bupropion and mirtazapine are more often prescribed in men (bupropion, females: 3.61%, males: 12.89%; $p = 0.001$; mirtazapine, females: 5.15%, males: 13.40%; $p = 0.005$) as these medications have fewer reports for sexual dysfunction, adverse reaction, or weight gain (Schwalsberger et al. 2022). The impact of the side effect profile strongly influences patient compliance to their medication, in turn influencing their outcome of the treatment.

5 What Is Next?

Given the current challenges in the treatment and the understanding of the etiology of MDD, new perspectives are needed. These include new ways to follow the disease progression and effectiveness of pharmacological treatments, new targets for treatments, and a better understanding of the pathological processes that govern MDD. One strategy involves non-invasive imaging, as it allows a researcher to follow a patient longitudinally and assess progress through the treatment course.

Co-registration of Magnetic Resonance Imaging (MRI) and Positron Emission Tomography (PET) was demonstrated to be a valuable tool in diagnosing and following patients undergoing MDD treatment. Importantly, the use of resting state FDG-PET imaging has been influential in guiding MDD treatment, though it has not been fully translated in the clinic to predict treatment outcome (Hill et al. 2021), nor has the ratio of glutamate and glutamine (Glx) to GABA (Glx/GABA) been used (Narayan et al. 2022), underlying the paucity of available biomarkers that will allow the stratification of proposed treatment. Nonetheless, recent investigations suggest that elevated hippocampal 5-$HT_{1A}R$ binding potential (using the partial agonist positron emission tomography tracer [^{11}C]CUMI-101) may serve as a promising biomarker through which to investigate the neurobiological link between childhood adversity and depression (Bartlett et al. 2023).

Other methodologies could involve using non-invasive brain surgeries. A recent study reported on the treatment of three patients with refractory depression using non-invasive anterior capsulotomy, a procedure typically used to remove the anterior limb of the internal capsule in the white matter (Khattab et al. 2022). The authors performed bilateral ablation of the anterior limb of the internal capsule using a mask-based linear accelerator. All three patients reported improvement of MDD symptoms (depression symptoms improving at 12-month and 18-month follow-ups). One of the patients discontinued his ketamine therapy, the second discontinued electroconvulsive therapy, and the third one reported global improvement in symptoms and function at 3 months. Another variation is non-invasive brain stimulation (NBS), as studies have shown that repetitive transcranial magnetic stimulation (rTMS) and transcranial direct current stimulation (tDCS) may impact mood dysregulation when applied over the prefrontal cortex (Liu et al. 2017). In general, the efficacy of NBS depends on the sites stimulated and the accuracy of the stimulation. NBS has been applied either as a monotherapy approach or in combination with pharmacotherapy (with sertraline, escitalopram, or amitriptyline), showing preliminarily success (Liu et al. 2017). Side effects include skin irritation, headache, and nausea, but there is a lack of data on how NBS efficacy and side effect profile is affected by sex.

Many reports have also indicated that MDD is not just a mental health disease, but rather that it affects the whole body. This argument asserts that MDD promotes disturbances in the enteric nervous system and along the gut-brain axis, which interacts with a variety of organ systems (e.g., CNS, gut, immune system, the HPA axis) (Fig. 3). In line with this, one of the contributing environmental factors to MDD is malnutrition and changes in the gut microbiome (Otte et al. 2016). Experiments that have involved transplantation of fecal microbiota from depressed patients to germ-free mice resulted in depressive symptoms in the relevant recipient mice, while the animals who received microbiota from healthy individuals did not exhibit depressive symptoms (Zheng et al. 2016). Moreover, patients with MDD have high rates of co-occurring gastrointestinal symptoms, many of which are related to impaired gastrointestinal motility (Kamran et al. 2022; Rajkumar 2021). These associations open a new set of targets for sex- and gender-specific pharmacological interventions that should be considered in the future (Holingue et al. 2020; Shobeiri et al. 2022).

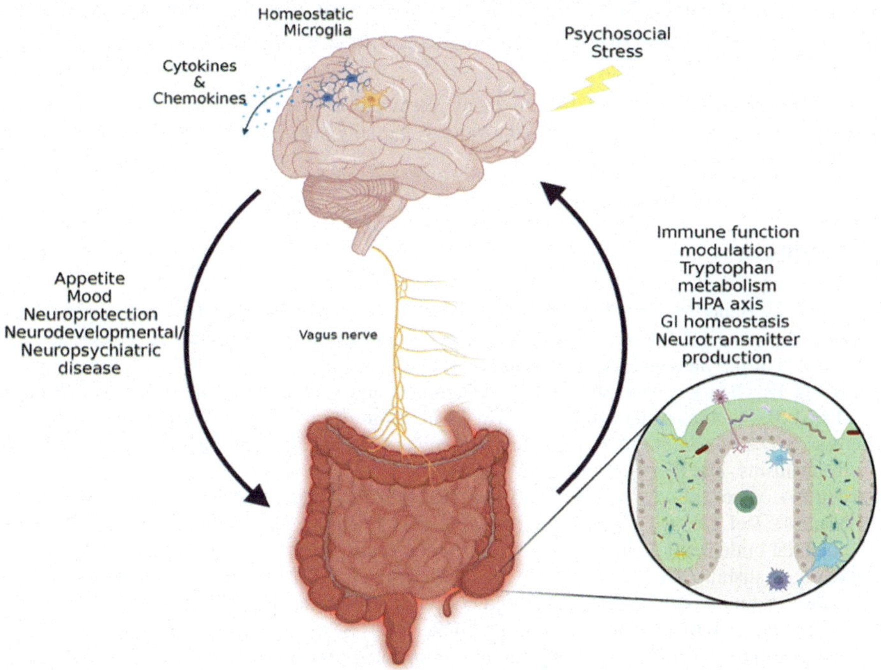

Fig. 3 Bidirectional relationship between the brain and gastrointestinal tract – the gut-brain axis is a link between the CNS and the enteric nervous system (ENS). Homeostatic microglia, the resident innate immune cells of the CNS, become reactive to psychosocial stress and secrete cytokines such as IL1-β, monocyte chemoattractant protein 1 (CCL2), and TNF-α, which in turn affect appetite, mood, and the development of neuro-developmental and psychiatric disease. This dysregulation affects the gastrointestinal tract. Within the gut, microbiota synthesize macromolecules [e.g., short chain fatty acids (SCFAs), bile acids, and neurotransmitters]. Enteric neurons and dendritic cells function to transport these products through the vagus nerve to the brain. The gut also sends signals to the brain that influence metabolism of tryptophan, balance of the HPA axis, and neurotransmitter synthesis. In pathophysiological states such as depression, this bidirectional communication causes a negative feedback loop in which production of neurotoxic cytokines and chemokines can cause dysregulation in the gut, and dysfunction within the gut can affect immune function within the brain. Figure adapted from Kokkosis and Tsirka 2020 and Created with BioRender.com

6 Conclusions

MDD etiology is still not understood, with sex/gender, genetic and environmental factors contributing to symptom development. The available pharmacological treatment options are not optimal or highly effective for a large proportion of patients. Side effects reported by patients, men or women, drive the category of medications prescribed. Experimental data from human and animal studies identify new cellular and molecular targets. Novel approaches to treatment as well as the consideration of MDD as a whole body disease warrant further investigation.

Acknowledgments We would like to thank members of the Tsirka lab, especially Miguel Madeira, for his input to this review. This work is partially supported by T32GM135746 (KKN) and R01MH123093W1.

References

Altshuler LL, Bauer M, Frye MA, Gitlin MJ, Mintz J, Szuba MP, Leight KL, Whybrow PC (2001) Does thyroid supplementation accelerate tricyclic antidepressant response? A review and meta-analysis of the literature. Am J Psychiatry 158:1617–1622

American Psychiatric Association (2013) Diagnostic and statistical manual of mental disorders (DSM-5), 5th edn. American Psychiatric Association

Bangasser DA, Cuarenta A (2021) Sex differences in anxiety and depression: circuits and mechanisms. Nat Rev Neurosci 22:674–684

Bartlett EA, Yttredahl AA, Boldrini M, Tyrer AE, Hill KR, Ananth MR, Milak MS, Oquendo MA, Mann JJ, DeLorenzo C, Parsey RV (2023) In vivo serotonin 1A receptor hippocampal binding potential in depression and reported childhood adversity. Eur Psychiatry 66:e17

Battle CL, Salisbury AL, Schofield CA, Ortiz-Hernandez S (2013) Perinatal antidepressant use: understanding women's preferences and concerns. J Psychiatr Pract 19:443–453

Bigos KL, Pollock BG, Stankevich BA, Bies RR (2009) Sex differences in the pharmacokinetics and pharmacodynamics of antidepressants: an updated review. Gend Med 6:522–543

Bjorkholm C, Monteggia LM (2016) BDNF – a key transducer of antidepressant effects. Neuropharmacology 102:72–79

Budni J, Moretti M, Freitas AE, Neis VB, Ribeiro CM, de Oliveira Balen G, Rieger DK, Leal RB, Rodrigues ALS (2021) Behavioral and neurochemical effects of folic acid in a mouse model of depression induced by TNF-alpha. Behav Brain Res 414:113512

Cahill B, Poelker-Wells S, Prather JF, Li Y (2021) A glimpse into the sexual dimorphisms in major depressive disorder through epigenetic studies. Front Neural Circuits 15:768571

Chan J, Natekar A, Einarson A, Koren G (2014) Risks of untreated depression in pregnancy. Can Fam Physician 60:242–243

Ciuculete DM, Voisin S, Kular L, Welihinda N, Jonsson J, Jagodic M, Mwinyi J, Schioth HB (2020) Longitudinal DNA methylation changes at MET may alter HGF/c-MET signalling in adolescents at risk for depression. Epigenetics 15:646–663

Conway CR, George MS, Sackeim HA (2017) Toward an evidence-based, operational definition of treatment-resistant depression: when enough is enough. JAMA Psychiatry 74:9–10

Coppen A (1967) The biochemistry of affective disorders. Br J Psychiatry 113:1237–1264

Damoiseaux VA, Proost JH, Jiawan VC, Melgert BN (2014) Sex differences in the pharmacokinetics of antidepressants: influence of female sex hormones and oral contraceptives. Clin Pharmacokinet 53:509–519

Davidson J, Turnbull CD, Strickland R, Miller R, Graves K (1986) The Montgomery-Asberg depression scale: reliability and validity. Acta Psychiatr Scand 73:544–548

De Long NE, Hyslop JR, Raha S, Hardy DB, Holloway AC (2014) Fluoxetine-induced pancreatic beta cell dysfunction: new insight into the benefits of folic acid in the treatment of depression. J Affect Disord 166:6–13

Delgado PL (2000) Depression: the case for a monoamine deficiency. J Clin Psychiatry 61(Suppl 6):7–11

Deligiannidis KM, Byatt N, Freeman MP (2014) Pharmacotherapy for mood disorders in pregnancy: a review of pharmacokinetic changes and clinical recommendations for therapeutic drug monitoring. J Clin Psychopharmacol 34:244–255

Devlin NJ, Brooks R (2017) EQ-5D and the EuroQol group: past, present and future. Appl Health Econ Health Policy 15:127–137

Diseases GBD, Injuries C (2020) Global burden of 369 diseases and injuries in 204 countries and territories, 1990-2019: a systematic analysis for the Global Burden of Disease Study 2019. Lancet 396:1204–1222

Ekhart C, van Hunsel F, Scholl J, de Vries S, van Puijenbroek E (2018) Sex differences in reported adverse drug reactions of selective serotonin reuptake inhibitors. Drug Saf 41:677–683

Evaluation, I.o.H.M.a (2021) Global Health Data Exchange (GHDx). http://ghdx.healthdata.org/gbd-results-tool?params=gbd-api-2019-permalink/d780dffbe8a381b25e1416884959e88b

Ferguson JM, Hill H (2006) Pharmacokinetics of fluoxetine in elderly men and women. Gerontology 52:45–50

Giakoumatos CI, Osser D (2019) The psychopharmacology algorithm project at the Harvard South Shore program: an update on unipolar nonpsychotic depression. Harv Rev Psychiatry 27:33–52

Gimeno D, Delclos GL, Ferrie JE, De Vogli R, Elovainio M, Marmot MG, Kivimaki M (2011) Association of CRP and IL-6 with lung function in a middle-aged population initially free from self-reported respiratory problems: the Whitehall II study. Eur J Epidemiol 26:135–144

Greil W, de Bardeci M, Seifert J, Bernegger X, Cattapan K, Stassen H, Wagner AL, Sieberer M, Grohmann R, Toto S (2022) Treatment of depression: are psychotropic drugs appropriately dosed in women and in the elderly? Dosages of psychotropic drugs by sex and age in routine clinical practice. Hum Psychopharmacol 37:e2809

Haley CL, Sung SC, Rush AJ, Trivedi MH, Wisniewski SR, Luther JF, Kornstein SG (2013) The clinical relevance of self-reported premenstrual worsening of depressive symptoms in the management of depressed outpatients: a STAR*D report. J Womens Health (Larchmt) 22: 219–229

Hill J, Pickles A, Wright N, Quinn JP, Murgatroyd C, Sharp H (2019) Mismatched prenatal and postnatal maternal depressive symptoms and child behaviours: a sex-dependent role for NR3C1 DNA methylation in the wirral child health and development study. Cell 8

Hill KR, Gardus JD, Bartlett EA, Perlman G, Parsey RV, DeLorenzo C (2021) Measuring brain glucose metabolism in order to predict response to antidepressant or placebo: a randomized clinical trial. Neuroimage Clin 32:102858

Holingue C, Budavari AC, Rodriguez KM, Zisman CR, Windheim G, Fallin MD (2020) Sex differences in the gut-brain axis: implications for mental health. Curr Psychiatry Rep 22:83

Horst WD, Preskorn SH (1998) Mechanisms of action and clinical characteristics of three atypical antidepressants: venlafaxine, nefazodone, bupropion. J Affect Disord 51:237–254

Hyde JS, Mezulis AH (2020) Gender differences in depression: biological, affective, cognitive, and sociocultural factors. Harv Rev Psychiatry 28:4–13

Iurescia S, Seripa D, Rinaldi M (2016) Role of the 5-HTTLPR and SNP promoter polymorphisms on serotonin transporter gene expression: a closer look at genetic architecture and in vitro functional studies of common and uncommon allelic variants. Mol Neurobiol 53:5510–5526

Jiang X, Chen Z, Yu X, Chen J, Sun C, Jing C, Xu L, Liu F, Ni W, Chen L (2021) Lipopolysaccharide-induced depression is associated with estrogen receptor-alpha/SIRT1/NF-kappaB signaling pathway in old female mice. Neurochem Int 148:105097

Kamran M, Bibi F, Ur Rehman A, Morris DW (2022) Major depressive disorder: existing hypotheses about pathophysiological mechanisms and new genetic findings. Genes (Basel) 13

Kendrick T, Taylor D, Johnson CF (2019) Which first-line antidepressant? Br J Gen Pract 69:114–115

Kessler RC (2012) The costs of depression. Psychiatr Clin North Am 35:1–14

Khan A, Brodhead AE, Schwartz KA, Kolts RL, Brown WA (2005) Sex differences in antidepressant response in recent antidepressant clinical trials. J Clin Psychopharmacol 25:318–324

Khattab MH, Sherry AD, Devan SP, Luo G, Chaballout BH, Jean-Baptiste S, Xu J, Bick S, Petrie WM, Cmelak AJ (2022) Noninvasive capsulotomy for refractory depression by frameless stereotactic radiosurgery. Int J Radiat Oncol Biol Phys 113:960–966

Kim JM, Kim SW, Stewart R, Kim SY, Yoon JS, Jung SW, Lee MS, Yim HW, Jun TY (2011) Predictors of 12-week remission in a nationwide cohort of people with depressive disorders: the CRESCEND study. Hum Psychopharmacol 26:41–50
Kim DW, Yao Z, Graybuck LT, Kim TK, Nguyen TN, Smith KA, Fong O, Yi L, Koulena N, Pierson N, Shah S, Lo L, Pool AH, Oka Y, Pachter L, Cai L, Tasic B, Zeng H, Anderson DJ (2019) Multimodal analysis of cell types in a hypothalamic node controlling social behavior. Cell 179:713–728 e717
Kroenke K, Spitzer RL, Williams JB (2001) The PHQ-9: validity of a brief depression severity measure. J Gen Intern Med 16:606–613
Kuehner C (2017) Why is depression more common among women than among men? Lancet Psychiatry 4:146–158
LeGates TA, Kvarta MD, Thompson SM (2019) Sex differences in antidepressant efficacy. Neuropsychopharmacology 44:140–154
Lei Y, Wang J, Wang D, Li C, Liu B, Fang X, You J, Guo M, Lu XY (2020) SIRT1 in forebrain excitatory neurons produces sexually dimorphic effects on depression-related behaviors and modulates neuronal excitability and synaptic transmission in the medial prefrontal cortex. Mol Psychiatry 25:1094–1111
Liu S, Sheng J, Li B, Zhang X (2017) Recent advances in non-invasive brain stimulation for major depressive disorder. Front Hum Neurosci 11:526
Lopez-Munoz F, Alamo C (2009) Monoaminergic neurotransmission: the history of the discovery of antidepressants from 1950s until today. Curr Pharm Des 15:1563–1586
Marazziti D, Baroni S, Picchetti M, Piccinni A, Carlini M, Vatteroni E, Falaschi V, Lombardi A, Dell'Osso L (2013) Pharmacokinetics and pharmacodynamics of psychotropic drugs: effect of sex. CNS Spectr 18:118–127
Maul S, Giegling I, Fabbri C, Corponi F, Serretti A, Rujescu D (2020) Genetics of resilience: implications from genome-wide association studies and candidate genes of the stress response system in posttraumatic stress disorder and depression. Am J Med Genet B Neuropsychiatr Genet 183:77–94
Miller AH, Raison CL (2016) The role of inflammation in depression: from evolutionary imperative to modern treatment target. Nat Rev Immunol 16:22–34
Misztak P, Panczyszyn-Trzewik P, Nowak G, Sowa-Kucma M (2020) Epigenetic marks and their relationship with BDNF in the brain of suicide victims. PLoS One 15:e0239335
Moncrieff J, Cooper RE, Stockmann T, Amendola S, Hengartner MP, Horowitz MA (2022) The serotonin theory of depression: a systematic umbrella review of the evidence. Mol Psychiatry
Moore TJ, Mattison DR (2017) Adult utilization of psychiatric drugs and differences by sex, age, and race. JAMA Intern Med 177:274–275
Narayan GA, Hill KR, Wengler K, He X, Wang J, Yang J, Parsey RV, DeLorenzo C (2022) Does the change in glutamate to GABA ratio correlate with change in depression severity? A randomized, double-blind clinical trial. Mol Psychiatry 27:3833–3841
Nemeroff CB (2020) The state of our understanding of the pathophysiology and optimal treatment of depression: glass half full or half empty? Am J Psychiatry 177:671–685
Osman A, Kopper BA, Barrios F, Gutierrez PM, Bagge CL (2004) Reliability and validity of the Beck depression inventory–II with adolescent psychiatric inpatients. Psychol Assess 16:120–132
Otte C, Gold SM, Penninx BW, Pariante CM, Etkin A, Fava M, Mohr DC, Schatzberg AF (2016) Major depressive disorder. Nat Rev Dis Primers 2:16065
Pae CU, Mandelli L, Kim TS, Han C, Masand PS, Marks DM, Patkar AA, Steffens DC, De Ronchi D, Serretti A (2009) Effectiveness of antidepressant treatments in pre-menopausal versus post-menopausal women: a pilot study on differential effects of sex hormones on antidepressant effects. Biomed Pharmacother 63:228–235
Price RB, Iosifescu DV, Murrough JW, Chang LC, Al Jurdi RK, Iqbal SZ, Soleimani L, Charney DS, Foulkes AL, Mathew SJ (2014) Effects of ketamine on explicit and implicit suicidal

cognition: a randomized controlled trial in treatment-resistant depression. Depress Anxiety 31: 335–343

Priess-Groben HA, Hyde JS (2013) 5-HTTLPR X stress in adolescent depression: moderation by MAOA and gender. J Abnorm Child Psychol 41:281–294

Radloff LS (1977) The CES-D scale: a self-report depression scale for research in the general population. Appl Psychol Meas 1:385–401

Rajkumar RP (2021) Gut hormones as potential therapeutic targets or biomarkers of response in depression: the case of motilin. Life (Basel) 11

Rawat R, Tunc-Ozcan E, McGuire TL, Peng CY, Kessler JA (2022) Ketamine activates adult-born immature granule neurons to rapidly alleviate depression-like behaviors in mice. Nat Commun 13:2650

Rosa PB, Ribeiro CM, Bettio LE, Colla A, Lieberknecht V, Moretti M, Rodrigues AL (2014) Folic acid prevents depressive-like behavior induced by chronic corticosterone treatment in mice. Pharmacol Biochem Behav 127:1–6

Ryan J, Burger HG, Szoeke C, Lehert P, Ancelin ML, Henderson VW, Dennerstein L (2009) A prospective study of the association between endogenous hormones and depressive symptoms in postmenopausal women. Menopause 16:509–517

Santomauro D, Mantilla Herrera A, Shadid J, Collaborators C-MD (2021) Global prevalence and burden of depressive and anxiety disorders in 204 countries and territories in 2020 due to the COVID-19 pandemic. Lancet 398:1700–1712

Sanwald S, Gahr M, Widenhorn-Muller K, Schonfeldt-Lecuona C, Richter K, Connemann BJ, Kammer T, Montag C, Kiefer M (2020) Relation of promoter methylation of the oxytocin gene to stressful life events and depression severity. J Mol Neurosci 70:201–211

Scarpa JR, Fatma M, Loh YE, Traore SR, Stefan T, Chen TH, Nestler EJ, Labonte B (2020) Shared transcriptional signatures in major depressive disorder and mouse chronic stress models. Biol Psychiatry 88:159–168

Schwalsberger K, Reininghaus B, Reiter A, Dalkner N, Fleischmann E, Fellendorf F, Platzer M, Reininghaus EZ (2022) Sex-related differences in the pharmacological treatment of major depression – are women and men treated differently? Psychiatr Danub 34:219–228

Shobeiri P, Kalantari A, Teixeira AL, Rezaei N (2022) Shedding light on biological sex differences and microbiota-gut-brain axis: a comprehensive review of its roles in neuropsychiatric disorders. Biol Sex Differ 13:12

Sit DK, Perel JM, Helsel JC, Wisner KL (2008) Changes in antidepressant metabolism and dosing across pregnancy and early postpartum. J Clin Psychiatry 69:652–658

Strawbridge R, Javed RR, Cave J, Jauhar S, Young AH (2022) The effects of reserpine on depression: a systematic review. J Psychopharmacol:2698811221115762

Thase ME, Entsuah R, Cantillon M, Kornstein SG (2005) Relative antidepressant efficacy of venlafaxine and SSRIs: sex-age interactions. J Womens Health (Larchmt) 14:609–616

Tordoff DM, Wanta JW, Collin A, Stepney C, Inwards-Breland DJ, Ahrens K (2022) Mental health outcomes in transgender and nonbinary youths receiving gender-affirming care. JAMA Netw Open 5:e220978

Trajkovic G, Starcevic V, Latas M, Lestarevic M, Ille T, Bukumiric Z, Marinkovic J (2011) Reliability of the Hamilton rating scale for depression: a meta-analysis over a period of 49 years. Psychiatry Res 189:1–9

Venkatasubramanian R, Kumar CN, Pandey RS (2013) A randomized double-blind comparison of fluoxetine augmentation by high and low dosage folic acid in patients with depressive episodes. J Affect Disord 150:644–648

Watkins CC, Pieper AA, Treisman GJ (2011) Safety considerations in drug treatment of depression in HIV-positive patients: an updated review. Drug Saf 34:623–639

Wiechmann T, Roh S, Sauer S, Czamara D, Arloth J, Kodel M, Beintner M, Knop L, Menke A, Binder EB, Provencal N (2019) Identification of dynamic glucocorticoid-induced methylation changes at the FKBP5 locus. Clin Epigenetics 11:83

Williams AV, Trainor BC (2018) The impact of sex as a biological variable in the search for novel antidepressants. Front Neuroendocrinol 50:107–117

Wissman AM, May RM, Woolley CS (2012) Ultrastructural analysis of sex differences in nucleus accumbens synaptic connectivity. Brain Struct Funct 217:181–190

Yao W, Cao Q, Luo S, He L, Yang C, Chen J, Qi Q, Hashimoto K, Zhang JC (2022) Microglial ERK-NRBP1-CREB-BDNF signaling in sustained antidepressant actions of (R)-ketamine. Mol Psychiatry 27:1618–1629

Yu M, Cullen N, Linn KA, Oathes DJ, Seok D, Cook PA, Duprat R, Aselcioglu I, Moore TM, Davatzikos C, Oquendo MA, Weissman MM, Shinohara RT, Sheline YI (2021) Structural brain measures linked to clinical phenotypes in major depression replicate across clinical centres. Mol Psychiatry 26:2764–2775

Zarate CA Jr, Singh JB, Carlson PJ, Brutsche NE, Ameli R, Luckenbaugh DA, Charney DS, Manji HK (2006) A randomized trial of an N-methyl-D-aspartate antagonist in treatment-resistant major depression. Arch Gen Psychiatry 63:856–864

Zhao L, Han G, Zhao Y, Jin Y, Ge T, Yang W, Cui R, Xu S, Li B (2020) Gender differences in depression: evidence from genetics. Front Genet 11:562316

Zheng P, Zeng B, Zhou C, Liu M, Fang Z, Xu X, Zeng L, Chen J, Fan S, Du X, Zhang X, Yang D, Yang Y, Meng H, Li W, Melgiri ND, Licinio J, Wei H, Xie P (2016) Gut microbiome remodeling induces depressive-like behaviors through a pathway mediated by the host's metabolism. Mol Psychiatry 21:786–796

Biological and Clinical Implications of Sex-Specific Differences in Alzheimer's Disease

Jose A. Santiago and Judith A. Potashkin

Contents

Abstract

Mounting evidence indicates that the female sex is a risk factor for Alzheimer's disease (AD), the most common cause of dementia worldwide. Decades of research suggest that sex-specific differences in genetics, environmental factors, hormones, comorbidities, and brain structure and function may contribute to AD development. However, although significant progress has been made in uncovering specific genetic factors and biological pathways, the precise mechanisms underlying sex-biased differences are not fully characterized. Here, we review several lines of evidence, including epidemiological, clinical, and

J. A. Santiago
NeuroHub Analytics, LLC, Chicago, IL, USA

J. A. Potashkin (✉)
Cellular and Molecular Pharmacology Department, Center for Neurodegenerative Diseases and Therapeutics, The Chicago Medical School, Rosalind Franklin University of Medicine and Science, North Chicago, IL, USA
e-mail: judy.potashkin@rosalindfranklin.edu

S. E. Tsirka, M. Acosta-Martinez (eds.), *Sex and Gender Effects in Pharmacology*, Handbook of Experimental Pharmacology 282,
https://doi.org/10.1007/164_2023_672

molecular studies addressing sex differences in AD. In addition, we discuss the challenges and future directions in advancing personalized treatments for AD.

Keywords

Alzheimer's disease · Dementia · Personalized medicine · Sex-differences

1 Alzheimer's Disease: A Major Global Health Threat to the Aging Population

Alzheimer's disease (AD) is the most common neurodegenerative disease worldwide. According to the World Health Organization, it is estimated that 55 million people live with dementia globally, and 60–70% of the cases are attributed to AD. The Alzheimer's Disease Association estimates that 6.5 million Americans aged 65 and older suffer from AD, and almost two-thirds are women (Rajan et al. 2021).

Pathologically, AD is characterized by the accumulation of extracellular β amyloid plaques and intraneuronal neurofibrillary tangles. Clinically, AD patients suffer from progressive cognitive and memory impairments leading to dementia and the deterioration of executive functions. Over 50 genetic loci are implicated in early and late-onset disease forms (Masters et al. 2015). Nevertheless, more than 95% of the cases are sporadic in which genetic, epigenetic, and environmental factors play a role in the disease pathogenesis. In this regard, environmental factors and lifestyle choices appear to be prime determinants of the disease. Type 2 diabetes mellitus (T2DM), obesity, cardiovascular disease, depression, and inflammatory bowel disease are commonly observed comorbidities in AD patients (Santiago and Potashkin 2021). Some chronic conditions, such as T2DM and depression, have been documented as risk factors for the disease (Santiago and Potashkin 2021).

The lack of diagnostic and prognostic biomarkers to identify patients at early stages and follow disease progression has been a significant hurdle in the design of clinical trials. In the absence of disease-modifying drugs, research efforts have directed their attention toward investigating modifiable factors in AD, physical activity, diet, and cognitive training to slow disease progression or prevent the disease. Unfortunately, AD remains an incurable disease, and most clinical trials testing potential drugs have proven futile.

While strategies focusing on modifiable risk factors have shown promise, the study of sex-specific influences in disease pathogenesis and progression still needs to be better understood. This chapter focuses on the studies that have identified sex-specific differences in AD patients, emphasizing epidemiological, genetics, biomarkers, and personalized therapeutic strategies.

2 Epidemiological Studies Indicate Women Are at Higher Risk of Alzheimer's Disease

Numerous epidemiological studies have reported a disproportionately higher incidence of AD among women compared to men (Fratiglioni et al. 1997; Ott et al. 1998; Andersen et al. 1999; Letenneur et al. 1999; Ruitenberg et al. 2001; Di Carlo et al. 2002; Yoshitake et al. 1995; Liu et al. 1998). For example, data from the Kungsholmen Project in Sweden found a higher risk of dementia in women, especially at very old ages (Fratiglioni et al. 1997). The Rotterdam Study determined that the incidence rate of AD for men and women up to 85 was similar, but the lifetime risk for 55-year-old women was twice as high as for men (Ott et al. 1998). The EURODEM studies showed a similar trend with women having an increased risk for AD after age 85 (Andersen et al. 1999). The incidence data from the PAQUID project showed that the incidence of AD was higher in men than in women before the age of 80 but higher in women after this age (Letenneur et al. 1999). Similarly, in the ILSA study in Italy, women had a greater risk of AD and men of vascular dementia (Di Carlo et al. 2002). These results are consistent with those of the Hisayama Study in Japan that determined a higher incidence of AD in women and vascular dementia in men (Yoshitake et al. 1995). Additionally, the female sex was associated with a marginally increased risk of AD in a Taiwanese population study (Liu et al. 1998).

Despite these findings, sex-specific interactions in AD are still extensively debated. Several explanations have been posited for the observed sex-biased in epidemiological studies of AD. One may argue that genetic and cultural differences may explain population discrepancies since these studies were mainly derived from data collected in European and Asian countries. In contrast, studies from North and South America have not reached statistical significance of sex in AD (Bachman et al. 1993; Rocca et al. 1998). Indeed, one study showed a higher incidence rate of all-cause dementia among men than women (Ganguli et al. 2000). In addition to the inherent genetic and cultural differences, emerging studies claim that sex, gender, and sexual orientation are equally important factors that warrant a more profound investigation (Mielke et al. 2022). Since advanced age is the most significant risk factor for AD (Guerreiro and Bras 2015), it is plausible to hypothesize that the higher prevalence of AD in females is due to their greater longevity compared to men (Barford et al. 2006; Hebert et al. 2001). Differences in study design, ascertainment of AD cases and controls, and comorbidities may also explain the discrepancies among the studies.

Sex-based differences have been reported in symptoms and disease progression in patients at risk for AD. For example, women with mild cognitive impairment (MCI) displayed greater longitudinal cognitive and functional decline than men (Lin et al. 2015). Similarly, women with MCI and AD showed greater memory impairment than men, including verbal learning, delayed recall, and visual memory (Gale et al. 2016). Other investigations have supported these findings (Chapman et al. 2011; Skup et al. 2011). For example, a meta-analysis of 15 studies revealed a consistently better performance in males over females on verbal, visuospatial, episodic, and semantic memory independent of age, education level, and disease severity (Irvine et al. 2012).

While the mechanisms underlying sex differences in AD remain elusive, several lines of evidence suggest that AD progression affects the female brain differently than men. Earlier postmortem studies found that women had more affected brain regions with more extensive senile plaques and neurofibrillary tangles than men in the early stages of the disease (Corder et al. 2004). Subsequent studies using magnetic resonance imaging (MRI) showed greater loss of gray matter in brain regions, including the bilateral precuneus, caudate nucleus, entorhinal gyrus, thalamus, middle temporal gyrus, insula, and amygdala in females with AD and MCI compared to males and healthy controls (Skup et al. 2011). Furthermore, neuroimaging studies showed that the rate of hippocampal atrophy affects the progression of AD in females more than in males (Williamson et al. 2022). This study demonstrated that hippocampus-brain stem connectivity was more robust in males than females. Indeed, hippocampal atrophy, as determined by hippocampal volume, has been an indicator of progression to AD only in women (Burke et al. 2019). This finding is of critical importance since the hippocampus is one of the brain structures affected in the earliest stages of AD (Braak and Braak 1995).

Recently, a neuroimaging study showed that post-menopausal women exhibited higher tau and global Aβ deposition than men in the inferior parietal, rostral middle-frontal, and lateral-occipital regions compared to age-matched men (Buckley et al. 2022). In addition, sex- and menopause-related changes were observed in the middle-frontal and parieto-occipital regions, independently of Aβ burden or APOEε4 genotype, further reinforcing the notion that menopause modulates tau vulnerability. Collectively, these findings indicate sex-specific vulnerability to AD in different brain regions and that menopause may be a critical timepoint in disease pathogenesis.

3 Sex Differences in Biomarkers for Alzheimer's Disease

Finding useful biomarkers to identify patients at risk and monitor disease progression remains an unmet goal in the field and a significant setback in the design of clinical trials. Several biomarkers have shown promise, but a definitive diagnostic test is yet to be found. Sex differences have been identified using neuroimaging modalities, including ^{11}C-Pittsburgh compound B [PiB] positron emission tomography (PET), ^{18}F-fluorodeoxyglucose, and structural MRI. For example, PET imaging revealed that cognitively intact men, compared with women, exhibited higher anterior cingulate cortex amyloid load, glucose hypometabolism, and lower resting state functional connectivity in the default mode network (Cavedo et al. 2018). Similarly, females showed higher PiB amyloid deposition, lower FDG glucose metabolism, and lower MRI gray and white matter volumes than males. These studies suggest that men are more resilient to the pathophysiological processes underlying AD.

In addition to imaging-based biomarkers, sex-specific differences have been noted in biofluid biomarkers for AD. For example, *APOEε4* women carriers showed higher CSF levels of phosphorylated tau (p-tau) in the subjective cognitive decline and MCI groups compared to men but not in AD dementia (Babapour Mofrad et al. 2020). Baseline CSF $A\beta_{1-42}$ and tau accumulation were higher in female *APOEε4* carriers compared to other groups (Buckley et al. 2019). In contrast, several studies have not found sex differences in CSF $A\beta_{1-42}$, p-tau, and total tau levels (Schoonenboom et al. 2004; Bouter et al. 2019; Mielke et al. 2019). Males with AD had higher CSF levels of VCAM1 and E-selectin than females (Hall 1986). The latter study suggested that female *APOEε4* carriers were at higher risk of AD after age 50, whereas men may have a higher rate of cerebrovascular disease. A meta-analysis of data collected from over 10,000 subjects revealed that CSF levels of neurofilament light protein (NfL), a marker of axonal degeneration, were higher in men than women (Bridel et al. 2019). Notably, CSF levels of NfL were increased in several neurodegenerative diseases, limiting its specificity for AD.

Similarly, the synaptic protein neurogranin (Ng), involved in synaptogenesis, has been associated with several neurodegenerative diseases, including AD, Parkinson's disease, frontotemporal dementia, and Huntington's disease. In contrast to NfL, there was a trend of lower levels of CSF Ng in men compared to women (Mielke et al. 2019). In another study, CSF Ng levels correlated with brain atrophy and future cognitive impairment, but no significant sex differences were observed (Tarawneh et al. 2016).

Another potential biomarker with sex-specific findings in AD is MMP9, a matrix metalloproteinase whose dysregulated expression is associated with blood-brain barrier disruption, neuroinflammation, and demyelination (Rempe et al. 2016). For instance, higher total and free MMP9 correlated with higher CSF t-tau in women and lower CSF t-tau in men. Further, higher free MMP9 was associated with worse Alzheimer's Disease Assessment Scale-Cognitive Subscale (ADA-cognitive) scores in women but not in men with AD dementia cross-sectionally (Tsiknia et al. 2022). These findings suggest that MMP9 may be a potential biomarker of disease severity in women with AD.

4 Sex-Specific Differences in Genetic Factors and Molecular Pathways in Alzheimer's Disease

The ε4 allele of the apolipoprotein E (*APOE*) gene is the strongest genetic risk factor for developing late-onset AD. In the context of sex differences, women who carry copies of the *APOE ε4* have a greater risk of developing AD than men (Farrer et al. 1997). Despite numerous studies suggesting a sex-specific biased among *APOE ε4* carriers, mixed results have sparked debate. A meta-analysis of 27 independent studies with women and men with one copy of *APOE ε4* did not find a sex-specific difference from age 55 to 85 but an increased risk at younger ages between 65 and 75 (Neu et al. 2017). The sex-specific discrepancies have also been noted in first-degree relatives, with females having nearly twice the risk of AD compared to men (Farrer et al. 1997). These findings suggest that sex-specific treatment should be initiated at younger ages in female *APOE ε4* carriers. Nonetheless, a more extensive meta-analysis confirmed the sex-specific interaction between *APOE ε4* and AD and suggested that the *APOE ε4* allele represents a significant risk factor for AD in both men and women from all ethnic groups studied (Farrer et al. 1997).

Another study investigating the interactions of sex, *APOE ε4*, Aβ burden, and AD found that cognitive decline was greater in females with higher Aβ burden (Buckley et al. 2018). The same study suggested that females' carriers of *APOE ε4* and positive for Aβ had a faster cognitive decline than males despite the finding that APOE ε4 prevalence and Aβ did not show sex differences. An imaging study revealed that in several brain regions, female heterozygotes for *APOE ε4* showed significantly increased tau deposition than male heterozygotes (Yan et al. 2021). Notably, the same study found an *APOE ε4* dosage effect observed in males but not females showing males homozygotes with a greater tau deposition than heterozygotes or non-carriers. It remains unclear, however, whether *APOE ε4* and Aβ independently account for the increased vulnerability to AD in females. The mechanisms underlying the effects of *APOE ε4*, Aβ burden, and sex interactions in the risk of AD warrant further research.

In addition to *APOE ε4*, other investigations have explored sex-specific genetic differences in AD. For instance, genetic variants within genetic risk factors for AD, including *DNAJA2*, *FERMT2*, and *TYW5* associated with tau deposition in women, independently of *APOE* and Aβ status, whereas genetic variants in CR1 are associated with tau deposition in men (Wang et al. 2022). Other sex-dependent polygenic effects have been documented in recent investigations. For example, the effect sizes of risk variants in *BIN1*, *MS4A6A*, *DNAJA2*, and *FERMT2* were larger among females, whereas *FAM193B*, *C2ORF47*, and *TYW5* showed larger effect sizes on males (Fan et al. 2020). Furthermore, *MAPT* showed stronger effects on males with AD than on females.

Another proposed genetic mechanism underlying sex-specific differences in AD is the X chromosome inactivation, a process by which mammals compensate for the unequal number of sex chromosomes. Dysregulated expression of genes involved in X chromosome inactivation has been found in several studies in AD. For instance, *XIST*, an RNA gene key in X chromosome inactivation, is upregulated in brain samples from AD patients (Wang et al. 2018). Similarly, a second X chromosome conferred resilience to AD in mice through kdm6a, an X chromosome encoded demethylase (Davis et al. 2020). Interestingly, *KDM6A* mRNA was significantly upregulated in women with and without AD compared to males, and a genetic variant in this gene was associated with a lesser extent of cognitive impairment (Davis et al. 2020).

Recent bioinformatic studies have revealed sex-specific gene expression signatures associated with AD. Co-expression network analysis identified sex-specific "switch genes" responsible for drastic transcriptional changes in the entorhinal cortex of AD patients postmortem (Santiago et al. 2022). In males, switch genes were associated with nicotine addiction, cell adhesion molecules, oxytocin and prolactin signaling, adipocytokine signaling, and alcoholism. In this regard, oxytocin and prolactin hormones have been implicated in neuroprotection and AD. Intranasal delivery of oxytocin improved cognitive functions, Aβ burden, and tau deposition in female rats with AD (El-Ganainy et al. 2022). Similarly, the pituitary hormone prolactin has been shown to promote neuroprotection via increased synaptogenesis, axon growth, neuronal plasticity, and memory consolidation (Carretero et al. 2019). Further evaluation in larger clinical studies is needed to verify these findings.

In the context of nicotine and alcohol addiction, epidemiological studies have yielded mixed results. Excessive alcohol consumption and cigarette smoking have been associated with cognitive decline and the risk of dementia. For example, alcohol use disorder is associated with smaller hippocampal volume and dementia severity in AD patients (Zhornitsky et al. 2021). It has been suggested that chronic alcohol consumption leads to the generation of reactive oxygen species and neurotoxic effects, leading to white matter atrophy and demyelination (Kamal et al. 2020). Nevertheless, a recent study indicated that low to moderate alcohol consumption correlated with a reduced risk of AD and related dementias (Yang et al. 2022). Likewise, cigarette smoking increased oxidative stress and Aβ pathology in a mouse mode of AD (Moreno-Gonzalez et al. 2013). A functional MRI study showed that cigarette smoking could affect the function of cortico-striatal circuits in patients with MCI (Qiu et al. 2022). Similarly, several studies have indicated that smoking may confer neuroprotection. The risk of AD increased by 50% every ten years of smoking cessation (Aggarwal et al. 2006). Nicotine may confer neuroprotection via the inhibition of NMDA neurotoxicity and the inhibition of Aβ aggregation (Aggarwal et al. 2006; Zamani et al. 1997). While there are numerous studies indicating sex-specific differences in reward and addiction (Orsini et al. 2022), the interaction between alcohol and smoking in driving sex differences in the risk of AD is a subject of extensive debate, and larger prospective studies are needed to clarify these findings. Additionally, differences in hormonal regulation may also explain addictive behaviors (Orsini et al. 2022).

In contrast, female switch genes were involved in myocarditis, endometrial cancer, insulin signaling, and the PI3K-AKT signaling pathway. In this context, impaired insulin signaling, diabetes, and PI3K-AKT signaling pathway have been reported as shared dysregulated pathways between diabetes and neurodegenerative diseases (Santiago and Potashkin 2013a, b, 2014, 2015a, b; Santiago et al. 2019). It is now established that diabetes increases the risk of AD in several populations, and patients with AD with comorbid diabetes may experience a faster disease progression and worsening symptoms (Santiago and Potashkin 2021; Marseglia et al. 2019). Adding to this complexity are the sex-specific differences observed in diabetes. For instance, diabetes is more prevalent in men than women, and women with diabetes have a greater risk of developing cardiovascular complications than men (Nordstrom et al. 2016; Kautzky-Willer et al. 2016). Therefore, a better understanding of the impact of disease comorbidities on disease pathogenesis and progression is critical for developing personalized treatments for AD patients.

5 Hormonal Differences May Underlie Sex-Specific Differences in Alzheimer's Disease

Hormonal differences have been posited to underlie a sex-specific vulnerability in AD. This hypothesis gained interest since several studies have shown a higher incidence of AD in women after menopause (Fisher et al. 2018). Decreased estrogen levels are characteristic of menopause and aging. Estrogen, an essential hormone in female reproduction, has been shown to play a role in emotions, memory, and cognitive functions (Luine 2014). It is, therefore, unsurprising that estrogen decline during menopause is associated with cognitive impairment and neurodegeneration (Matyi et al. 2019). A population-based study of over 2000 older adult women found that endogenous estrogen exposure and hormone replacement therapy correlated positively with cognitive status in late life (Anastas'eva et al. 1985). Furthermore, oral contraceptives and hormone replacement therapy decreased the risk of AD in post-menopausal women (Shumaker et al. 2004).

Like menopause, age-related decline of sex male hormones, best known as andropause, may be associated with AD. Depletion of both serum and brain androgen levels in males has been implicated in the accumulation of Aβ (Lei and Renyuan 2018). Evidence from animal models suggests that androgen-based hormone therapy may afford neuroprotection (Rosario et al. 2006, 2010). Recently, a cohort study in Sweden determined that males receiving 5α-reductase inhibitors showed a higher risk of dementia (Garcia-Argibay et al. 2022).

In addition to estrogen and testosterone, other hormones, including oxytocin, prolactin, and follicle-stimulating hormone (FSH), have been implicated in processes related to AD and neurodegeneration. Oxytocin and prolactin may be involved in neuroprotection and the regulation of inflammation (El-Ganainy et al. 2022; Costanza and Pedotti 2016). Recently, the blockade of FSH improved cognition in mice with AD (Xiong et al. 2022). Epidemiological studies indicate that higher levels of FSH are related to lipid metabolism, obesity, and cognitive decline in menopausal women (Mao et al. 2022). While hormonal differences may explain sex vulnerability in AD, more detailed mechanistic studies and more extensive prospective trials are needed to verify findings obtained from preclinical models.

6 Personalized Treatments for AD

The sex differences observed in the prevalence, genetic, and environmental factors in AD suggest that drugs and neuroprotective agents may act differently in men and women. Given the pivotal role of impaired insulin signaling in AD (Chatterjee and Mudher 2018), insulin delivery has been investigated as a potential disease-modifying treatment. Intranasal insulin has been demonstrated to be effective in improving memory deficits in human studies. Notably, sex-dependent insulin effects have been observed in several studies. Intranasal insulin delivery improved hippocampus-dependent memory and working memory in healthy women but not men (Benedict et al. 2008). Interestingly, insulin administration decreased food intake in men but not in women. A follow-up study of intranasal insulin found that healthy females displayed enhanced memory for interfering declarative contents, whereas men showed memory impairments (Feld et al. 2016). Notably, all female subjects in this study were taking estrogen-dominant oral contraceptives; thus, additional studies considering medication effect and sex hormones are needed to further validate these findings. In the context of AD, the potential role of insulin as a neuroprotective agent is currently debated due to mixed results observed in clinical trials. For example, a randomized double-blinded and placebo-controlled trial showed that intranasal insulin therapy improved memory and preserved general cognition in adults with amnestic MCI (Craft et al. 2012). Nevertheless, follow-up studies failed to find a beneficial effect of insulin in cognition, mood, and functional abilities in MCI or probable AD patients (Craft et al. 2020; Rosenbloom et al. 2021). A smaller trial showed improved memory in subjects treated with regular insulin, but no effect was observed in the group treated with long-acting insulin (Craft et al. 2017). Sex differences in insulin signaling, different insulin formulations, and sex hormones may explain these discrepancies. For instance, males have more visceral fat and are more likely to develop obesity than females. It has been proposed that the male brain is more sensitive to the catabolic action of insulin and that estrogen decreases insulin sensitivity (Clegg et al. 2006). Furthermore, women are more likely to develop insulin resistance than men (Mittendorfer 2005). In addition to these discrepancies, clinical trials examining the potential of intranasal insulin in MCI and AD patients have not yielded positive outcomes on cognition or disease modification (Craft et al. 2020; Rosenbloom et al. 2021). These findings suggest that intrinsic sex differences in regulating sex hormones and insulin may be responsible for the positive effects of intranasal insulin in women. Nevertheless, these findings warrant further investigations in future clinical trials involving populations at risk for AD.

Statins, the most prescribed drug for lowering cholesterol, have shown neuroprotective effects in AD patients. Sex and race differences have been documented in epidemiological investigations on the use of statins. A study on statins users showed that high exposure to statins was associated with a 15% lower risk of AD in women and 12% in men (Zissimopoulos et al. 2017). Interestingly, pravastatin and rosuvastatin were associated with a lower risk of AD in white women only. Furthermore, high statin exposure did not show benefit in reducing the risk of AD among black men. Differences in race and ethnicity imply that inherent genetic differences may also play a role in the health outcomes of statin use. For example, genetic variants in *APOE* have been shown to affect responses to statins (Bi et al. 2022). Similarly, genetic and racial differences in drug-metabolizing enzymes and transporters may also explain different responses to statins (Warnich et al. 2011). Furthermore, differences in diet may have biased the results, as these were not accounted in the studies discussed above. These findings reinforce the importance of carefully assessing sex, genetic, and racial differences in designing clinical trials for AD. Personalized medicine strategies should include factors beyond genetics, including comorbidities and lifestyle choices (Fig. 1).

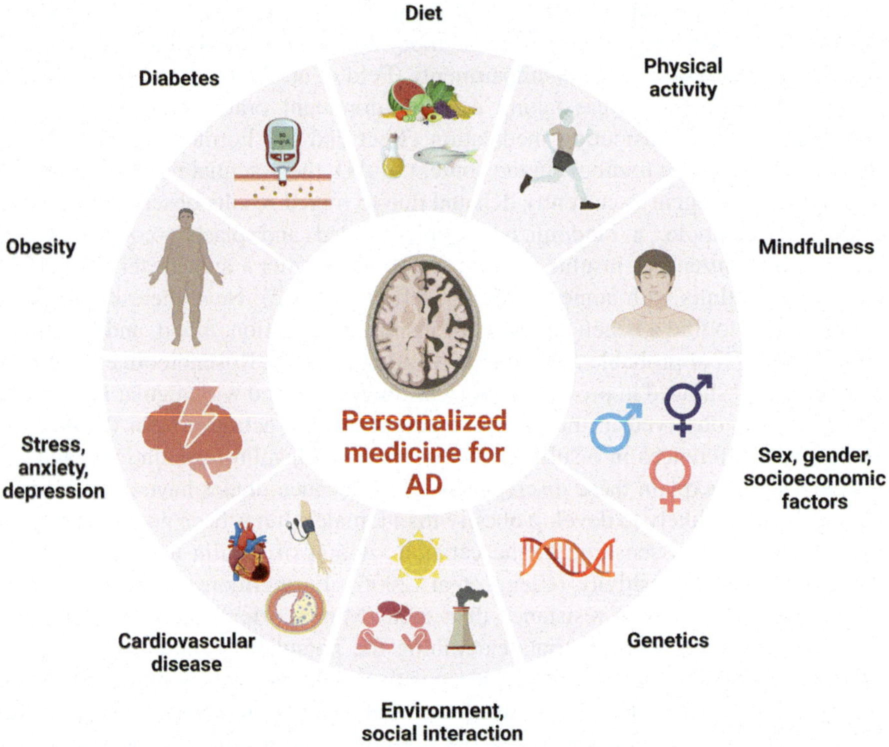

Fig. 1 Personalized medicine in AD. Personalized medicine therapeutic strategies should take into consideration factors beyond genetics, including comorbidities such as diabetes, obesity, depression, and cardiovascular disease. Lifestyle choices including diet, physical activity, mindfulness, and social interaction are important determinants of brain health that should be included in future studies

7 Conclusions and Future Directions

AD is a highly complex disease wherein the interplay of genetic and environmental factors is the prime contributor of disease pathogenesis and progression. Preclinical and clinical studies in AD have identified sex-related differences in risk factors, comorbidities, genetic variants, sex hormones, brain structure, and function, response to treatment, and biomarkers (Fig. 2). The overwhelming evidence supporting a sex-specific vulnerability in AD has raised cautionary flags in our current view and treatment strategies for AD. Women display a more accelerated cognitive decline and phenotypic conversion from MCI to AD. Despite numerous studies reporting sex differences, to date there are no sufficient data on sex-specific differences on the efficacy of drugs tested in clinical trials for AD. Larger randomized trials considering the impact of sex, gender and socioeconomic factors,

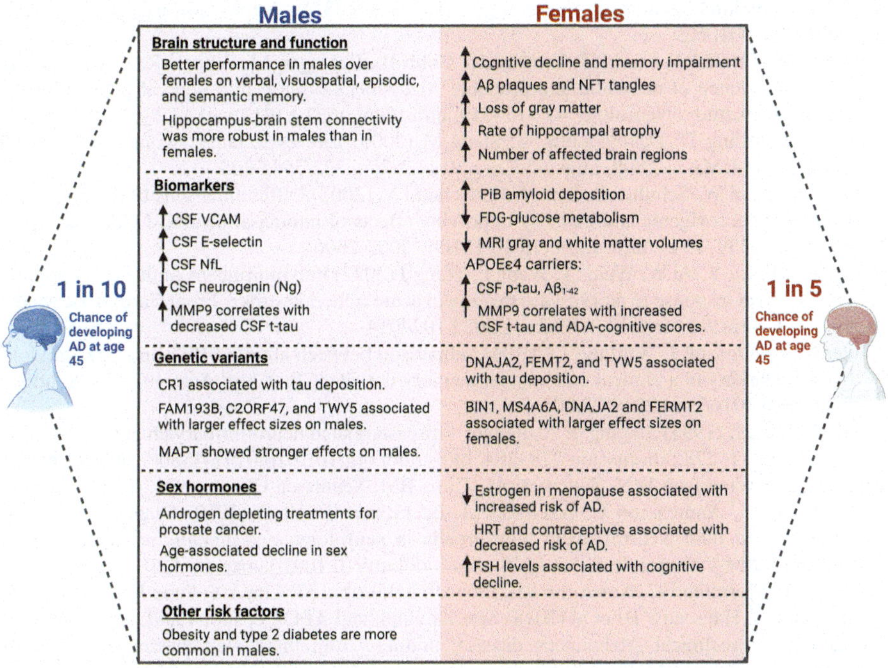

Fig. 2 Sex-related differences in Alzheimer's disease. Epidemiological evidence has consistently shown a disproportionately greater incidence of AD among women compared to men. Preclinical and clinical studies have identified potential sex-specific differences in brain structure and function, biofluid and imaging biomarkers, genetic variants, sex hormones, and other potential risk factors. *CSF* cerebrospinal fluid, ^{11}C-Pittsburgh compound B: PiB, *ADA* Alzheimer's Disease Assessment Scale-Cognitive Subscale

race, comorbidities, and risk factors for AD will help delineate new personalized medicine strategies.

References

Aggarwal NT, Bienias JL, Bennett DA, Wilson RS, Morris MC, Schneider JA, Shah RC, Evans DA (2006) The relation of cigarette smoking to incident Alzheimer's disease in a biracial urban community population. Neuroepidemiology 26:140–146. https://doi.org/10.1159/000091654

Anastas'eva NV, Pasman NM, Soboleva MK, Loseva MI (1985) Morphological and functional characteristics of erythrocytes of mothers with late pregnancy toxemias and their newborn infants. Akush Ginekol (Mosk):18–21

Andersen K, Launer LJ, Dewey ME, Letenneur L, Ott A, Copeland JR, Dartigues JF, Kragh-Sorensen P, Baldereschi M, Brayne C et al (1999) Gender differences in the incidence of AD and vascular dementia: the EURODEM studies. EURODEM Incidence Research Group. Neurology 53:1992–1997. https://doi.org/10.1212/wnl.53.9.1992

Babapour Mofrad R, Tijms BM, Scheltens P, Barkhof F, van der Flier WM, Sikkes SAM, Teunissen CE (2020) Sex differences in CSF biomarkers vary by Alzheimer disease stage and

APOE epsilon4 genotype. Neurology 95:e2378–e2388. https://doi.org/10.1212/WNL.0000000000010629
Bachman DL, Wolf PA, Linn RT, Knoefel JE, Cobb JL, Belanger AJ, White LR, D'Agostino RB (1993) Incidence of dementia and probable Alzheimer's disease in a general population: the Framingham study. Neurology 43:515–519. https://doi.org/10.1212/wnl.43.3_part_1.515
Barford A, Dorling D, Davey Smith G, Shaw M (2006) Life expectancy: women now on top everywhere. BMJ 332:808. https://doi.org/10.1136/bmj.332.7545.808
Benedict C, Kern W, Schultes B, Born J, Hallschmid M (2008) Differential sensitivity of men and women to anorexigenic and memory-improving effects of intranasal insulin. J Clin Endocrinol Metab 93:1339–1344. https://doi.org/10.1210/jc.2007-2606
Bi Q, Zhou X, Lu Y, Fu W, Wang Y, Wang F, Wang J (2022) Polymorphisms of the apolipoprotein E gene affect response to atorvastatin therapy in acute ischemic stroke. Front Cardiovasc Med 9: 1024014. https://doi.org/10.3389/fcvm.2022.1024014
Bouter C, Vogelgsang J, Wiltfang J (2019) Comparison between amyloid-PET and CSF amyloid-beta biomarkers in a clinical cohort with memory deficits. Clin Chim Acta 492:62–68. https://doi.org/10.1016/j.cca.2019.02.005
Braak H, Braak E (1995) Staging of Alzheimer's disease-related neurofibrillary changes. Neurobiol Aging 16:271–278.; discussion 278–284. https://doi.org/10.1016/0197-4580(95)00021-6
Bridel C, van Wieringen WN, Zetterberg H, Tijms BM, Teunissen CE, the NFL Group, Alvarez-Cermeno JC, Andreasson U, Axelsson M, Backstrom DC et al (2019) Diagnostic value of cerebrospinal fluid Neurofilament light protein in neurology: a systematic review and meta-analysis. JAMA Neurol 76:1035–1048. https://doi.org/10.1001/jamaneurol.2019.1534
Buckley RF, Mormino EC, Amariglio RE, Properzi MJ, Rabin JS, Lim YY, Papp KV, Jacobs HIL, Burnham S, Hanseeuw BJ et al (2018) Sex, amyloid, and APOE epsilon4 and risk of cognitive decline in preclinical Alzheimer's disease: findings from three well-characterized cohorts. Alzheimers Dement 14:1193–1203. https://doi.org/10.1016/j.jalz.2018.04.010
Buckley RF, Mormino EC, Chhatwal J, Schultz AP, Rabin JS, Rentz DM, Acar D, Properzi MJ, Dumurgier J, Jacobs H et al (2019) Associations between baseline amyloid, sex, and APOE on subsequent tau accumulation in cerebrospinal fluid. Neurobiol Aging 78:178–185. https://doi.org/10.1016/j.neurobiolaging.2019.02.019
Buckley RF, O'Donnell A, McGrath ER, Jacobs HIL, Lois C, Satizabal CL, Ghosh S, Rubinstein ZB, Murabito JM, Sperling RA et al (2022) Menopause status moderates sex differences in tau burden: a Framingham PET study. Ann Neurol 92:11–22. https://doi.org/10.1002/ana.26382
Burke SL, Hu T, Fava NM, Li T, Rodriguez MJ, Schuldiner KL, Burgess A, Laird A (2019) Sex differences in the development of mild cognitive impairment and probable Alzheimer's disease as predicted by hippocampal volume or white matter hyperintensities. J Women Aging 31:140–164. https://doi.org/10.1080/08952841.2018.1419476
Carretero J, Sanchez-Robledo V, Carretero-Hernandez M, Catalano-Iniesta L, Garcia-Barrado MJ, Iglesias-Osma MC, Blanco EJ (2019) Prolactin system in the hippocampus. Cell Tissue Res 375:193–199. https://doi.org/10.1007/s00441-018-2858-2
Cavedo E, Chiesa PA, Houot M, Ferretti MT, Grothe MJ, Teipel SJ, Lista S, Habert MO, Potier MC, Dubois B et al (2018) Sex differences in functional and molecular neuroimaging biomarkers of Alzheimer's disease in cognitively normal older adults with subjective memory complaints. Alzheimers Dement 14:1204–1215. https://doi.org/10.1016/j.jalz.2018.05.014
Chapman RM, Mapstone M, Gardner MN, Sandoval TC, McCrary JW, Guillily MD, Reilly LA, DeGrush E (2011) Women have farther to fall: gender differences between normal elderly and Alzheimer's disease in verbal memory engender better detection of Alzheimer's disease in women. J Int Neuropsychol Soc 17:654–662. https://doi.org/10.1017/S1355617711000452
Chatterjee S, Mudher A (2018) Alzheimer's disease and type 2 diabetes: a critical assessment of the shared pathological traits. Front Neurosci 12:383. https://doi.org/10.3389/fnins.2018.00383
Clegg DJ, Brown LM, Woods SC, Benoit SC (2006) Gonadal hormones determine sensitivity to central leptin and insulin. Diabetes 55:978–987. https://doi.org/10.2337/diabetes.55.04.06.db05-1339

Corder EH, Ghebremedhin E, Taylor MG, Thal DR, Ohm TG, Braak H (2004) The biphasic relationship between regional brain senile plaque and neurofibrillary tangle distributions: modification by age, sex, and APOE polymorphism. Ann N Y Acad Sci 1019:24–28. https://doi.org/10.1196/annals.1297.005

Costanza M, Pedotti R (2016) Prolactin: friend or foe in central nervous system autoimmune inflammation? Int J Mol Sci 17. https://doi.org/10.3390/ijms17122026

Craft S, Baker LD, Montine TJ, Minoshima S, Watson GS, Claxton A, Arbuckle M, Callaghan M, Tsai E, Plymate SR et al (2012) Intranasal insulin therapy for Alzheimer disease and amnestic mild cognitive impairment: a pilot clinical trial. Arch Neurol 69:29–38. https://doi.org/10.1001/archneurol.2011.233

Craft S, Claxton A, Baker LD, Hanson AJ, Cholerton B, Trittschuh EH, Dahl D, Caulder E, Neth B, Montine TJ et al (2017) Effects of regular and long-acting insulin on cognition and Alzheimer's disease biomarkers: a pilot clinical trial. J Alzheimers Dis 57:1325–1334. https://doi.org/10.3233/JAD-161256

Craft S, Raman R, Chow TW, Rafii MS, Sun CK, Rissman RA, Donohue MC, Brewer JB, Jenkins C, Harless K et al (2020) Safety, efficacy, and feasibility of intranasal insulin for the treatment of mild cognitive impairment and Alzheimer disease dementia: a randomized clinical trial. JAMA Neurol 77:1099–1109. https://doi.org/10.1001/jamaneurol.2020.1840

Davis EJ, Broestl L, Abdulai-Saiku S, Worden K, Bonham LW, Minones-Moyano E, Moreno AJ, Wang D, Chang K, Williams G et al (2020) A second X chromosome contributes to resilience in a mouse model of Alzheimer's disease. Sci Transl Med 12. https://doi.org/10.1126/scitranslmed.aaz5677

Di Carlo A, Baldereschi M, Amaducci L, Lepore V, Bracco L, Maggi S, Bonaiuto S, Perissinotto E, Scarlato G, Farchi G et al (2002) Incidence of dementia, Alzheimer's disease, and vascular dementia in Italy. The ILSA study. J Am Geriatr Soc 50:41–48. https://doi.org/10.1046/j.1532-5415.2002.50006.x

El-Ganainy SO, Soliman OA, Ghazy AA, Allam M, Elbahnasi AI, Mansour AM, Gowayed MA (2022) Intranasal oxytocin attenuates cognitive impairment, beta-amyloid burden and tau deposition in female rats with Alzheimer's disease: interplay of ERK1/2/GSK3beta/Caspase-3. Neurochem Res. https://doi.org/10.1007/s11064-022-03624-x

Fan CC, Banks SJ, Thompson WK, Chen CH, McEvoy LK, Tan CH, Kukull W, Bennett DA, Farrer LA, Mayeux R et al (2020) Sex-dependent autosomal effects on clinical progression of Alzheimer's disease. Brain 143:2272–2280. https://doi.org/10.1093/brain/awaa164

Farrer LA, Cupples LA, Haines JL, Hyman B, Kukull WA, Mayeux R, Myers RH, Pericak-Vance MA, Risch N, van Duijn CM (1997) Effects of age, sex, and ethnicity on the association between apolipoprotein E genotype and Alzheimer disease. A meta-analysis. APOE and Alzheimer disease meta analysis consortium. JAMA 278:1349–1356

Feld GB, Wilhem I, Benedict C, Rudel B, Klameth C, Born J, Hallschmid M (2016) Central nervous insulin signaling in sleep-associated memory formation and neuroendocrine regulation. Neuropsychopharmacology 41:1540–1550. https://doi.org/10.1038/npp.2015.312

Fisher DW, Bennett DA, Dong H (2018) Sexual dimorphism in predisposition to Alzheimer's disease. Neurobiol Aging 70:308–324. https://doi.org/10.1016/j.neurobiolaging.2018.04.004

Fratiglioni L, Viitanen M, von Strauss E, Tontodonati V, Herlitz A, Winblad B (1997) Very old women at highest risk of dementia and Alzheimer's disease: incidence data from the Kungsholmen project, Stockholm. Neurology 48:132–138. https://doi.org/10.1212/wnl.48.1.132

Gale SD, Baxter L, Thompson J (2016) Greater memory impairment in dementing females than males relative to sex-matched healthy controls. J Clin Exp Neuropsychol 38:527–533. https://doi.org/10.1080/13803395.2015.1132298

Ganguli M, Dodge HH, Chen P, Belle S, DeKosky ST (2000) Ten-year incidence of dementia in a rural elderly US community population: the MoVIES project. Neurology 54:1109–1116. https://doi.org/10.1212/wnl.54.5.1109

Garcia-Argibay M, Hiyoshi A, Fall K, Montgomery S (2022) Association of 5alpha-reductase inhibitors with dementia, depression, and suicide. JAMA Netw Open 5:e2248135. https://doi.org/10.1001/jamanetworkopen.2022.48135

Guerreiro R, Bras J (2015) The age factor in Alzheimer's disease. Genome Med 7:106. https://doi.org/10.1186/s13073-015-0232-5

Hall MJ (1986) Cassava toxicity. Lancet 1:95. https://doi.org/10.1016/s0140-6736(86)90742-7

Hebert LE, Scherr PA, McCann JJ, Beckett LA, Evans DA (2001) Is the risk of developing Alzheimer's disease greater for women than for men? Am J Epidemiol 153:132–136. https://doi.org/10.1093/aje/153.2.132

Irvine K, Laws KR, Gale TM, Kondel TK (2012) Greater cognitive deterioration in women than men with Alzheimer's disease: a meta analysis. J Clin Exp Neuropsychol 34:989–998. https://doi.org/10.1080/13803395.2012.712676

Kamal H, Tan GC, Ibrahim SF, Shaikh MF, Mohamed IN, Mohamed RMP, Hamid AA, Ugusman A, Kumar J (2020) Alcohol use disorder, neurodegeneration, Alzheimer's and Parkinson's disease: interplay between oxidative stress, neuroimmune response and excitotoxicity. Front Cell Neurosci 14:282. https://doi.org/10.3389/fncel.2020.00282

Kautzky-Willer A, Harreiter J, Pacini G (2016) Sex and gender differences in risk, pathophysiology and complications of type 2 diabetes mellitus. Endocr Rev 37:278–316. https://doi.org/10.1210/er.2015-1137

Lei Y, Renyuan Z (2018) Effects of androgens on the amyloid-beta protein in Alzheimer's disease. Endocrinology 159:3885–3894. https://doi.org/10.1210/en.2018-00660

Letenneur L, Gilleron V, Commenges D, Helmer C, Orgogozo JM, Dartigues JF (1999) Are sex and educational level independent predictors of dementia and Alzheimer's disease? Incidence data from the PAQUID project. J Neurol Neurosurg Psychiatry 66:177–183. https://doi.org/10.1136/jnnp.66.2.177

Lin KA, Choudhury KR, Rathakrishnan BG, Marks DM, Petrella JR, Doraiswamy PM, Alzheimer's Disease Neuroimaging Initiative (2015) Marked gender differences in progression of mild cognitive impairment over 8 years. Alzheimers Dement (N Y) 1:103–110. https://doi.org/10.1016/j.trci.2015.07.001

Liu CK, Lai CL, Tai CT, Lin RT, Yen YY, Howng SL (1998) Incidence and subtypes of dementia in southern Taiwan: impact of socio-demographic factors. Neurology 50:1572–1579. https://doi.org/10.1212/wnl.50.6.1572

Luine VN (2014) Estradiol and cognitive function: past, present and future. Horm Behav 66:602–618. https://doi.org/10.1016/j.yhbeh.2014.08.011

Mao L, Wang L, Bennett S, Xu J, Zou J (2022) Effects of follicle-stimulating hormone on fat metabolism and cognitive impairment in women during menopause. Front Physiol 13:1043237. https://doi.org/10.3389/fphys.2022.1043237

Marseglia A, Fratiglioni L, Kalpouzos G, Wang R, Backman L, Xu W (2019) Prediabetes and diabetes accelerate cognitive decline and predict microvascular lesions: a population-based cohort study. Alzheimers Dement 15:25–33. https://doi.org/10.1016/j.jalz.2018.06.3060

Masters CL, Bateman R, Blennow K, Rowe CC, Sperling RA, Cummings JL (2015) Alzheimer's disease. Nat Rev Dis Primers 1:15056. https://doi.org/10.1038/nrdp.2015.56

Matyi JM, Rattinger GB, Schwartz S, Buhusi M, Tschanz JT (2019) Lifetime estrogen exposure and cognition in late life: the Cache County study. Menopause 26:1366–1374. https://doi.org/10.1097/GME.0000000000001405

Mielke MM, Syrjanen JA, Blennow K, Zetterberg H, Skoog I, Vemuri P, Machulda MM, Graff-Radford J, Knopman DS, Jack CR Jr et al (2019) Comparison of variables associated with cerebrospinal fluid neurofilament, total-tau, and neurogranin. Alzheimers Dement 15:1437–1447. https://doi.org/10.1016/j.jalz.2019.07.009

Mielke MM, Aggarwal NT, Vila-Castelar C, Agarwal P, Arenaza-Urquijo EM, Brett B, Brugulat-Serrat A, DuBose LE, Eikelboom WS, Flatt J et al (2022) Consideration of sex and gender in Alzheimer's disease and related disorders from a global perspective. Alzheimers Dement. https://doi.org/10.1002/alz.12662

Mittendorfer B (2005) Insulin resistance: sex matters. Curr Opin Clin Nutr Metab Care 8:367–372. https://doi.org/10.1097/01.mco.0000172574.64019.98

Moreno-Gonzalez I, Estrada LD, Sanchez-Mejias E, Soto C (2013) Smoking exacerbates amyloid pathology in a mouse model of Alzheimer's disease. Nat Commun 4:1495. https://doi.org/10.1038/ncomms2494

Neu SC, Pa J, Kukull W, Beekly D, Kuzma A, Gangadharan P, Wang LS, Romero K, Arneric SP, Redolfi A et al (2017) Apolipoprotein E genotype and sex risk factors for Alzheimer disease: a meta-analysis. JAMA Neurol 74:1178–1189. https://doi.org/10.1001/jamaneurol.2017.2188

Nordstrom A, Hadrevi J, Olsson T, Franks PW, Nordstrom P (2016) Higher prevalence of type 2 diabetes in men than in women is associated with differences in visceral fat mass. J Clin Endocrinol Metab 101:3740–3746. https://doi.org/10.1210/jc.2016-1915

Orsini CA, Brown TE, Hodges TE, Alonso-Caraballo Y, Winstanley CA, Becker JB (2022) Neural mechanisms mediating sex differences in motivation for reward: cognitive bias, food, gambling, and drugs of abuse. J Neurosci 42:8477–8487. https://doi.org/10.1523/JNEUROSCI.1378-22.2022

Ott A, Breteler MM, van Harskamp F, Stijnen T, Hofman A (1998) Incidence and risk of dementia. The Rotterdam Study. Am J Epidemiol 147:574–580. https://doi.org/10.1093/oxfordjournals.aje.a009489

Qiu T, Xie F, Zeng Q, Shen Z, Du G, Xu X, Wang C, Li X, Luo X, Li K et al (2022) Interactions between cigarette smoking and cognitive status on functional connectivity of the cortico-striatal circuits in individuals without dementia: a resting-state functional MRI study. CNS Neurosci Ther 28:1195–1204. https://doi.org/10.1111/cns.13852

Rajan KB, Weuve J, Barnes LL, McAninch EA, Wilson RS, Evans DA (2021) Population estimate of people with clinical Alzheimer's disease and mild cognitive impairment in the United States (2020-2060). Alzheimers Dement 17:1966–1975. https://doi.org/10.1002/alz.12362

Rempe RG, Hartz AMS, Bauer B (2016) Matrix metalloproteinases in the brain and blood-brain barrier: versatile breakers and makers. J Cereb Blood Flow Metab 36:1481–1507. https://doi.org/10.1177/0271678X16655551

Rocca WA, Cha RH, Waring SC, Kokmen E (1998) Incidence of dementia and Alzheimer's disease: a reanalysis of data from Rochester, Minnesota, 1975-1984. Am J Epidemiol 148:51–62. https://doi.org/10.1093/oxfordjournals.aje.a009560

Rosario ER, Carroll JC, Oddo S, LaFerla FM, Pike CJ (2006) Androgens regulate the development of neuropathology in a triple transgenic mouse model of Alzheimer's disease. J Neurosci 26:13384–13389. https://doi.org/10.1523/JNEUROSCI.2514-06.2006

Rosario ER, Carroll J, Pike CJ (2010) Testosterone regulation of Alzheimer-like neuropathology in male 3xTg-AD mice involves both estrogen and androgen pathways. Brain Res 1359:281–290. https://doi.org/10.1016/j.brainres.2010.08.068

Rosenbloom M, Barclay TR, Kashyap B, Hage L, O'Keefe LR, Svitak A, Pyle M, Frey W, Hanson LR (2021) A phase II, single-center, randomized, double-blind, placebo-controlled study of the safety and therapeutic efficacy of intranasal Glulisine in amnestic mild cognitive impairment and probable mild Alzheimer's disease. Drugs Aging 38:407–415. https://doi.org/10.1007/s40266-021-00845-7

Ruitenberg A, Ott A, van Swieten JC, Hofman A, Breteler MM (2001) Incidence of dementia: does gender make a difference? Neurobiol Aging 22:575–580. https://doi.org/10.1016/s0197-4580(01)00231-7

Santiago JA, Potashkin JA (2013a) Shared dysregulated pathways lead to Parkinson's disease and diabetes. Trends Mol Med 19:176–186. https://doi.org/10.1016/j.molmed.2013.01.002

Santiago JA, Potashkin JA (2013b) Integrative network analysis unveils convergent molecular pathways in Parkinson's disease and diabetes. PloS One 8:e83940. https://doi.org/10.1371/journal.pone.0083940

Santiago JA, Potashkin JA (2014) System-based approaches to decode the molecular links in Parkinson's disease and diabetes. Neurobiol Dis 72(Pt A):84–91. https://doi.org/10.1016/j.nbd.2014.03.019

Santiago JA, Potashkin JA (2015a) Network-based metaanalysis identifies HNF4A and PTBP1 as longitudinally dynamic biomarkers for Parkinson's disease. Proc Natl Acad Sci U S A 112: 2257–2262. https://doi.org/10.1073/pnas.1423573112

Santiago JA, Potashkin JA (2015b) Blood biomarkers associated with cognitive decline in early stage and drug-naive Parkinson's disease patients. PloS One 10:e0142582. https://doi.org/10.1371/journal.pone.0142582

Santiago JA, Potashkin JA (2021) The impact of disease comorbidities in Alzheimer's disease. Front Aging Neurosci 13:631770. https://doi.org/10.3389/fnagi.2021.631770

Santiago JA, Bottero V, Potashkin JA (2019) Transcriptomic and network analysis highlight the association of diabetes at different stages of Alzheimer's disease. Front Neurosci 13:1273. https://doi.org/10.3389/fnins.2019.01273

Santiago JA, Quinn JP, Potashkin JA (2022) Sex-specific transcriptional rewiring in the brain of Alzheimer's disease patients. Front Aging Neurosci 14:1009368. https://doi.org/10.3389/fnagi.2022.1009368

Schoonenboom NS, Pijnenburg YA, Mulder C, Rosso SM, Van Elk EJ, Van Kamp GJ, Van Swieten JC, Scheltens P (2004) Amyloid beta(1-42) and phosphorylated tau in CSF as markers for early-onset Alzheimer disease. Neurology 62:1580–1584. https://doi.org/10.1212/01.wnl.0000123249.58898.e0

Shumaker SA, Legault C, Kuller L, Rapp SR, Thal L, Lane DS, Fillit H, Stefanick ML, Hendrix SL, Lewis CE et al (2004) Conjugated equine estrogens and incidence of probable dementia and mild cognitive impairment in postmenopausal women: women's health initiative memory study. JAMA 291:2947–2958. https://doi.org/10.1001/jama.291.24.2947

Skup M, Zhu H, Wang Y, Giovanello KS, Lin JA, Shen D, Shi F, Gao W, Lin W, Fan Y et al (2011) Sex differences in grey matter atrophy patterns among AD and aMCI patients: results from ADNI. Neuroimage 56:890–906. https://doi.org/10.1016/j.neuroimage.2011.02.060

Tarawneh R, D'Angelo G, Crimmins D, Herries E, Griest T, Fagan AM, Zipfel GJ, Ladenson JH, Morris JC, Holtzman DM (2016) Diagnostic and prognostic utility of the synaptic marker neurogranin in Alzheimer disease. JAMA Neurol 73:561–571. https://doi.org/10.1001/jamaneurol.2016.0086

Tsiknia AA, Sundermann EE, Reas ET, Edland SD, Brewer JB, Galasko D, Banks SJ, Alzheimer's Disease Neuroimaging Initiative (2022) Sex differences in Alzheimer's disease: plasma MMP-9 and markers of disease severity. Alzheimers Res Ther 14:160. https://doi.org/10.1186/s13195-022-01106-4

Wang X, Wang C, Geng C, Zhao K (2018) LncRNA XIST knockdown attenuates Abeta(25-35)-induced toxicity, oxidative stress, and apoptosis in primary cultured rat hippocampal neurons by targeting miR-132. Int J Clin Exp Pathol 11:3915–3924

Wang X, Broce I, Deters KD, Fan CC, Banks SJ (2022) Identification of sex-specific genetic variants associated with Tau PET. Neurol Genet 8:e200043. https://doi.org/10.1212/NXG.0000000000200043

Warnich L, Drogemoller BI, Pepper MS, Dandara C, Wright GE (2011) Pharmacogenomic research in South Africa: lessons learned and future opportunities in the rainbow nation. Curr Pharmacogenomics Person Med 9:191–207. https://doi.org/10.2174/187569211796957575

Williamson J, Yabluchanskiy A, Mukli P, Wu DH, Sonntag W, Ciro C, Yang Y (2022) Sex differences in brain functional connectivity of hippocampus in mild cognitive impairment. Front Aging Neurosci 14:959394. https://doi.org/10.3389/fnagi.2022.959394

Xiong J, Kang SS, Wang Z, Liu X, Kuo TC, Korkmaz F, Padilla A, Miyashita S, Chan P, Zhang Z et al (2022) FSH blockade improves cognition in mice with Alzheimer's disease. Nature 603: 470–476. https://doi.org/10.1038/s41586-022-04463-0

Yan S, Zheng C, Paranjpe MD, Li Y, Li W, Wang X, Benzinger TLS, Lu J, Zhou Y (2021) Sex modifies APOE epsilon4 dose effect on brain tau deposition in cognitively impaired individuals. Brain 144:3201–3211. https://doi.org/10.1093/brain/awab160

Yang JJ, Keohane LM, Pan X, Qu R, Shu XO, Lipworth LP, Braun K, Steinwandel MD, Dai Q, Shrubsole M et al (2022) Association of Healthy Lifestyles with risk of Alzheimer disease and

related dementias in low-income black and White Americans. Neurology. https://doi.org/10.1212/WNL.0000000000200774
Yoshitake T, Kiyohara Y, Kato I, Ohmura T, Iwamoto H, Nakayama K, Ohmori S, Nomiyama K, Kawano H, Ueda K et al (1995) Incidence and risk factors of vascular dementia and Alzheimer's disease in a defined elderly Japanese population: the Hisayama study. Neurology 45:1161–1168. https://doi.org/10.1212/wnl.45.6.1161
Zamani MR, Allen YS, Owen GP, Gray JA (1997) Nicotine modulates the neurotoxic effect of beta-amyloid protein(25-35) in hippocampal cultures. Neuroreport 8:513–517. https://doi.org/10.1097/00001756-199701200-00027
Zhornitsky S, Chaudhary S, Le TM, Chen Y, Zhang S, Potvin S, Chao HH, van Dyck CH, Li CR (2021) Cognitive dysfunction and cerebral volumetric deficits in individuals with Alzheimer's disease, alcohol use disorder, and dual diagnosis. Psychiatry Res Neuroimaging 317:111380. https://doi.org/10.1016/j.pscychresns.2021.111380
Zissimopoulos JM, Barthold D, Brinton RD, Joyce G (2017) Sex and race differences in the association between statin use and the incidence of Alzheimer disease. JAMA Neurol 74:225–232. https://doi.org/10.1001/jamaneurol.2016.3783

Part III

Diabetes, Metabolic Diseases & Cardiovascular Risk

Gender Differences in Cardiovascular Health: Hormonal Effects on Cardiovascular Risk and Management

Anna Tsirka

Contents

A. Tsirka (✉)
University of Connecticut School of Medicine, Farmington, CT, USA

Connecticut Children's Medical Center, Hartford, CT, USA

St Christopher's Children's Hospital, Drexel University Medical School, Philadelphia, PA, USA
e-mail: Tsirka@uchc.edu; Atsirka@connecticutchildrens.org

S. E. Tsirka, M. Acosta-Martinez (eds.), *Sex and Gender Effects in Pharmacology*, Handbook of Experimental Pharmacology 282,
https://doi.org/10.1007/164_2023_668

Abstract

Cardiovascular disease is the number one cause of death worldwide both in men and women. Significant differences however exist in the age of onset, type of cardiovascular disease (CVD), and treatment response among the genders. These differences are due to both gender societal effects and biological differences from the influence of the hormonal and metabolic milieu in the two sexes.

Estrogens are the main female hormone. They impact signaling in almost every body organ and thus affect cardiovascular risk factors. These result in differential expression of CVD. The differential effect of treatment modalities is only recently being evaluated.

Research is ongoing regarding the pathophysiology of these differences. Our current level of knowledge is described in this chapter.

Keywords

Sex differences in cardiovascular disease · Sex and lipid metabolism · Sex pharmacology in cardiovascular disease · Sex differences in heart failure · Sex hormones and the heart

1 Introduction

It has been known for decades that women are less commonly diagnosed with heart disease than men, as women are somewhat protected from atherosclerosis during their premenopausal years. The age of onset of the first myocardial infarction is estimated as occurring 10 years later in women than in men (Leening et al. 2014). The risk for new onset of cardiovascular disease (CVD) increases dramatically post menopause, however still, women at any given age carry about half the risk of CVD disease than men (Leening et al. 2014). Despite that, the World Health Organization states that cardiovascular disease is the leading cause of death in women worldwide.

Differences in cardiovascular disease among men and women derive from both biological and societal or environmental factors. Gender differences is a general term and may refer to those that could be attributed to socially constructed roles, behaviors, expressions, and identities. In contrast, biological variances among women and men are called sex differences. The fundamental origin of all sex differences in health and disease is conferred by the presence of the sex chromosomes (XX for female and XY for males). Genes on these chromosomes influence expression of other genes, the development of the reproductive organs, and ultimately gonadal production of sex hormones. These result in differential gene expression and function (Garcia et al. 2016) and are frequently reproducible in experimental models. Women carry risk factors for development of cardiovascular disease that are unique to females: they suffer from pregnancy-associated conditions, have diseases that are either absent or very infrequent in males (polycystic ovary syndrome or breast cancer), and go through menopause. They also carry a significantly higher predisposition to autoimmune diseases, which in turn play a role in the development of CVD.

The most common condition that leads to cardiac death and CVD is atherosclerosis, the development of plaque in the blood vessels. There is an intricate link between atherosclerosis and circulating lipids that has been known to science for over a century. In 1910, German chemist Adolf Windaus showed that atheromatous lesions in the diseased aorta contained 6 times as much free cholesterol and 20 times as much esterified cholesterol as the wall of normal aortas. Soon after, in 1913, Nikolai Anichkov showed that cholesterol was the cause of the atheromatous changes in the vascular wall (Nicholls 2019). Since then over a century of research has solidly established the role of both endogenous and exogenous cholesterol on atherosclerosis.

Cholesterol is an essential component of higher eukaryotic membranes and plays an important role in cell membrane organization, dynamics, and function. It is the end product of a long, multi-step, sterol biosynthetic pathway involving more than 20 enzymes (Cerqueira et al. 2016) (Fig. 1). Its biosynthesis and degradation depend on a very fine-tuned feedback network (Singh et al. 2013). Cholesterol is insoluble in plasma and thus, transported by lipoproteins, which consist of a hydrophobic core, containing mainly cholesteryl esters and triglycerides, and a hydrophilic coat consisting of phospholipids, free cholesterol, and apolipoproteins. The major cholesterol-carrying lipoproteins are low-density lipoprotein (LDL) and high-density lipoprotein (HDL). An imbalance in cholesterol or lipoprotein metabolism can lead to atherosclerosis and endothelial dysfunction, resulting in cardiovascular disease.

Sex-steroid hormones and their receptors are critical determinants of cardiovascular gender differences. Sex hormones are synthesized from cholesterol. Cholesterol is first converted into progestogens, followed by production of androgens and subsequently estrogens (Fig. 1). It is essential when considering expression of various cardiovascular diseases to recall that: (1) receptors for the sex steroids are present in most tissue of the body, but their relative expression may vary; (2) estrogen is a metabolic product of testosterone, thus both testosterone and estrogen are present in men and women but in different proportions; (3) concentrations of the sex steroids vary across the life span.

2 Mechanisms of Sex Hormone Signaling on Lipid Metabolism

2.1 Estrogens in Lipid Metabolism

Estrogens are lipophilic steroid hormones mostly made in the ovaries that regulate female differentiation. They carry a number of effects on cardiovascular function and disease. Estrogens affect vascular function, the inflammatory response, metabolism, insulin sensitivity, cardiac myocyte and stem cell survival, and the development of hypertrophy. They are thought to be circulating in the plasma and passively

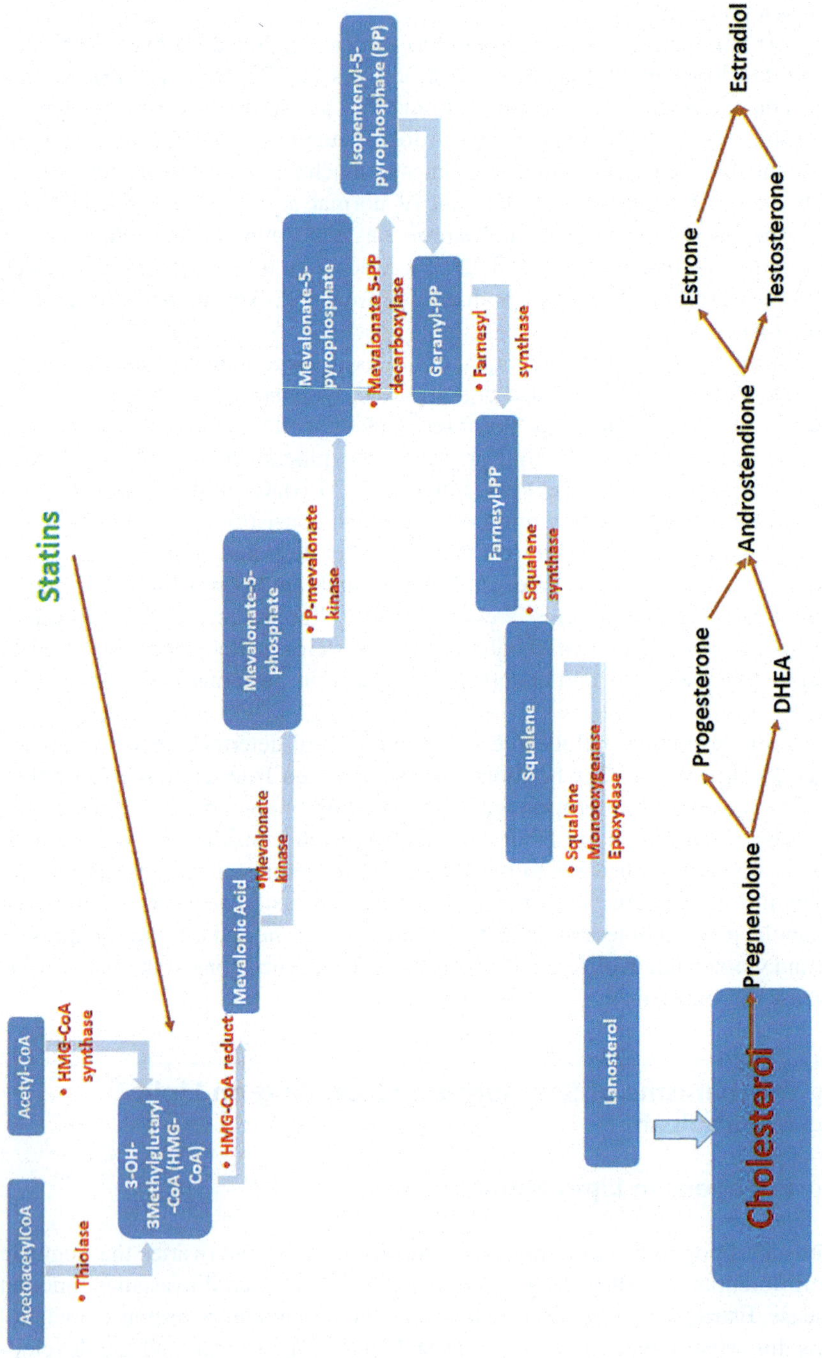

Fig. 1 The biosynthesis of cholesterol involves multiple enzymatic steps that are subject to biofeedback

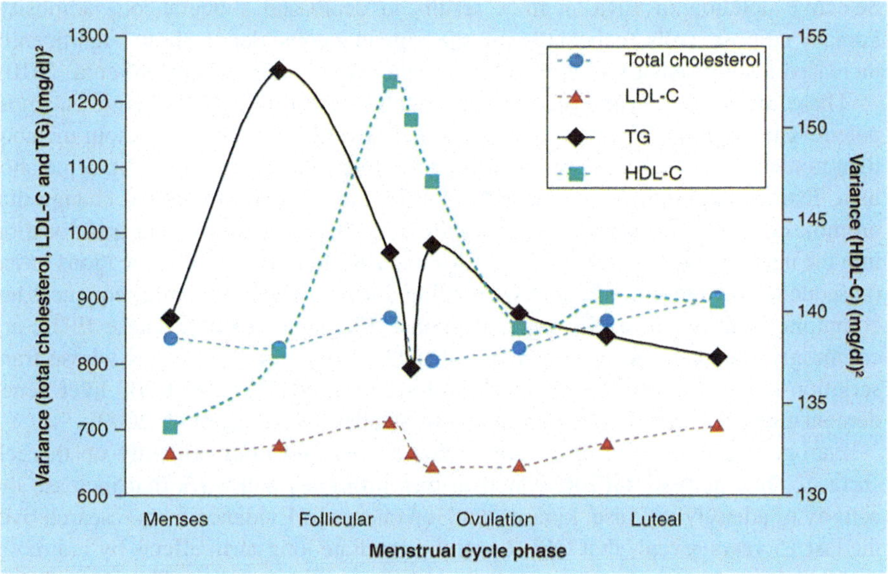

Fig. 2 Variation of cholesterol, LDL, HDL, and triglycerides during the menstrual cycle (figure from Memford et al. (2011))

pass through the cell membrane into the cytoplasm and the cell nucleus. In the nucleus, estrogens bind to activate nuclear receptors which can alter gene transcription in the nucleus or acutely activate kinase signaling in the cytosol (Murphy 2011). Many of these effects are mediated via the estrogen receptors (ER), ERα and ERβ, as well as the more recently recognized G-protein coupled Estrogen Receptor (GPER) (Palmisano et al. 2018). Following estrogen binding, the ER undergoes a conformational change, which facilitates chromatin binding and the modulation of estrogen responsive gene expression.

Menopause is characterized by low estrogen levels and subsequently heralds the onset of low levels of high-density lipoprotein cholesterol, high levels of total cholesterol, low-density lipoprotein cholesterol, very-low-density lipoprotein cholesterol (VLDL), triglycerides (TG), and lipoprotein(a) (Lp(a)), which are strongly predictive of an increasing risk for cardiovascular disease (Fig. 2).

Studies in mice have revealed variation in lipid metabolism during the different phases of the menstrual cycle (Palmisano et al. 2017). In addition, studies in humans have revealed variation in the levels of total cholesterol, triglycerides, and lipoproteins during the menstrual cycle, giving further evidence that estrogens play a major role in lipid metabolism (Zhang et al. 2011; Villa et al. 2012).

A key component of gender differences in lipid metabolism lies in the different body fat distribution among males and females. Visceral adiposity, as measured by the waist to hip ratio, increases the risk of CVD. Estrogens promote subcutaneous adipose storage, while testosterone promotes visceral adipose tissue storage.

Selective deletion of ERα in mice results in decreased subcutaneous adiposity. Female adipose cells, especially of the subcutaneous depot show significantly increased insulin sensitivity compared to male adipose cells (Mumford et al. 2010).

There are several types of estrogens, with 17β-estradiol (E2) being the most potent. They regulate signaling pathways that govern lipid and lipoprotein metabolism in many tissues, most prominently in the liver, the major site of lipid metabolism. Estrogens binding to either ERα or ERβ cause a conformational change that promotes dissociation from Heat Shock Protein 90, dimerization, and translocation into the nucleus. Once in the nucleus, ERα and ERβ bind to genomic locations based on sequence recognition of the DNA binding domain. These genomic sequences are commonly referred to as Estrogen Response Elements (EREs). These EREs are commonly found in the promoter or enhancer regions of liver genes whose transcription is regulated by estrogens (Mumford et al. 2011). Over 1,000 liver genes demonstrate differential gene expression by gender (Macotela et al. 2009).

Estrogens can also act on receptors that are located predominantly on the cell surface. They activate GPER, which in turn promotes pathways that increase the activity of adenylyl cyclase, kinases, and ion channels. Evidence from research over the last 15 years reveals that GPER can also mediate long-term effects by indirectly regulating expression of target genes, secondary to rapid signaling. Therefore, GPER is a novel estrogen receptor that mediates both rapid and genomic responses.

2.2 Testosterone in Lipid Metabolism

Testosterone is the main male sex hormone. Its role in cardiovascular disease is of high debate. Observational studies to investigate the association between circulating testosterone concentrations and cardiovascular disease (CVD) risk have yielded inconsistent findings. Several studies have reported an inverse association between endogenous testosterone levels and adverse CVD outcomes, independent of traditional risk factors. In contrast, testosterone therapy has been associated with increased mortality of CVD. Over the last decade, evidence is mounting that testosterone deficiency is associated with increased risk of coronary artery disease in multiple cohort studies, however it remains unclear whether this is a causal relationship or due to low testosterone level being a biomarker of poor overall health (Elagizi et al. 2018).

Ongoing research efforts have been focused on better understanding the mechanisms by which testosterone may influence lipid metabolism. Lower endogenous testosterone levels are associated with a pro-atherogenic lipid profile. A positive correlation exists between HDL and circulating testosterone concentrations, while there is an inverse relationship between testosterone levels and both plasma triglycerides and LDL (Mäkinen et al. 2008).

Testosterone affects lipid metabolism through effects on gene transcription via the androgen receptor (AR). Similarly to estrogen, testosterone bound to AR enters the nucleus and regulates gene transcription by recognizing Androgen Response elements (AREs) of target genes. Mice with a global AR knockout (ARKO) had increased adiposity, plasma cholesterol, and triglycerides relative to controls. This data suggests that AR signaling reduces atherosclerosis. While the signaling mechanisms of estrogen on lipid metabolism have been studied extensively, the effects of androgens are much less well understood (Fagman et al. 2015).

3 Mechanisms of Sex Hormone Signaling on Endothelial Function

The normal vascular endothelium is effectively one cell layer that separates the blood and vascular smooth muscle. The normal vascular endothelium regulates arterial tone, platelet and leukocyte interactions, coagulation, fibrinolysis, and vascular growth. Measurement of endothelial function in the systemic arteries has become established as an important method for the detection of early arterial abnormalities in humans. The endothelium responds to physical and chemical stimuli via the synthesis and release of regulatory substances affecting vascular tone and growth, thrombosis, and thrombolysis. Such substances include nitric oxide (NO), prostacyclins, and the endothelium-derived relaxing factor (EDRF).

NO synthesis and EDRF are increased by estrogen. Estradiol binds to ER α or β activating the phosphoinositide-3-kinase/protein kinase B pathway, leading to increased eNOS activity and production of NO (Duckles and Miller 2010). It is postulated that endothelial inflammation and microvascular dysfunction may be the common link among heart failure syndromes that present most commonly in women.

The effect of testosterone on endothelial function is not well understood and may be bimodal. Several studies suggest that low testosterone levels are associated with endothelial dysfunction. Conversely however, administration of supra-physiologic doses of testosterone to rats caused endothelial dysfunction in the aorta (Kataoka et al. 2022).

4 Hormone Therapy and Cardiovascular Disease

The decreased risk of developing CVD in premenopausal women is attributed to the high levels of estrogen during the menstruating period in a woman's life. Conversely, it has been suggested that metabolic changes due to estrogen depletion after menopause lead to an increased CVD risk in postmenopausal women.

Menopausal hormone therapy (MHT) was suggested as a means to reduce CVD risk based on the hypothesis of cardioprotection by estrogen. Many randomized controlled trials (RCTs) and observational studies investigated the association between MHT and CVD risk. The Women's Health Initiative Trial was the first large-scale one that sought to evaluate this hypothesis (Manson et al. 2017). The trial randomized postmenopausal women into groups – taking conjugated equine estrogens (CEE) plus medroxyprogesterone acetate (MPA), CEE alone, or placebo. Among postmenopausal women, hormone therapy with CEE plus MPA versus placebo for a median of 5.6 years or with CEE alone versus placebo for a median of 7.2 years was not associated with risk of all-cause, cardiovascular, or cancer mortality during a cumulative follow-up of 18 years. However, when morbidity and not mortality was considered, the CEE plus MPA versus placebo trial revealed a higher risk of stroke, myocardial infarction, and venous thromboembolism, while the CEE versus placebo trial was also terminated early due to increased risk for stroke. After discontinuation of the intervention phase, the risk returned to baseline.

The Women's Health Initiative trial enrolled mostly older women. This led to the hypothesis that MHT initiated closer to the time of estrogen depletion may reduce the progression of atherosclerosis. This, in turn, led to multiple trials that evaluated this timing hypothesis. While several of the studies revealed decrease in atherosclerosis in the early menopausal treatment groups, unfortunately, the results have been controversial, at best. A meta-analysis of all observational and randomized clinical trials of MHT (Kim et al. 2020) did not find any effect of MHT on all-cause death or cardiovascular death. Contrary to the expectations, RCTs and observational studies both showed that MHT was associated with an increased risk of venous thromboembolism and pulmonary embolism, and RCTs revealed an increased risk of stroke among those administered MHT. The general conclusions are that established atherosclerotic CVD is a contra-indication to MHT, the only clear indication for MHT is in the clinical situation of premature menopause, and in the absence of contraindications, MHT can be used if administered early primarily for menopausal symptom relief.

Oral contraceptives (OC) are another form of exogenous hormone therapy frequently used in otherwise healthy, young, premenopausal women. Several studies of the first or second generation oral contraceptive use found an increase in the risk for thromboembolism and myocardial infarction with the use of oral contraception. More recent large-scale studies using third generation OC have not found such an association (Lam et al. 2019). A prospective study from Sweden followed 48,321 women age 30 to 49 years over an average of 11 years. When adjusted for age as well as cardiac risk factors such as hypertension, smoking status, and diabetes, the study found no increased risk of MI in both former and current users of OCs (Margolis et al. 2007). Interestingly however, the concomitant presence of other risk factors for CVD (such as smoking, diabetes, or hypertension) increases the risk for myocardial infarction or thromboembolism even in those on third generation contraception.

It is theorized that the endogenous, cyclic estrogen and progesterone have a differential effect than exogenous formulations.

5 Gender and Hypertension

Hypertension is the leading modifiable risk factor for the development of cardiovascular disease (CVD) and mortality. It is much less common in females in the premenopausal years, while by the age of 60, the prevalence of hypertension is similar in both genders (Connelly et al. 2022). Interestingly however, women develop heart failure and cardiovascular disease at lower levels of blood pressure than men. The incremental increase in the risk of development of CVD is higher in

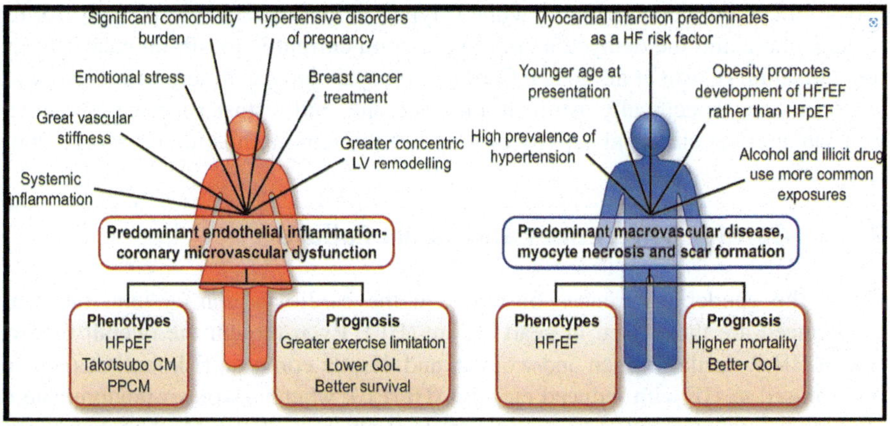

Fig. 3 Sex differeces in heart failure (copyright from Lam CSP et al. (2019))

women than in men (Connelly et al. 2022). These differences arise from a combination of biological and psychosocial mediated factors.

The effect of sex on hypertension is complex and insufficiently understood. It appears to involve numerous systems, a main component being the renin angiotensin aldosterone system (RAAS).

In females, plasma renin fluctuates with the menstrual cycle. Chidambaram et al. found that renin and aldosterone levels are increased in the luteal phase of the cycle compared to the follicular phase (Chidambaram et al. 2002). It has also been demonstrated that the vasodilatory effects of angiotensin are more potent in females and are believed to be modulated by estrogen, as the response becomes less robust in postmenopausal females. Therefore, in females the RAAS is influenced significantly by estrogen status.

In experimental models, androgens stimulate the RAAS system while estrogens reduce plasma renin activity, angiotensin converting enzyme activity, and aldosterone levels (Kalibala et al. 2020).

The reason why hypertension is a more potent risk factor for CVD in females than in males is not well understood. It is believed that lower treatment thresholds may be necessary for women compared to men and that societal disparities may play a role as well (Fig. 3).

6 Sex and Arrhythmogenesis

Biologic sex is an independent risk factor for some types of cardiac arrhythmias. For example, males have a greater prevalence of atrial fibrillation and the Brugada syndrome. In contrast, females are at increased risk for the Long QT syndrome. Cardiac repolarization and depolarization depend on the action of voltage-gated channels. In the myocardium, the rapidly activating sodium channel is the principal driver for cellular depolarization, while L-type calcium current is responsible for the plateau phase and the delayed rectifier potassium current is mostly in charge of the repolarization (Costa et al. 2021). Cardiac myocytes have a variety of receptors for sex hormones, specifically estrogen, progesterone, and testosterone, whose activation can alter the electrical activity of the heart through modulation of ion channels.

7 Gender Differences and Heart Failure

Of all the gender differences observed in the cardiovascular system, the most pronounced are those seen in heart failure (HF). Even though the overall lifetime risk of HF is similar in men and women, and despite common risk factors, men are predisposed to HF with reduced ejection (HFrEF), whereas women predominate in HF with preserved ejection fraction (HFpEF) (Lam et al. 2019). Most epidemiologic studies have revealed that men carry an almost two-fold higher risk than women for HFrEF but not for HFpEF, while in contrast, women have an almost two-fold risk of HFpEF. The presence of cardiovascular risk factors affects the cardiovascular health of women differently than men. Diabetes is a more potent risk factor for the development of HF in women than in men (five-fold increase in risk in women vs. two-fold in men). Similarly, obesity is a stronger risk factor for the development of HFpEF than HFrEF, and to a more pronounced extent in women than in men. This relationship is modified by sex, where women are more likely to develop HFpEF compared to HFrEF if obese, compared to men (Lam et al. 2019).

The contribution of hormonal and reproductive factors to HF risk is still incompletely understood. Peripartum cardiomyopathy presents as a potentially life-threatening condition in the last month of pregnancy or in the months following delivery in women without other known causes of HF. It is unclear if the heart failure in peripartum cardiomyopathy is the result of the hormonal milieu of pregnancy versus an immune reaction, or pure volume load in predisposed individuals.

In human cardiomyocytes, estrogens exert anti-hypertrophic effects mediated by myocyte-enriched calcineurin-interacting protein, histone deacetylases, and natriuretic peptide precursor A (Willemars et al. 2022). Additionally, they improve mitochondrial efficiency, by increasing ATP synthesis. They exert antiapoptotic effects on cardiomyocytes (Willemars et al. 2022). In addition, estrogens promote nitric oxide synthesis, therefore increasing vasodilation (Duckles and Miller 2010).

Testosterone also acts directly on cardiac cells. Testosterone binds to androgen receptors and regulated intracellular calcium homeostasis, increasing contractility.

As heart failure is seen more frequently in some conditions of hormonal abnormalities, conversely, sex hormone levels may be altered by the presence of heart failure. In fact, several studies have found that the levels of anabolic steroids/androgens in the blood are decreased in men with heart failure, and testosterone levels are inversely associated with mortality in men. Testosterone supplementation however was not associated with improvement in symptoms of heart failure, exercise capacity, or mortality in either sex (Tao et al. 2020).

In summary, the effect of sex hormones on the cardiovascular system is multifaceted and complex. Sex hormones influence atherogenesis and coronary artery

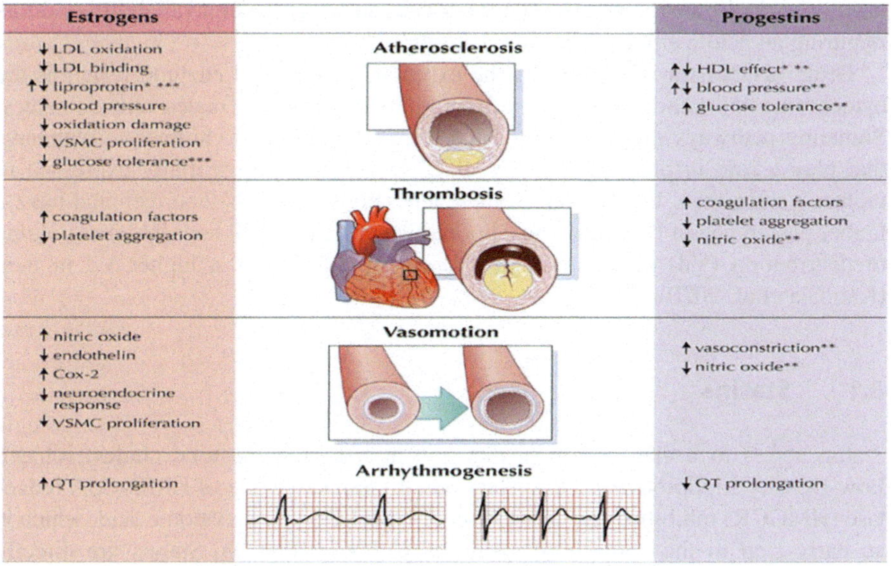

Fig. 4 Impact of exogenous hormones on mechanisms of cardiovascular disease (copyright from Shufelt and Bairey Merz (2009))

disease, endothelial function, thrombogenesis, and the cardiac electrical cycle, as shown in Fig. 4 (Shufelt and Bairey Merz 2009).

8 Gender Differences in the Effects of Cardiovascular Pharmacotherapy

For a long time, the risk of CVD in women was underestimated. Although considerable progress has been made over the last two decades, the effects of cardiovascular pharmacotherapy on women are still frequently understudied, and women often remain undertreated. A recent study in a large population sample of American adults found that women were less likely to receive preventive treatments and were treated less aggressively with guideline-recommended medication than men at similar cardiovascular risk. They are also less adherent to their medication regimen (Chou et al. 2007).

Pharmacokinetics of medications differ among genders. There are important differences in body composition, with women having significantly lower weight and height, a higher proportion of body fat, and a lower peripheral distribution volume. These result in lower glomerular and hepatic filtration rate, which can slow down drug clearance and further elevates plasma concentrations. In addition, women are believed to have a higher gastric pH, slower gastric emptying, and a longer total gastrointestinal transit time. These differences can affect the bioavailability of drugs requiring an acidic environment for absorption.

Drug metabolism is affected by the expression of several enzymes, such as the cytochrome 450 family, which are differentially expressed in males versus females. Signaling pathways that involve the RAAS, adrenergic and cholinergic pathways that play a role in pharmacotherapy of CVD are also differentially expressed in women versus men. In addition, women generally weigh less than men and have a higher percentage of body fat. Thus, lipophilic substances will have a higher volume of distribution (Vd) in women and hydrophilic substances a higher Vd in men (Kalibala et al. 2020).

8.1 Statins

Statins refers to a class of drugs that aim at lowering the total cholesterol and Low-Density Lipoprotein (LDL). They bind to the active site of HMG-CoA reductase (HMGCR) inhibiting the conversion of HMG-CoA to mevalonic acid, which is an early step in the cholesterol synthesis pathway (Fig. 1). Statins are directly absorbed by the intestines. Several statins, such as simvastatin, atorvastatin, and lovastatin, are partially metabolized by CYP3A4/5 enzymes within the intestinal cell. Statins are then transported through the portal bloodstream and into hepatocytes. As estrogens are metabolized in the liver, it is conceivable that statins may result in differential effect in males versus females.

Statins are widely used worldwide and have been found to have effects on multiple organ systems and functions. Until recently, many of the statin trials predominantly involved men with the results extrapolated to women and without regard to potential interactions of the drugs with sex-steroid action or metabolism. Plasma concentrations of statins are generally 15–20% higher in women than in men.

Data from a national database in the Netherlands, looking at gender differences in the response to statins revealed that statins resulted in significantly increased HDL level in women compared to men, however the differences in the mean percentage change of total cholesterol, LDL, and triglycerides from baseline between the sexes were not statistically significant. The proportion of men and women who attained the LDL treatment target was similar, only 37% for both groups (Hunt et al. 2022). Despite the bigger increase in levels of HDL in women, a meta-analysis of clinical trials did not reveal any reduction in the risk from CVD in women using statins, while other trials revealed similar decrease in CVD in men and women using statins (Petretta et al. 2010; Downs et al. 1998).

Regarding the side effects of statins in women versus men, studies have shown a statistically significant increase in myalgia, transaminases, and new onset diabetes in women taking statins, the differences however were very small and not clinically significant.

8.2 Angiotensin Converting Enzyme (ACE) Inhibitors and Angiotensin Receptor Blockers (ARB)

ACE inhibitors and ARBs are the most commonly used medications in CVD. They target the RAAS and are used both for treatment of hypertension and for management of cardiac dysfunction and heart failure. Both drug classes reduce systemic BP, risk of stroke and improve heart failure outcomes. Sex-specific data are limited.

A small pharmacologic study in healthy volunteers found no sex differences in the pharmacokinetics of enalapril (Zapater et al. 2004). Women however had lower ACE inhibition than men at low doses of the medication, while the inhibition was equivalent at higher doses. Pharmacologic studies on ARBs did not reveal differential pharmacokinetics or pharmacodynamics by sex (Cabaleiro et al. 2013).

In terms of the clinical effect of those medications, there is very limited data. The CALIBREX trial found that both drug classes reduce systemic BP equally in men and women, however postmenopausal women had significant improvement in arterial stiffness with an ACE inhibitor, but not with an ARB, while no change in arterial stiffness was observed among men with either agent (Rogers et al. 2022). These findings may partially be explained by the observations that a loss of estrogen in the postmenopausal period increases angiotensin-1 receptor expression and angiotensin II levels and may make ARBs less effective in postmenopausal women.

8.3 Digoxin

Digoxin is a cardiac glycoside that has been used in heart failure for many decades. Women have higher serum digoxin concentrations due to reduced volume of distributions and lower drug clearance. The Digoxin Investigation Group trial was not specifically designed to evaluate sex differences. A post-trial analysis of subgroups however found that digoxin therapy was associated with a small, non-significant reduction in the risk of death from any cause among and a significantly increased risk of death from any cause among women. It is therefore recommended that women receive lower doses to achieve pharmacologic benefit without risk of adverse reactions (Rathore et al. 2002).

8.4 Beta-Blockers

The cardiovascular system is controlled and regulated by the noradrenergic system. Premenopausal women have lower sympathetic nerve activity than age-matched men and also appear to be less sensitive to sympathetic vasoconstrictor activity. Beta adrenergic blockade is considered one of the cornerstones of treatment of heart failure both with reduced and preserved ejection fraction.

While women were underrepresented in the large trials of beta blockade in heart failure, it appears that the survival benefit is similar in women and men. However, optimal doses for beta-blockers are lower in women than in men. The BIOSTAT

European study in Chronic HF found that women with HFrEF needed lower doses of beta-blockers men for optimal effects and increasing the doses further did not improve the outcomes. This may be explained by sex differences in the pharmacokinetics of beta-blockers. Metoprolol and propranolol are primarily metabolized by liver cytochrome CYP2D6 which has a lower activity in women than in men (Santema et al. 2019).

8.5 Calcium Channel Blockers

Calcium channel antagonists are used in cardiology for several indications, including hypertension, arrhythmias, pulmonary hypertension, and hypertrophic cardiomyopathy. Pharmacokinetic sex differences are common with calcium channel blockers due to the higher activity of CYP3A4 or lower activity of P-glycoprotein in females. In addition, the Amlodipine Cardiovascular Community Trial Study Group found a greater BP response to amlodipine in women versus men, along with higher incidence of edema as a side effect (Kloner et al. 1996).

8.6 Mineralocorticoid Receptor Antagonists (MRA)

Current guidelines recommend the use of mineralocorticoid receptor antagonists in patients with symptomatic heart failure and left ventricular dysfunction. As all of the large trials using MRA were underpowered to evaluate sex differences in the pharmacologic response, a pooled meta-analysis assessed the sex-specific responses to MRA treatment in individuals with heart failure (Rossello et al. 2020). MRA consistently reduced the risk for cardiovascular death and HF hospitalization without any evidence of interaction between treatment effect and sex. In addition, there was no sex-specific impact of MRA on hyperkalemia, worsening renal function or other adverse effects.

8.7 Angiotensin Receptor/Neprilysin Inhibitors (ARNI)

The combination of sacubitril and valsartan is a newer medication that combines an ARB with neprilysin inhibition. The exact mechanism underlying the therapeutic benefit of neprilysin inhibition is not well understood. It appears that sacubitril causes vasodilation, decreased sympathetic and increased parasympathetic system activity, as well as natriuresis. Several large clinical trials have shown evidence of decreased mortality and improved quality of life in heart failure patients both with reduced and preserved ejection fraction (McMurray et al. 2014; Solomon et al. 2019) to the point that nowadays ARNIs are the first-line medications in the management of heart failure.

The pharmacokinetics of sacubitril-valsartan and its metabolites do not differ in women versus men. Comparison of treatment effect in women versus men with

HFrEF did not reveal any differential effect on morbidity, mortality, or adverse events (Nuechterlein et al. 2021). In fact, women with HFrEF treated with ARNI had similar all-cause mortality, CV mortality, hyperkalemia, and hypotension as men with HFrEF treated with sacubitril-valsartan. In contrast, in the PARAGON-HF trial of HFpEF, sex appeared to modify the effect of sacubitril-valsartan on heart failure hospitalizations and cardiovascular death, with a more favorable treatment effect in women than in men (rate ratio, 0.73 [95% CI, 0.59–0.90] in women; 1.03 [95% CI, 0.84–1.25] in men; P interaction = 0.017) (McMurray et al. 2020). The pathophysiological mechanism of this difference is not well understood. Sex hormones play a role in natriuretic peptide physiology. It is possible that by augmenting natriuretic peptides, sacubitril-valsartan may be of greater benefit in women than in men, if women are viewed as having deficient cGMP-protein kinase G signaling. Further studies are needed in order to understand the molecular mechanisms implicated in the differential action of ARNI.

9 Conclusion

In summary, sex plays a significant role in every aspect of CVD, from epidemiology and risk factors to pathophysiology, response to therapy, and outcomes. Sex modifies the association of several traditional risk factors with development of coronary artery disease, atherosclerosis, and heart failure. Pharmacokinetics and pharmacodynamics differ significantly among women and men. Despite that, till very recently, there was a paucity of women recruited to clinical trials and thus treatment guidelines are predominantly based on male-derived data. Large gaps in knowledge exist in sex-specific mechanisms, optimal drug doses for women with CVD. It is imperative the research community commits to performing robust sex-specific translational and clinical trials powered to perform sex-disaggregated analyses and thus report on sex-specific outcomes and efficacy.

References

Cabaleiro T, Román M, Ochoa D, Talegón M, Prieto-Pérez R, Wojnicz A, López-Rodríguez R, Novalbos J, Abad-Santos F (2013) Evaluation of the relationship between sex, polymorphisms in CYP2C8 and CYP2C9, and pharmacokinetics of angiotensin receptor blockers. Drug Metab Dispos 41(1):224–229. https://doi.org/10.1124/dmd.112.046292

Cerqueira NM, Oliveira EF, Gesto DS, Santos-Martins D, Moreira C, Moorthy HN, Ramos MJ, Fernandes PA (2016) Cholesterol biosynthesis: a mechanistic overview. Biochemistry 55(39): 5483–5506. https://doi.org/10.1021/acs.biochem.6b00342

Chidambaram M, Duncan JA, Lai VS, Cattran DC, Floras JS, Scholey JW, Miller JA (2002) Variation in the renin angiotensin system throughout the normal menstrual cycle. J Am Soc Nephrol 13(2):446–452. https://doi.org/10.1681/ASN.V132446

Chou AF, Scholle SH, Weisman CS, Bierman AS, Correa-de-Araujo R, Mosca L (2007) Gender disparities in the quality of cardiovascular disease care in private managed care plans. Womens Health Issues 17(3):120–130. https://doi.org/10.1016/j.whi.2007.03.002

Connelly PJ, Currie G, Delles C (2022) Sex differences in the prevalence, outcomes and management of hypertension. Curr Hypertens Rep 24(6):185–192. https://doi.org/10.1007/s11906-022-01183-8

Costa S, Saguner AM, Gasperetti A, Akdis D, Brunckhorst C, Duru F (2021) The link between sex hormones and susceptibility to cardiac arrhythmias: from molecular basis to clinical implications. Front Cardiovasc Med 8:644279. https://doi.org/10.3389/fcvm.2021.644279

Downs JR, Clearfield M, Weis S, Whitney E, Shapiro DR, Beere PA, Langendorfer A, Stein EA, Kruyer W, Gotto AM Jr (1998) Primary prevention of acute coronary events with lovastatin in men and women with average cholesterol levels: results of AFCAPS/TexCAPS. Air force/Texas coronary atherosclerosis prevention study. JAMA 279(20):1615–1622. https://doi.org/10.1001/jama.279.20.1615

Duckles SP, Miller VM (2010) Hormonal modulation of endothelial NO production. Pflugers Arch 459(6):841–851. https://doi.org/10.1007/s00424-010-0797-1

Elagizi A, Köhler TS, Lavie CJ (2018) Testosterone and cardiovascular health. Mayo Clin Proc 93(1):83–100. https://doi.org/10.1016/j.mayocp.2017.11.006

Fagman JB, Wilhelmson AS, Motta BM, Pirazzi C, Alexanderson C, De Gendt K, Verhoeven G, Holmäng A, Anesten F, Jansson JO, Levin M, Borén J, Ohlsson C, Krettek A, Romeo S, Tivesten Å (2015) The androgen receptor confers protection against diet-induced atherosclerosis, obesity, and dyslipidemia in female mice. FASEB J 29(4):1540–1550. https://doi.org/10.1096/fj.14-259234

Garcia M, Mulvagh SL, Merz CN, Buring JE, Manson JE (2016) Cardiovascular disease in women: clinical perspectives. Circ Res 118(8):1273–1293. https://doi.org/10.1161/CIRCRESAHA.116.307547

Hunt NB, Emmens JE, Irawati S, de Vos S, Bos JHJ, Wilffert B, Hak E, de Boer RA (2022) Sex disparities in the effect of statins on lipid parameters: the PharmLines initiative. Medicine (Baltimore) 101(2):e28394. https://doi.org/10.1097/MD.0000000000028394

Kalibala J, Pechère-Bertschi A, Desmeules J (2020) Gender differences in cardiovascular pharmacotherapy – the example of hypertension: a mini review. Front Pharmacol 11:564. https://doi.org/10.3389/fphar.2020.00564

Kataoka T, Fukamoto A, Hotta Y, Sanagawa A, Maeda Y, Furukawa-Hibi Y, Kimura K (2022) Effect of high testosterone levels on endothelial function in aorta and erectile function in rats. Sex Med 10(5):100550. https://doi.org/10.1016/j.esxm.2022.100550

Kim JE, Chang JH, Jeong MJ et al (2020) A systematic review and meta-analysis of effects of menopausal hormone therapy on cardiovascular diseases. Sci Rep 10:20631. https://doi.org/10.1038/s41598-020-77534-9

Kloner RA, Sowers JR, DiBona GF, Gaffney M, Wein M (1996) Sex- and age-related antihypertensive effects of amlodipine. The amlodipine cardiovascular community trial study group. Am J Cardiol 77(9):713–722. https://doi.org/10.1016/s0002-9149(97)89205-3

Lam CSP, Arnott C, Beale AL, Chandramouli C, Hilfiker-Kleiner D, Kaye DM, Ky B, Santema BT, Sliwa K, Voors AA (2019) Sex differences in heart failure. Eur Heart J 40(47):3859–3868c. https://doi.org/10.1093/eurheartj/ehz835

Leening MJ, Ferket BS, Steyerberg EW, Kavousi M, Deckers JW, Nieboer D, Heeringa J, Portegies ML, Hofman A, Ikram MA, Hunink MG, Franco OH, Stricker BH, Witteman JC, Roos-Hesselink JW (2014) Sex differences in lifetime risk and first manifestation of cardiovascular disease: prospective population based cohort study. BMJ 349:g5992. https://doi.org/10.1136/bmj.g5992

Macotela Y, Boucher J, Tran TT, Kahn CR (2009) Sex and depot differences in adipocyte insulin sensitivity and glucose metabolism. Diabetes 58(4):803–812. https://doi.org/10.2337/db08-1054

Mäkinen JI, Perheentupa A, Irjala K, Pöllänen P, Mäkinen J, Huhtaniemi I, Raitakari OT (2008) Endogenous testosterone and serum lipids in middle-aged men. Atherosclerosis 197(2):688–693. https://doi.org/10.1016/j.atherosclerosis.2007.05.009

Manson JE, Aragaki AK, Rossouw JE et al (2017) Menopausal hormone therapy and long-term all-cause and cause-specific mortality: the women's health initiative randomized trials. JAMA 318(10):927–938. https://doi.org/10.1001/jama.2017.11217

Margolis KL, Adami HO, Luo J, Ye W, Weiderpass E (2007) A prospective study of oral contraceptive use and risk of myocardial infarction among Swedish women. Fertil Steril 88(2):310–316. https://doi.org/10.1016/j.fertnstert.2006.11.206

McMurray JJ, Packer M, Desai AS, Gong J, Lefkowitz MP, Rizkala AR, Rouleau JL, Shi VC, Solomon SD, Swedberg K, Zile MR, PARADIGM-HF Investigators and Committees (2014) Angiotensin-neprilysin inhibition versus enalapril in heart failure. N Engl J Med 371(11): 993–1004. https://doi.org/10.1056/NEJMoa1409077

McMurray JJV, Jackson AM, Lam CSP, Redfield MM, Anand IS, Ge J, Lefkowitz MP, Maggioni AP, Martinez F, Packer M, Pfeffer MA, Pieske B, Rizkala AR, Sabarwal SV, Shah AM, Shah SJ, Shi VC, van Veldhuisen DJ, Zannad F, Zile MR, Cikes M, Goncalvesova E, Katova T, Kosztin A, Lelonek M, Sweitzer N, Vardeny O, Claggett B, Jhund PS, Solomon SD (2020) Effects of Sacubitril-valsartan versus valsartan in women compared with men with Heart Failure and Preserved Ejection Fraction: insights from PARAGON-HF. Circulation 141(5):338–351. https://doi.org/10.1161/CIRCULATIONAHA.119.044491

Mumford SL, Schisterman EF, Siega-Riz AM, Browne RW, Gaskins AJ, Trevisan M, Steiner AZ, Daniels JL, Zhang C, Perkins NJ, Wactawski-Wende J (2010) A longitudinal study of serum lipoproteins in relation to endogenous reproductive hormones during the menstrual cycle: findings from the BioCycle study. J Clin Endocrinol Metab 95(9):E80–E85. https://doi.org/10.1210/jc.2010-0109

Mumford SL, Dasharathy S, Pollack AZ, Schisterman EF (2011) Variations in lipid levels according to menstrual cycle phase: clinical implications. Clin Lipidol 6(2):225–234. https://doi.org/10.2217/clp.11.9

Murphy E (2011) Estrogen signaling and cardiovascular disease. Circ Res 109(6):687–696. https://doi.org/10.1161/CIRCRESAHA.110.236687

Nicholls, M. Adolf Otto Reinhold Windaus: German chemist Adolf Otto Reinhold Windaus received the 1928 Nobel prize in chemistry for his contribution to research into the structure of sterols and their connections with vitamins, Eur Heart J, Volume 40, Issue 32, 21 August 2019, Pages 2659–2660, https://doi.org/10.1093/eurheartj/ehz573

Nuechterlein K, AlTurki A, Ni J, Martínez-Sellés M, Martens P, Russo V, Backelin CN, Huynh T (2021) Real-world safety of Sacubitril/valsartan in women and men with Heart Failure and reduced Ejection Fraction: a meta-analysis. CJC Open 3(12 Suppl):S202–S208. https://doi.org/10.1016/j.cjco.2021.09.009

Palmisano BT, Zhu L, Stafford JM (2017) Role of estrogens in the regulation of liver lipid metabolism. Adv Exp Med Biol 1043:227–256. https://doi.org/10.1007/978-3-319-70178-3_12

Palmisano BT, Zhu L, Eckel RH, Stafford JM (2018) Sex differences in lipid and lipoprotein metabolism. Mol Metab 15:45–55. https://doi.org/10.1016/j.molmet.2018.05.008

Petretta M, Costanzo P, Perrone-Filardi P, Chiariello M (2010) Impact of gender in primary prevention of coronary heart disease with statin therapy: a meta-analysis. Int J Cardiol 138(1): 25–31. https://doi.org/10.1016/j.ijcard.2008.08.001

Rathore SS, Wang Y, Krumholz HM (2002) Sex-based differences in the effect of digoxin for the treatment of heart failure. N Engl J Med 347(18):1403–1411. https://doi.org/10.1056/NEJMoa021266

Rogers SC, Ko YA, Quyyumi AA, Hajjar I (2022) Differential sex-specific effects of angiotensin-converting enzyme Inhibition and Angiotensin receptor blocker therapy on arterial function in hypertension: CALIBREX trial. Hypertension 79(10):2316–2327. https://doi.org/10.1161/HYPERTENSIONAHA.122.19105

Rossello X, Ferreira JP, Pocock SJ, McMurray JJV, Solomon SD, Lam CSP, Girerd N, Pitt B, Rossignol P, Zannad F (2020) Sex differences in mineralocorticoid receptor antagonist trials: a pooled analysis of three large clinical trials. Eur J Heart Fail 22(5):834–844. https://doi.org/10.1002/ejhf.1740

Santema BT, Ouwerkerk W, Tromp J, Sama IE, Ravera A, Regitz-Zagrosek V, Hillege H, Samani NJ, Zannad F, Dickstein K, Lang CC, Cleland JG, Ter Maaten JM, Metra M, Anker SD, van der Harst P, Ng LL, van der Meer P, van Veldhuisen DJ, Meyer S, Lam CSP, ASIAN-HF investigators; Voors AA. (2019) Identifying optimal doses of heart failure medications in men compared with women: a prospective, observational, cohort study. Lancet 394(10205): 1254–1263. https://doi.org/10.1016/S0140-6736(19)31792-1

Shufelt CL, Bairey Merz CN (2009) Contraceptive hormone use and cardiovascular disease. J Am Coll Cardiol 53(3):221–231. https://doi.org/10.1016/j.jacc.2008.09.042. Erratum in: J Am Coll Cardiol;53(10):904

Singh P, Saxena R, Srinivas G, Pande G, Chattopadhyay A (2013) Cholesterol biosynthesis and homeostasis in regulation of the cell cycle. PLoS One 8(3):e58833. https://doi.org/10.1371/journal.pone.0058833

Solomon SD, McMurray JJV, Anand IS, Ge J, Lam CSP, Maggioni AP, Martinez F, Packer M, Pfeffer MA, Pieske B, Redfield MM, Rouleau JL, van Veldhuisen DJ, Zannad F, Zile MR, Desai AS, Claggett B, Jhund PS, Boytsov SA, Comin-Colet J, Cleland J, Düngen HD, Goncalvesova E, Katova T, Kerr Saraiva JF, Lelonek M, Merkely B, Senni M, Shah SJ, Zhou J, Rizkala AR, Gong J, Shi VC, Lefkowitz MP, PARAGON-HF Investigators and Committees (2019) Angiotensin-Neprilysin inhibition in heart failure with preserved ejection fraction. N Engl J Med 381(17):1609–1620. https://doi.org/10.1056/NEJMoa1908655

Tao J, Liu X, Bai W (2020) Testosterone supplementation in patients with chronic heart failure: a meta-analysis of randomized controlled trials. Front Endocrinol (Lausanne) 11:110. https://doi.org/10.3389/fendo.2020.00110

Villa A, Della Torre S, Stell A, Cook J, Brown M, Maggi A (2012) Tetradian oscillation of estrogen receptor α is necessary to prevent liver lipid deposition. Proc Natl Acad Sci U S A 109(29): 11806–11811. https://doi.org/10.1073/pnas.1205797109

Willemars MMA, Nabben M, Verdonschot JAJ, Hoes MF (2022) Evaluation of the interaction of sex hormones and cardiovascular function and health. Curr Heart Fail Rep 19(4):200–212. https://doi.org/10.1007/s11897-022-00555-0

Zapater P, Novalbos J, Gallego-Sandín S, Hernández FT, Abad-Santos F (2004) Gender differences in angiotensin-converting enzyme (ACE) activity and inhibition by enalaprilat in healthy volunteers. J Cardiovasc Pharmacol 43(5):737–744. https://doi.org/10.1097/00005344-200405000-00018

Zhang Y, Klein K, Sugathan A, Nassery N, Dombkowski A, Zanger UM, Waxman DJ (2011) Transcriptional profiling of human liver identifies sex-biased genes associated with polygenic dyslipidemia and coronary artery disease. PLoS One 6(8):e23506. https://doi.org/10.1371/journal.pone.0023506

Sex Differences in Glucose Homeostasis

Ebru Arioglu-Inan and Gizem Kayki-Mutlu

Contents

Abstract

Sexual dimorphism has been demonstrated to have an effect on various physiological functions. In this regard, researchers have investigated its impact on glucose homeostasis in both preclinical and clinical studies. Sex differences mainly arise from physiological factors such as sex hormones, body fat and muscle distribution, and sex chromosomes. The sexual dimorphism has also been studied in the context of diabetes. Reflecting the prevalence of the disease among the population, studies focusing on the sex difference in type 1 diabetes (T1D) are not common as the ones in type 2 diabetes (T2D). T1D is reported as the only major specific autoimmune disease that exhibits a male predominance. Clinical studies have demonstrated that impaired fasting glucose is more frequent in men whereas women more commonly exhibit impaired glucose tolerance. Understanding the sex difference in glucose homeostasis becomes more attractive when focusing on the findings that highlight sexual dimorphism on the efficacy or adverse effect profile of antidiabetic medications. Thus, in this chapter, we aimed

E. Arioglu-Inan (✉) · G. Kayki-Mutlu
Department of Pharmacology, Faculty of Pharmacy, Ankara University, Ankara, Turkey
e-mail: arioglu@ankara.edu.tr

S. E. Tsirka, M. Acosta-Martinez (eds.), *Sex and Gender Effects in Pharmacology*,
Handbook of Experimental Pharmacology 282,
https://doi.org/10.1007/164_2023_664

to discuss the impact of sex on the glucose homeostasis both in health and in diabetes.

Keywords

Blood glucose · Diabetes · Insulin · Insulin resistance · Sex difference

1 Overview of the Effects of Sex on Glucose Homeostasis

Both preclinical and clinical studies so far have demonstrated that many physiological systems in the body exhibit a sex-specific pattern. In this regard, researchers have investigated the effect of sexual dimorphism on glucose homeostasis. Many aspects of glucose homeostasis, including fasting blood glucose levels, glucose tolerance, and insulin sensitivity, are modulated differentially between men and women. These parameters have been shown to be influenced by various factors, including sex hormones, body fat and muscle distribution, and sex chromosomes.

It has been reported that men have higher frequency of type 2 diabetes (T2D) (Aregbesola et al. 2017; Wild et al. 2004). Nonetheless, its prevalence is estimated to be same or higher in women when one takes into consideration the longer lifespan of women (Gale and Gillespie 2001; Szalat and Raz 2008). The findings of clinical studies indicate that the fasting glucose levels are impaired (elevated) in men while women exhibit a disrupted glucose tolerance (Glümer et al. 2003; Regitz-Zagrosek et al. 2006; Sicree et al. 2008; Szalat and Raz 2008). The effect of sex hormones on glucose homeostasis has been suggested as a contributing factor to the sex differences in diabetes or insulin resistance (Mauvais-Jarvis 2017).

Understanding sex differences in glucose homeostasis has been of special interest as it may help to optimize therapeutic approaches for the prevention and treatment of diabetes (Tramunt et al. 2020). The finding that insulin naive type 2 diabetic women had smaller improvements in Hemoglobin A1C (HbA1c) and more hypoglycemia highlights the importance of considering sex differences in treatment (Kautzky-Willer et al. 2015). Similarly, Rossi et al. evaluated the data of 415,294 patients from 236 diabetes outpatient centers and indicated that the prevalence of women with an HbA1c value higher than 9% was 14% higher than that of men, despite insulin treatment (Rossi et al. 2013). Furthermore, the proportion of males who reached a target 1-year glycemic response of HbA1c $\leq$ 7% by Glucagon like peptide-1 (GLP-1) agonist exenatide therapy was higher compared to females (Anichini et al. 2013). In addition to its effect on the efficacy of antidiabetic drugs, sexual dimorphism also contributes to the adverse effects seen with these drugs. The incidence of elevated plasma lactate levels was higher in women, pointing to the increased risk of lactic acidosis in this sex (Li et al. 2010). The risk of bone fracture with thiazolidinediones (Kahn et al. 2006) and the incidence of gastrointestinal adverse effects of GLP-1 receptor agonists (Anichini et al. 2013) were also higher in women. Furthermore, Sodium Glucose Cotransporter 2 Inhibitors (SGLT2Is) more commonly cause urinary infections in women (Dave et al. 2019). Based on these findings, sex-based strategies may increase the effectiveness of treatment and reduce the risk of adverse effects in the treatment of diabetes.

2 Regulation of Glucose Homeostasis

The islets of Langerhans in pancreas contain different cell types, including insulin-secreting beta cells, glucagon-secreting alpha cells, somatostatin-secreting delta cells, and pancreatic polypeptide-secreting P (F) cells (Susan 2004). Insulin, a hormone composed of 51 amino acids arranged in A and B chains, is secreted from beta cells of Langerhans islets as a response to elevated blood glucose. Other factors such as amino acids and free fatty acids can also stimulate glucose-induced insulin secretion. Furthermore, several hormones such as GLP-1, estrogen, leptin, growth hormone, and melatonin also have a role in the regulation of insulin secretion (Fu et al. 2013). Glucose is taken up into beta cell through glucose transporter 2 (GLUT2) and is converted to ATP. The increase in ATP levels leads to the closing of ATP-sensitive K+ channels, which in turn depolarizes the membrane. Subsequently, voltage-dependent Ca^{++} channels open, leading to an increase in intracellular Ca^{++} levels in beta cells and results in insulin secretion via exocytosis (Ashcroft and Rorsman 2012).

Insulin secretion exhibits a biphasic pattern, consisting of a transient first phase and a sustained second phase (Kashyap et al. 2003). The readily releasable pool (RRP), that makes up only 1% of insulin granules, enables rapid insulin release in response to glucose (Olofsson et al. 2002). The reserve pool containing 99% of insulin granules refills RRP when it is depleted. Impaired regulation of insulin secretion due to beta cell dysfunction leads to diabetes or hypoglycemia, as insulin is essential for maintaining glucose homeostasis (Seino 2012). It has been reported that the first phase of insulin secretion is lost and the second phase of secretion is characteristically decreased in T2D (Porte 1991). After being secreted, insulin is directed to target tissues such as liver, skeletal muscle, and adipose tissue. In these target tissues, insulin binds to its receptors (IRs) on the membrane. IR is composed of two extracellular alpha units and two membrane spanning beta subunits which have a tyrosine kinase domain (Hubbard 2013). Insulin binds to the alpha subunit, and then the tyrosine kinase becomes activated and phosphorylates insulin receptor substrate (IRS). Thereby, IRS molecules activate two different pathways. The phosphatidylinositol 3-kinase/protein kinase B (PI3K/Akt) pathway regulates the effect of insulin on cellular function and energy metabolism (Haeusler et al. 2018). Activated IRS stimulates PI3K which enables the conversion of phosphatidylinositol 4,5-bisphosphate (PIP2) to phosphatidylinositol 3,4,5-trisphosphate (PIP3) (Ho et al. 2016). PIP3 activates protein kinases such as Akt, which in turn lead to the translocation of glucose transporter GLUT4 to the membrane, allowing glucose to enter the cells (Haeusler et al. 2018). The second pathway, mitogen-activated protein kinase (MAPK) signaling pathway, includes the activation of extracellular signal-regulated kinases 1 and 2 (ERK1 and ERK2), gene expression, protein translation, and cell growth (Niswender 2011).

The effects of insulin on carbohydrate, protein, and lipid metabolism have been well described. The main metabolic effects of insulin can be summarized as follows: stimulation of glycogen synthesis in the liver; adipose tissue and skeletal muscle; inhibition of glycogenolysis and gluconeogenesis in the liver; increased rate of glycolysis in the skeletal muscle and adipose tissue; inhibition of lipolysis in adipose tissue; stimulation of protein synthesis in the liver, adipose tissue, skeletal muscle, and other tissues (Newsholme and Dimitriadis 2001).

3 Sex Differences and Glucose Homeostasis

In recent years, research on sex differences has become increasingly prominent in the medical field. There is a mounting evidence indicating that such differences play crucial roles in a range of physiological and pathological metabolic processes, including glucose homeostasis and insulin secretion.

The term "sex differences" refers to the biological distinctions between males and females, which are driven by different sex hormones, sex-specific organ systems, sex chromosomes, sex-specific gene expressions, fetal/neonatal programming, and epigenetic modifications (Tramunt et al. 2020). The term "sexual dimorphism," originally referring to the morphological differences between males and females, is also increasingly used to describe differences between two sexes. The latest guidelines express the need to consider sex differences throughout the entire period from preclinical to clinical research and to avoid male predominance (Mauvais-Jarvis et al. 2017a).

Almost all aspects of glucose homeostasis, such as fasting blood glucose (FBG), glucose tolerance, and insulin sensitivity, are modulated in a sexually dimorphic manner (Mauvais-Jarvis 2018) (Fig. 1). For example, females generally have lower fasting blood glucose levels than males, but their blood glucose levels after 2-h oral glucose tolerance test (OGTT) remained higher than those of men (Faerch et al. 2010; Horie et al. 2018; Sicree et al. 2008). This may be due to a lower rate of

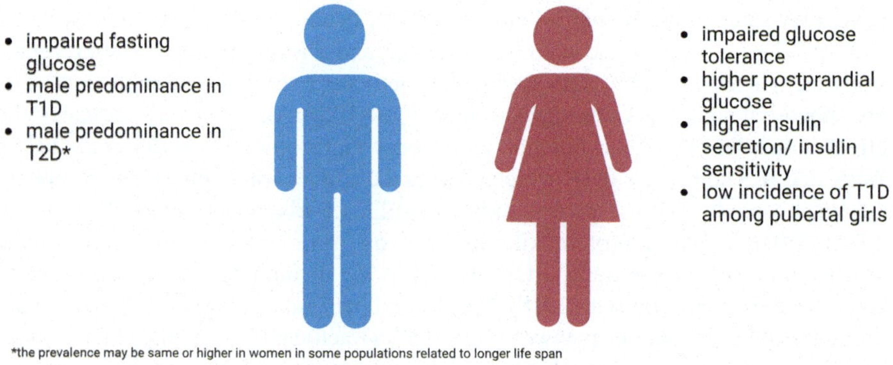

Fig. 1 Sex differences in glucose homeostasis

glucose uptake in women in response to the bolus glucose administration containing fixed glucose concentration during OGTT, which could be attributed to differences in body fat content and height. In fact, studies conducted in mice receiving glucose based on their body weight revealed that females exhibit improved glucose tolerance and insulin sensitivity (Macotela et al. 2009). Thus, measuring FPG and HbA1c levels have been proposed as more reliable assays than OGTT (Faerch et al. 2010). Insulin sensitivity is also differentially regulated between men and women, with women in the early reproductive years being more insulin sensitive than men and less likely to develop insulin resistance.

Women typically have lower fasting glucose levels than men, they tend to have higher postprandial glucose levels (Basu et al. 2017). Postprandial glucose concentration is balanced by the amount of glucose entering (rate of appearance, or Ra) and leaving (rate of disappearance, or Rd) the circulation (Basu et al. 2017). Ra depends on the rate of meal carbohydrate appearance and endogenous glucose production, whereas Rd depends on the rate of whole-body glucose uptake. After a meal, plasma glucose levels rise until Ra gets equal to Rd (Basu et al. 2017). Women had higher rate of meal glucose appearance, but a lower rate of glucose disappearance, evident particularly in young women compared to age-matched men. However, there was no difference in postprandial glucose levels between elderly men and women (Basu et al. 2017).

Sexual dimorphism in glucose homeostasis has been discussed through various mechanisms (Fig. 2). Sex chromosomes may play a role in sex-specific regulation of metabolism and insulin signaling, independently of their function in determining sexual characteristics. Studies have shown that X chromosomes are associated with increased body weight and adiposity, whereas Y chromosomes have negative effects on glucose metabolism (Chen et al. 2013). Furthermore, pancreas islets have also been found to have a sex-biased sensory modulation, likely through different sex hormone signaling and components controlled by sex chromosomes (McEwan et al. 2021).

Women are reported to have higher capacity for insulin secretion and insulin sensitivity (Kautzky-Willer et al. 2012). Pancreatic islets in females were shown to contain 6% more beta cells and have greater insulin secretion rates (Vital et al. 2006). Female mouse adipocytes were also reported to have higher levels of insulin-regulated glucose transporter (GLUT4) and thus make females more insulin sensitive than male mice (Macotela et al. 2009; Paloma Álvarez-Rendón et al. 2023).

Sex also impacts insulin signaling. For example, male mice with IRS-2 deletion develop diabetes at 12 weeks of age, whereas females with the same mutation only experience mild obesity and slower development of diabetes, possibly due to diverse alterations in pancreatic islets and adipocytes (Garcia-Barrado et al. 2011). A study has suggested that 4E-BP1 acts as a sex-specific obesity suppressor, since augmented expression of 4E-BP1 was shown to be protective in male mice but not in female (Tsai et al. 2016). Both male and female mice with AS160 knockout experienced insulin tolerance. However, only females showed impaired glucose tolerance (Lansey et al. 2012). In male mice with FOXO 1/3/4 triple knockout, insulin resistance was observed due to lower Akt phosphorylation and impaired

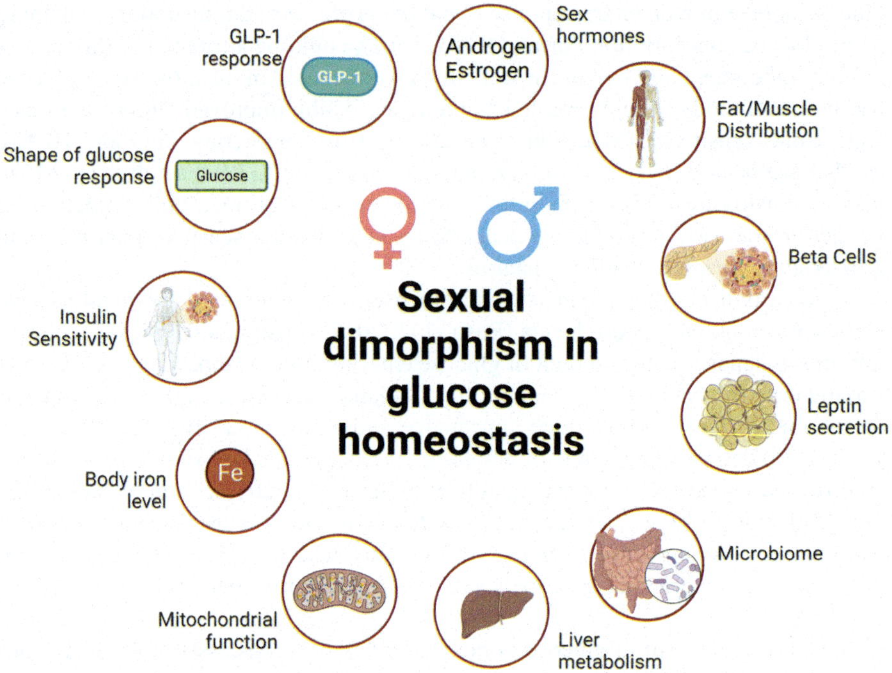

Fig. 2 Contributing factors of sexual dimorphism in glucose homeostasis

insulin-stimulated glucose uptake. However, female mice demonstrated normal levels of Akt phosphorylation and glucose uptake (Penniman et al. 2019).

Sex has a significant impact on body fat and muscle distribution, which in turn contribute to the observed differences between males and females. Women typically have higher global body fat and lower skeletal muscle mass compared to men. Fat tissue in women is typically stored in subcutaneous sites, especially in the gluteofemoral area, resulting in a "pear-shaped" fat distribution. In contrast, men tend to have visceral fat accumulation (Karastergiou et al. 2012; Kautzky-Willer et al. 2016). Additionally, women have lower ectopic fat deposition in organs, such as liver and myocardium, which can help to protect them from metabolic diseases (Tramunt et al. 2020). However, men with an abdominal fat accumulation are at greater risk for cardiovascular diseases than women (Bredella 2017; Karastergiou et al. 2012). This diverse fat distribution is claimed to be an evolutionary adaptation mechanism against undernutrition, enabling women to maintain reproduction through preferred energy storage, while males utilize energy stores to maintain physical activity (Kautzky-Willer et al. 2016). Subcutaneous fat distribution in females is suggested to mediate a better long-term storage (Tramunt et al. 2020). Similarly, skeletal muscle distribution differs between men and women and contributes to sex-specific regulation of glucose homeostasis. Women have greater insulin sensitivity due to higher glucose uptake and utilization in muscle compared to men (Paula et al. 1990).

Sex hormones certainly play significant roles revealing sex bias. Insulin sensitivity in women is correlated with estrogen levels. While young women have a lower incidence of insulin resistance, after menopause this incidence starts to match that of men, suggesting a protective role of estrogen (Mauvais-Jarvis et al. 2013; Shi et al. 2009). Estrogen is known to have a protective role in body composition and glucose metabolism, which is reversed after menopause resulting in an increased of metabolic diseases in women (Mauvais-Jarvis et al. 2013). Studies have shown that estrogen therapy during menopause can decrease fasting glucose and improve glucose tolerance (Mauvais-Jarvis et al. 2017b). Similarly, androgen deficiency in men increases metabolic risk, which can be reversed by testosterone supplementation (Yassin et al. 2019). On the other hand, excess androgen may lead to insulin resistance in women (Tramunt et al. 2020). The effect of testosterone was investigated in castrated rats, which are deficient in endogenous androgen (Muthusamy et al. 2009). Blood glucose levels were found to be elevated in these rats, and the glucose transporter, GLUT2 in the liver was upregulated. Of note, testosterone supplementation improved the increase in blood glucose and GLUT2 expression, suggesting that testosterone regulates hepatic glucose output (Muthusamy et al. 2009). Studies have shown that testosterone has a favorable effect on glucose homeostasis, including the upregulation of insulin receptor in the liver (Movérare-Skrtic et al. 2006), restoration of GLUT4, glucose uptake in the liver (Muthusamy et al. 2009), and stimulation of glycogen synthesis in skeletal muscle (Ramamani et al. 1999).

Steroid sex hormones also act on the tissues that produce insulin or are affected by insulin. Androgen receptors stimulate GLP-1-mediated insulin secretion (Mauvais-Jarvis 2016). On the other hand, estrogen receptors have been shown to improve beta cell function, while progesterone receptors have a role in adaptation to pregnancy. The role of ERα on glucose homeostasis has been shown in ERα knockout mice, where systemic insulin sensitivity was impaired (Manrique et al. 2012). Allard et al. (2019) further discussed the issue through nuclear ERα signaling in mice expressing either membrane ERα (MOER) or nuclear ERα (NOER) (Allard et al. 2019). They reported that both female and male MOER mice exhibited fasting and postprandial hyperglycemia and glucose intolerance. In female MOER mice, impaired central insulin signaling led to hyperinsulinemia and insulin resistance, resulting from unrestrained hepatic gluconeogenesis. In contrast, insulin resistance was not observed in male MOER mice, although glucose-stimulated insulin secretion was disrupted, along with decreased brain glucose sensing. Based on their findings, Allard et al. indicated that nuclear ERα signaling predominantly affects glucose homeostasis in both sexes, mainly through central control of insulin sensitivity and secretion in females and males, respectively (Allard et al. 2019).

Maintenance of glucose homeostasis is a finely tuned mechanism that is regulated by various tissues, including muscle, liver, and fat (Bredella 2017). The liver plays a significant role in maintaining glucose homeostasis, primarily through hepatic glucose synthesis via gluconeogenesis and glycogenolysis (Pilkis and Granner 1992).

Liver metabolism is also affected by sex differences. Estrogen receptor alpha (ERα) in the liver plays a key role in regulating sex-dependent hepatic metabolism. Female mice were shown to utilize amino acids to maintain energy storage, while males slow down anabolic processes (Della Torre et al. 2018).

Estrogen has also direct sexually dimorphic effects on central nervous system. Activation of hypothalamic estrogen receptors (ERα) has been reported to modulate food intake and energy homeostasis (Xu et al. 2011). ERα activation in the brain inhibits AMP-activated protein kinase (AMPK) leading to increased thermogenesis in brown adipose tissue (BAT) (Martínez de Morentin et al. 2014). Pro-opiomelanocortin (POMC) neurons in hypothalamus that are involved in the energy homeostasis are also sexually dimorphic. *Pro-opiomelanocortin* (POMC) neurons have an essential role in the glycemic control (Claret et al. 2011). The study conducted on Pomc-Cre, Lepr flox/flox mice, a mouse model with disrupted leptin action in POMC neurons, pointed the sex difference in leptin action in POMC neurons in regulating glucose homeostasis (Shi et al. 2008). Glucose intolerance and insulin resistance were observed in males lacking leptin receptor in POMC neurons. In contrast, glucose tolerance was not impaired during intraperitoneal GTT (ipGTT) in Pomc-Cre, Lepr flox/flox females. Similarly, the response to peripheral insulin was normal in high-fat diet-fed Pomc-Cre, Lepr flox/flox females whereas it was disrupted in males. Thus, it appears that leptin action in POMC neurons affected glucose homeostasis in males (Shi et al. 2008). The group then confirmed the effect of sexual dimorphism on glucose homeostasis using the same model with the addition of ovariectomized Pomc-Cre Lepr flox/flox mice (Shi et al. 2010). Interestingly, Lepr flox/flox females with or without ovariectomy had comparable glucose levels during ipGTT. Thus, it was suggested that the sex difference in leptin POMC signaling on glucose tolerance was not related to ovarian hormones (Shi et al. 2010). In addition, a study showed that the calcium-activated potassium channel (SK) in POMC neurons modulated energy metabolism in male mice and glucose homeostasis in female mice (Yu et al. 2022). Estrogen has been shown to increase leptin and reduce insulin sensitivity, leading to subcutaneous fat distribution (Clegg et al. 2006). Leptin secretion varies between sexes, with higher leptin secretion rates in females compared to males. Excess weight and obesity exacerbate leptin secretion. Obesity-associated hypertension is induced via different mechanisms: through sympathetic nervous system activation in males and aldosterone-mineralocorticoid receptor signaling activation in females. This finding could potentially lead to the development of sex-specific therapies (Belin de Chantemèle 2017).

Healthy women have greater GLP-1 concentrations following OGTT (Færch et al. 2015). Estrogen also enhances incretin response through proglucagon-derived peptide secretion (Handgraaf et al. 2018). Furthermore, the voltage-gated proton channel (Hv1), that regulates insulin secretion in pancreatic beta cells, has been shown to have sex-specific effects. Male mice with a knockout of Hv1 had higher blood glucose levels compared to females, possibly due to diverse sex hormones (Pang et al. 2021).

Lipid metabolism differs between male and females in several ways. Women have more fat mass, circulating free fatty acid (FFA) levels, and lipid content in myocytes than men (Tramunt et al. 2020). However, women are protected against FFA-induced insulin resistance and lipotoxicity (Frias et al. 2001). Unlike males who primarily produce energy through FFA oxidation, females tend to store FFAs in triglycerides. Additionally, predominant fuel sources during exercise are also different between sexes. For instance, lipid oxidation is preferred in females whereas glucose oxidation is dominant in males (Kautzky-Willer et al. 2016).

Energy expenditure is also differentially regulated between men and women. Females exhibit higher metabolic rate per kilogram of adipose tissue than males, along with increased expressions of genes regulating the function of mitochondrial function, including brown adipose tissue (BAT) marker UCP1 (Nookaew et al. 2013). In contrast, males display lower mitochondrial function in adipose tissues. These differences are linked to variations in gene expression related to adipose tissue beiging between sexes (Norheim et al. 2019). BAT and "beige" or BAT-like adipose tissues are regulated differentially. Pre-menopausal women possess more BAT that is more sensitive to activation. Selective activation of adipose tissue ERα promotes beiging via AMP-activated protein kinase (AMPK) and adipose triglyceride lipase (ATGL)-mediated lipolysis, leading to FFA production and UCP1 activation (Santos et al. 2018). Studies using PET-CT scanning reveals that adipose tissue of women is metabolically more active, contributing to higher energy expenditure (Cypess et al. 2009; Virtanen et al. 2009).

Growing evidence suggests that gut microbiota play a role in the sex-biased regulation of glucose and lipid homeostasis (Baars et al. 2018; Gao et al. 2021). Androgens have been shown to differentially regulate the gut microbiome between males and females. In fact, adult male mice exhibit worsened glucose tolerance and insulin sensitivity, along with a distinct gut microbiome composition compared to adult female mice (Gao et al. 2021). Depletion of the gut microbiome, however, eliminates sex-specific effects on glucose metabolism. When antibiotic-treated female mice received male donor microbiota, they displayed increased insulin resistance. Conversely, castration leading to androgen depletion resulted in a female-like gut microbiome in male mice, improving glucose metabolism which was reversed by dihydrotestosterone (DHT) reintroduction. Furthermore, when the gut microbiome was depleted, androgen effects were also abolished (Gao et al. 2021). The gut microbiome is known to be associated with amino acids, such as glutamine and glutamine/glutamate (Gln/Glu) ratio, which play roles in metabolic diseases (Gao et al. 2021). Androgens disrupt glucose metabolism by altering glutamine levels and Gln/glu ratio, depending on the gut microbiome (Gao et al. 2021).

4 Sex Differences in Diabetes

4.1 Sex Differences in Type 1 Diabetes

Type 1 Diabetes (T1D) is a chronic autoimmune disease that is characterized by a lack of endogenous insulin secretion due to the destruction of pancreatic beta cells. It is believed that T1D arises from the interaction of various factors such as genome, metabolism, microbiome, immune system, and environmental factors (DiMeglio et al. 2018). Although it is typically observed in children or young adults, it may occur at any age (Buzzetti et al. 2017).

The influence of sex on glucose homeostasis in T1D has been investigated in a limited number of preclinical studies. In STZ-diabetic rat model, blood glucose level was found higher in males compared to females (Rebolledo-Solleiro and Fernandez-Guasti 2018). Consistently, fasting blood glucose levels were significantly higher in male STZ-diabetic mice compared to females (Kim et al. 2020). In addition, HbA1c and the ratio of glucagon to insulin were also higher in male diabetic mice. Both male and female mice were found to have insulin resistance, determined by HOMA-IR, at the third week of STZ injection while it was only present in male diabetic mice at the sixth week. Therefore, the more favorable glucose homeostasis observed in females has been referred to the protective effects of estrogens (Kim et al. 2020).

Reflecting the low prevalence of the disease among the population, the clinical studies focusing on sexual dimorphism in T1D are limited. Actually, T1D is known as the only major organ-specific autoimmune disease without a female predominance (Gale and Gillespie 2001). Ostman et al. have reported a male predominance of T1D in a clinical study conducted among newly diagnosed T1D patients aged 15–34 years in Sweden (Ostman et al. 2008). On the other hand, female patients with T1D have higher levels of antibodies against glutamic acid decarboxylase and a more pronounced impairment in beta cell function compared to males of the same age at diagnosis (Tonolo 2021). Based on the reports indicating that the incidence of disease is lower in girls in puberty (Blohmé et al. 1992; Nyström et al. 1992), it is suggested that the female gonadal hormones may offer protection against T1D during this period (Mauvais-Jarvis 2017). Thus, T1D with adult onset is mostly male biased (Tonolo 2021).

4.2 Sex Differences in Type 2 Diabetes or Insulin Resistance

In Type 2 Diabetes (T2D), the main problem is insulin resistance which impairs insulin response in the target tissues and inhibits glucose uptake. As a result, the stimulation of insulin secretion from beta cells is enhanced to regulate glucose homeostasis leading to decreased insulin secretion over time (Goyal and Jialal 2022). T2D accounts for more than 85% of diabetes cases (Forouhi and Wareham 2014) and it is typically observed in individuals over the age of 45 (Goyal and Jialal 2022). However, insulin resistance is becoming increasingly common in children and adolescents as well (Al-Beltagi et al. 2022).

In contrast to the limited data on the impact of sex and gender in T1D, there are numerous preclinical and clinical studies reporting the effect of these factors in T2D and insulin resistance. In one such study, Nile Gras rats, an animal model of spontaneous metabolic syndrome (Noda et al. 2010), exhibited hyperinsulinemia to similar extent in both males and females (Schneider et al. 2020). On the other hand, female rats maintained normal fasting blood glucose levels, while males experienced impairment beginning at 6 months of age. As a result, only male rats in this study developed T2D on a standard rodent diet.

The impact of sex difference on glucose homeostasis has often been discussed through the role of sex hormones. For instance, male type 2 diabetic Goto-Kakizaki rats were found be more prone to develop T2D with age (Díaz et al. 2019). Glucose consumption in the brain, cerebellum, and heart determined by positron emission tomography (PET) was lower in males. Hence, these differences between the sexes were partly attributed to the protective effect of estrogens, which are thought to improve oxidative stress and contribute to favorable effects on glucose homeostasis. The role of sex hormones in sexual dimorphism has also been demonstrated in Mito-Ob mice, an animal model of obesity and insulin resistance (Xu et al. 2018). By comparing gonadectomized Mito-Ob and wild-type mice in both sexes, the study indicated that obesity-related glucose homeostasis impairment and insulin resistance occur in a male-specific manner.

Gao et al. have addressed the issue in the context of androgen-gut microbiome relation (Gao et al. 2021). They demonstrated that transferring male donor microbiota into antibiotics-treated female mice resulted in more pronounced insulin resistance. On the other hand, castration led to depletion of androgens which in turn changed the microbiome of male mice into a form similar to that of females. Androgen deficiency also improved glucose metabolism. Of note, the impact of androgens on glucose metabolism disappeared in the case of gut microbiome depletion. Furthermore, androgens also modulated the circulating glutamine level and glutamine/glutamate ratio, which was partially related to gut microbiome. Thus, it was suggested that the sexual dimorphism on glucose homeostasis may be associated with androgen-mediated effects on gut microbiome, circulating glutamine, and glutamine/glutamate ratio (Gao et al. 2021). The contribution of gut microbiota to the sex bias in diabetes is confirmed in NOD mice, as the higher incidence of females developing T1D was abolished in germ-free NOD mice (Yurkovetskiy et al. 2013). They also demonstrated the relationship between androgens and microbiota as the microbiota of females and castrated male mice were similar. In line with this finding, Markle et al. reported that transferring the gut microbiota of adult males to immature females provided protection against T1D by altering the microbiota and elevating testosterone levels (Markle et al. 2013). However, the results of two studies on NOD mice argue against the hypothesis of Gao et al. (2021) that androgen deficiency promotes glucose metabolism. This discrepancy might result from the fact that NOD mice are a model of autoimmune type 1 diabetes whereas the study by Gao et al. (2021) was conducted on mice fed a high-fat diet (HFD), which is a model of insulin resistance.

The impact of the T2D-associated gene C2cd4b on glucose homeostasis has also been investigated with regard to sexual dimorphism (Mousavy Gharavy et al. 2021). It was found that C2cd4b null female mice had abnormal glucose tolerance and impaired insulin secretion, which was associated with lower levels of follicle-stimulating hormone (Olivotto et al. 2020). On the other hand, C2cd4b null males displayed normal glucose tolerance but increased fasting blood glucose when put on a high-fat and sucrose diet.

Based on the findings, it has been suggested that insulin resistance and mitochondrial dysfunction may be related (Szendroedi et al. 2011), as subjects with T2D or insulin resistance show reduced mitochondrial content (Morino et al. 2005; Chomentowski et al. 2011; Heilbronn et al. 2007) or activity (Szendroedi et al. 2011; Petersen et al. 2003; Petersen et al. 2004; Szendroedi et al. 2007). In this regard, the effect of sexual dimorphism on insulin sensitivity has been investigated in terms of mitochondrial function in HFD fed rats (Szendroedi et al. 2011; Amengual-Cladera et al. 2012). The HOMA-IR values were higher in males, although serum glucose levels were comparable between HFD fed male and female rats. Insulin sensitivity was found to be better in HFD fed female rats, which was linked to highly differentiated mitochondria, a greater retroperitoneal white adipose tissue expandability capacity, and less mitochondrial dysfunction in this sex. Furthermore, the protein expression of the components in insulin signaling pathway, IRβ, pAkt, total Akt and GLUT4, was higher in white adipose tissue of control female rats compared to males. However, the expression of these genes was increased only in HFD fed males. The expression of IRS1 was not different among the groups (Amengual-Cladera et al. 2012).

In the study by Penniman et al. (2019), Forkhead box O transcription factors (FoxOs), which contribute to various processes in the body such as metabolism, cellular proliferation, apoptosis, and stress resistance (Wang et al. 2014), have been suggested to contribute to sexually dimorphic differences in insulin action (Penniman et al. 2019). Muscle-specific deletion of FoxOs in TKO mice resulted in equivalent muscle hypertrophy and alleviated glycemic abnormalities related to diet-induced obesity in both sexes. However, deletion of this gene reduced AKT2 expression only in males, which was associated with impaired insulin action and reduced glucose uptake in glycolytic muscles (Penniman et al. 2019).

Clinical studies confirm sex differences in insulin resistance and T2D. The metabolic syndrome is more commonly seen in men, however, its prevalence in young women has risen due to increased obesity (Regitz-Zagrosek et al. 2007). In addition, impaired fasting glucose and glucose tolerance were more frequent in men and women (Regitz-Zagrosek et al. 2006; Szalat and Raz 2008; Glumer et al. 2003; Sicree et al. 2008), respectively. Interestingly, men with impaired fasting glucose were more insulin resistant compared to women who have impaired glucose tolerance with disrupted insulin secretion in early and late phases (Hanefeld et al. 2003). Thus, sex differences in glucose homeostasis should be considered when choosing a preventive therapy (Szalat and Raz 2008). T2D is more often seen in men (Wild et al. 2004; Aregbesola et al. 2017). However, in some populations the prevalence may be same or higher in women related to longer life span (Szalat and Raz 2008; Gale and Gillespie 2001). Mauvais-Jarvis pointed to the significance of 2 h postprandial glucose level when estimating the prevalence of T2D between women and men (Mauvais-Jarvis 2017) as the exclusion of this parameter changes the prevalence of diabetes and prediabetes in women (Menke et al. 2015).

In a clinical study conducted on schoolchildren, the insulin resistance measured with HOMA-IR steadily increased in boys aged 6–18 years (Tsou et al. 2004). However, in girls, it increased with age, peaking at age 12–14 years and decreasing afterward. Fasting blood glucose levels were relatively stable and similar in both males and females. The authors indicated that insulin resistance and beta cell function exhibited a sex-specific pattern during puberty (Tsou et al. 2004).

On the other hand, Diaf et al. (2014) found that the parameters related to glycemic control such as HbA1c, fasting and postprandial glucose levels were comparable among women and men with T2D (Diaf et al. 2014). In line with these results, it has been demonstrated that insulin sensitivity, the degree of beta cell impairment, the level of HbA1c, and the severity of hyperglycemia were similar within a multiethnic cohort of patients with T2D (Hermans et al. 2020). Thus, it was indicated that no difference in glucose homeostasis or metabolic control was observed among this population, despite a lesser loss of beta cell function observed in Maghrebian women compared to men of the same ethnicity. Tura et al. investigated the sex-related difference in subjects with impaired glucose metabolism or T2D (Tura et al. 2018). In this clinical study, insulin sensitivity was similar in men and women in the impaired glucose metabolism group. Fasting glucose levels were comparable between elderly women and men. On the other hand, age-related worsening of early phase insulin release was more pronounced in women, which was attributed to metabolic deterioration after menopause at older ages. Furthermore, no difference on glucose metabolism between women and men was observed in patients with T2D.

The role of sex differences in the prevalence of insulin resistance or diabetes has been discussed over gonadal hormones. Testosterone levels were found to be associated with insulin resistance (Seidell et al. 1990) and T2D in males (Tibblin et al. 1996). It has been demonstrated that androgen deprivation therapy in cancer patients reduces pancreatic cell function and elevates blood glucose levels (Inaba et al. 2005). In line with this finding, testosterone replacement treatment has been shown to improve fasting blood glucose levels in men (Corona et al. 2011). On the contrary, women with increased androgen levels have been found to be at higher risk of developing insulin resistance and T2D (Ding et al. 2006; Andersson et al. 1994). Furthermore, postmenopausal women with higher plasma levels of estradiol and testosterone have been found to have an increased risk for the development of T2D (Ding et al. 2007). Increased estradiol levels may lead to insulin resistance in men, whereas the risk for impaired fasting glucose is higher in women after menopause due to the attenuated estrogen levels (Szalat and Raz 2008).

Sex differences in glucose homeostasis have also been discussed in the context of GLP-1 response during oral glucose loading (Færch et al. 2015). In the Danish ADDITION-Pro study, individuals with prediabetes or T2D presented 25% lower GLP-1 response to OGTT compared to those with normal glucose tolerance, and this difference was most prominent among women. However, this sex-related difference was partially attributed to higher GLP-1 response in normoglycemic women. Thus, the authors concluded that sex difference in GLP-1 response disappeared as glucose tolerance worsened (Færch et al. 2015).

In addition to the contributing factors of sex differences in diabetes, Aregbesola et al. have indicated that body iron also affects the incidence of T2D in male subjects, given that men tend to accumulate more iron compared to women (Aregbesola et al. 2017). This claim was supported by the role of adiponectin, an adipokine that regulates glucose and lipid metabolism. Iron has been found to reduce the production of adiponectin and thus impairs insulin sensitivity (Gabrielsen et al. 2012).

Georg et al. have investigated the sex differences in beta cell function using cells donated by subjects with or without T2D (Brownrigg et al. 2023). They demonstrated that female beta cells were more capable of maintaining glucose-stimulated insulin production and secretion. The shape of the glucose response curve has been suggested as a biomarker for beta cell function in T2D patients. The pattern of continuous rise in patients with T2D is considered an indicator of reduced beta cell function (Utzschneider et al. 2021). In this regard, the sex differences on the shape of glucose response curve have also been investigated. In the "Glycemia Reduction Approaches in Diabetes: A Comparative Effectiveness Study" (GRADE) study, women exhibited a continuous rise which interpreted as lower beta cell function in this sex (Utzschneider et al. 2021). However, previous studies reported either a common biphasic/multiphasic pattern among women with or without diabetes (Cheng et al. 2019; Tschritter et al. 2003) or no difference between women and men (de Andrade Mesquita et al. 2018; Kanauchi et al. 2005). Therefore, further investigation is needed to clarify the sex effect on the shape of glucose response curve.

References

Al-Beltagi M, Bediwy AS, Saeed NK (2022) Insulin-resistance in paediatric age: its magnitude and implications. World J Diabetes 13:282–307

Allard C, Morford JJ, Xu B et al (2019) Loss of nuclear and membrane estrogen receptor-a differentially impairs insulin secretion and action in male and female mice. Diabetes 68:490–501

Amengual-Cladera E, Lladó I, Gianotti M, Proenza AM (2012) Sex differences in the effect of high-fat diet feeding on rat White adipose tissue mitochondrial function and insulin sensitivity. Metabolism 61:1108–1117

Andersson B, Marin P, Lissner L, Vermeulen A, Bjorntorp P (1994) Testosterone concentrations in women and men with Niddm. Diabetes Care 17:405–411

Anichini R, Cosimi S, Di Carlo A, Orsini P, De Bellis A, Seghieri G, Franconi F, Baccetti F (2013) Gender difference in response predictors after 1-year exenatide therapy twice daily in type 2 diabetic patients: a real world experience. Diabetes Metab Syndr Obes 6:123–129

Aregbesola A, Voutilainen S, Virtanen JK, Mursu J, Tuomainen TP (2017) Gender difference in type 2 diabetes and the role of body iron stores. Ann Clin Biochem 54:113–120

Ashcroft FM, Rorsman P (2012) Diabetes mellitus and the B cell: the last ten years. Cell 148:1160–1171

Baars A, Oosting A, Lohuis M, Koehorst M, El Aidy S, Hugenholtz F, Smidt H, Mischke M, Boekschoten MV, Verkade HJ, Garssen J, Van Der Beek EM, Knol J, De Vos P, Van Bergenhenegouwen J, Fransen F (2018) Sex differences in lipid metabolism are affected by presence of the gut microbiota. Sci Rep 8:13426

Basu A, Dube S, Basu R (2017) Men are from Mars, women are from Venus: sex differences in insulin action and secretion. Adv Exp Med Biol 1043:53–64

Belin De Chantemèle EJ (2017) Sex differences in leptin control of cardiovascular function in health and metabolic diseases. Adv Exp Med Biol 1043:87–111

Blohmé G, Nyström L, Arnqvist HJ, Lithner F, Littorin B, Olsson PO, Scherstén B, Wibell L, Ostman J (1992) Male predominance of type 1 (insulin-dependent) Diabetes mellitus in young adults: results from A 5-year prospective Nationwide study of the 15-34-year age group in Sweden. Diabetologia 35:56–62

Bredella MA (2017) Sex differences in body composition. Adv Exp Med Biol 1043:9–27

Brownrigg GP, Xia YH, Chu CMJ, Wang S, Chao C, Zhang JA, Skovsø S, Panzhinskiy E, Hu X, Johnson JD, Rideout EJ (2023) Sex differences in islet stress responses support female B cell resilience. Mol Metab 69:101678

Buzzetti R, Zampetti S, Maddaloni E (2017) Adult-onset autoimmune diabetes: current knowledge and implications for management. Nat Rev Endocrinol 13:674–686

Chen X, Mcclusky R, Itoh Y, Reue K, Arnold AP (2013) X and Y chromosome complement influence adiposity and metabolism in mice. Endocrinology 154:1092–1104

Cheng X, Yang N, Li Y, Sun Q, Qiu L, Xu L, Ping F, Li W, Zhang H (2019) The shape of the glucose response curve during an oral glucose tolerance test heralds B-cell function in a large Chinese population. BMC Endocr Disord 19:119

Chomentowski P, Coen PM, Radiková Z, Goodpaster BH, Toledo FG (2011) Skeletal muscle mitochondria in insulin resistance: differences in Intermyofibrillar versus subsarcolemmal subpopulations and relationship to metabolic flexibility. J Clin Endocrinol Metab 96:494–503

Claret M, Smith MA, Knauf C, Al-Qassab H, Woods A, Heslegrave A, Piipari K, Emmanuel JJ, Colom A, Valet P, Cani PD, Begum G, White A, Mucket P, Peters M, Mizuno K, Batterham RL, Giese KP, Ashworth A, Burcelin R, Ashford ML, Carling D, Withers DJ (2011) Deletion of Lkb1 in pro-opiomelanocortin neurons impairs peripheral glucose homeostasis in mice. Diabetes 60:735–745

Clegg DJ, Brown LM, Woods SC, Benoit SC (2006) Gonadal hormones determine sensitivity to central leptin and insulin. Diabetes 55:978–987

Corona G, Monami M, Rastrelli G, Aversa A, Sforza A, Lenzi A, Forti G, Mannucci E, Maggi M (2011) Type 2 diabetes mellitus and testosterone: a meta-analysis study. Int J Androl 34:528–540

Cypess AM, Lehman S, Williams G, Tal I, Rodman D, Goldfine AB, Kuo FC, Palmer EL, Tseng Y-H, Doria A, Kolodny GM, Kahn CR (2009) Identification and importance of Brown adipose tissue in adult humans. N Engl J Med 360:1509–1517

Dave CV, Schneeweiss S, Kim D, Fralick M, Tong A, Patorno E (2019) Sodium-glucose Cotransporter-2 inhibitors and the risk For severe urinary tract infections: a population-based cohort study. Ann Intern Med 171:248–256

De Andrade Mesquita L, Pavan Antoniolli L, Cittolin-Santos GF, Gerchman F (2018) Distinct metabolic profile according to the shape of the oral glucose tolerance test curve is related to whole glucose excursion: a cross-sectional study. BMC Endocr Disord 18:56

De Morentin M, Pablo B, González-García I, Martins L, Lage R, Fernández-Mallo D, Martínez-Sánchez N, Ruíz-Pino F, Liu J, Morgan DA, Pinilla L, Gallego R, Saha AK, Kalsbeek A, Fliers E, Bisschop PH, Diéguez C, Nogueiras R, Rahmouni K, Tena-Sempere M, López M (2014) Estradiol regulates Brown adipose tissue thermogenesis via hypothalamic Ampk. Cell Metab 20:41–53

Della Torre S, Mitro N, Meda C, Lolli F, Pedretti S, Barcella M, Ottobrini L, Metzger D, Caruso D, Maggi A (2018) Short-term fasting reveals amino acid metabolism as a major sex-discriminating factor in the liver. Cell Metab 28:256–267.E5

Diaf M, Khaled BM, Habib HH, Belbraoued S (2014) Effect of gender and body weight on postprandial glucose and lipid metabolism in adults with type 2 diabetes. J Nepal Med Assoc 52:866–877

Díaz A, López-Grueso R, Gambini J, Monleón D, Mas-Bargues C, Abdelaziz KM, Viña J, Borrás C (2019) Sex differences in age-associated type 2 diabetes in rats-role of estrogens and oxidative stress. Oxid Med Cell Longev 2019:6734836

Dimeglio LA, Evans-Molina C, Oram RA (2018) Type 1 diabetes. Lancet 391:2449–2462

Ding EL, Song Y, Malik VS, Liu S (2006) Sex differences of endogenous sex hormones and risk of type 2 diabetes: a systematic review and meta-analysis. JAMA 295:1288–1299

Ding EL, Song Y, Manson JE, Rifai N, Buring JE, Liu S (2007) Plasma sex steroid hormones and risk of developing type 2 diabetes in women: a prospective study. Diabetologia 50:2076–2084
Faerch K, Borch-Johnsen K, Vaag A, Jørgensen T, Witte DR (2010) Sex differences in glucose levels: a consequence of physiology or methodological convenience? The Inter99 study. Diabetologia 53:858–865
Færch K, Torekov SS, Vistisen D, Johansen NB, Witte DR, Jonsson A, Pedersen O, Hansen T, Lauritzen T, Sandbæk A, Holst JJ, Jørgensen ME (2015) Glp-1 response to oral glucose is reduced in prediabetes, screen-detected type 2 diabetes, and obesity and influenced by sex: the addition-pro study. Diabetes 64:2513–2525
Forouhi NG, Wareham NJ (2014) Epidemiology of diabetes. Medicine (Abingdon) 42:698–702
Frias JP, Macaraeg GB, Ofrecio J, Yu JG, Olefsky JM, Kruszynska YT (2001) Decreased susceptibility to fatty acid-induced peripheral tissue insulin resistance in women. Diabetes 50: 1344–1350
Fu Z, Gilbert ER, Liu D (2013) Regulation of insulin synthesis and secretion and pancreatic beta-cell dysfunction in diabetes. Curr Diabetes Rev 9:25–53
Gabrielsen JS, Gao Y, Simcox JA, Huang J, Thorup D, Jones D, Cooksey RC, Gabrielsen D, Adams TD, Hunt SC, Hopkins PN, Cefalu WT, Mcclain DA (2012) Adipocyte iron regulates adiponectin and insulin sensitivity. J Clin Invest 122:3529–3540
Gale EA, Gillespie KM (2001) Diabetes and gender. Diabetologia 44:3–15
Gao A, Su J, Liu R, Zhao S, Li W, Xu X, Li D, Shi J, Gu B, Zhang J, Li Q, Wang X, Zhang Y, Xu Y, Lu J, Ning G, Hong J, Bi Y, Gu W, Wang J, Wang W (2021) Sexual dimorphism in glucose metabolism is shaped by androgen-driven gut microbiome. Nat Commun 12:7080
Garcia-Barrado MJ, Iglesias-Osma MC, Moreno-Viedma V, Pastor Mansilla MF, Gonzalez SS, Carretero J, Moratinos J, Burks DJ (2011) Differential sensitivity to adrenergic stimulation underlies the sexual dimorphism in the development of diabetes caused by Irs-2 deficiency. Biochem Pharmacol 81:279–288
Glumer C, Jorgensen T, Borch-Johnsen K, Inter S (2003) Prevalences of diabetes and impaired glucose regulation in a Danish population: the Inter99 study. Diabetes Care 26:2335–2340
Glümer C, Jørgensen T, Borch-Johnsen K (2003) Prevalences of diabetes and impaired glucose regulation in a Danish population: the Inter99 study. Diabetes Care 26:2335–2340
Goyal R, Jialal I (2022) Diabetes mellitus type 2. Statpearls Publishing, Treasure Island. Copyright © 2022
Haeusler RA, Mcgraw TE, Accili D (2018) Biochemical and cellular properties of insulin receptor signalling. Nat Rev Mol Cell Biol 19:31–44
Handgraaf S, Dusaulcy R, Visentin F, Philippe J, Gosmain Y (2018) 17-B estradiol regulates Proglucagon-derived peptide secretion in mouse and human A- and L cells. JCI Insight 3
Hanefeld M, Koehler C, Fuecker K, Henkel E, Schaper F, Temelkova-Kurktschiev T, Impaired Glucose Tolerance for Atherosclerosis and Diabetes Study (2003) Insulin secretion and insulin sensitivity pattern is different in isolated impaired glucose tolerance and impaired fasting glucose: the risk factor in impaired glucose tolerance for atherosclerosis and diabetes study. Diabetes Care 26:868–874
Heilbronn LK, Gan SK, Turner N, Campbell LV, Chisholm DJ (2007) Markers of mitochondrial biogenesis and metabolism are lower in overweight and obese insulin-resistant subjects. J Clin Endocrinol Metab 92:1467–1473
Hermans MP, Ahn SA, Sadikot S, Rousseau MF (2020) Established and novel gender dimorphisms in type 2 diabetes mellitus: insights from A multiethnic cohort. Diabetes Metab Syndr 14:1503–1509
Ho CK, Sriram G, Dipple KM (2016) Insulin sensitivity predictions in individuals with obesity and type ii diabetes mellitus using mathematical model of the insulin signal transduction pathway. Mol Genet Metab 119:288–292
Horie I, Abiru N, Eto M, Sako A, Akeshima J, Nakao T, Nakashima Y, Niri T, Ito A, Nozaki A, Haraguchi A, Akazawa S, Mori Y, Ando T, Kawakami A (2018) Sex differences in insulin and

glucagon responses for glucose homeostasis in young healthy Japanese adults. J Diabetes Investig 9:1283–1287

Hubbard SR (2013) The insulin receptor: both a prototypical and atypical receptor tyrosine kinase. Cold Spring Harb Perspect Biol 5:A008946

Inaba M, Otani Y, Nishimura K, Takaha N, Okuyama A, Koga M, Azuma J, Kawase I, Kasayama S (2005) Marked hyperglycemia after androgen-deprivation therapy for prostate cancer and usefulness of pioglitazone for its treatment. Metabolism 54:55–59

Kahn SE, Haffner SM, Heise MA, Herman WH, Holman RR, Jones NP, Kravitz BG, Lachin JM, O'neill MC, Zinman B, Viberti G (2006) Glycemic durability of rosiglitazone, metformin, or glyburide monotherapy. N Engl J Med 355:2427–2443

Kanauchi M, Kimura K, Kanauchi K, Saito Y (2005) Beta-cell function and insulin sensitivity contribute to the shape of plasma glucose curve during an oral glucose tolerance test in non-diabetic individuals. Int J Clin Pract 59:427–432

Karastergiou K, Smith SR, Greenberg AS, Fried SK (2012) Sex differences in human adipose tissues – the biology of pear shape. Biol Sex Differ 3:13

Kashyap S, Belfort R, Gastaldelli A, Pratipanawatr T, Berria R, Pratipanawatr W, Bajaj M, Mandarino L, Defronzo R, Cusi K (2003) A sustained increase in plasma free fatty acids impairs insulin secretion in nondiabetic subjects genetically predisposed to develop type 2 diabetes. Diabetes 52:2461–2474

Kautzky-Willer A, Brazzale AR, Moro E, Vrbíková J, Bendlova B, Sbrignadello S, Tura A, Pacini G (2012) Influence of increasing BMI on insulin sensitivity and secretion in normotolerant men and women of a wide age span. Obesity (Silver Spring) 20(10):1966–1973

Kautzky-Willer A, Kosi L, Lin J, Mihaljevic R (2015) Gender-based differences in glycaemic control and hypoglycaemia prevalence in patients with type 2 diabetes: results from patient-level pooled data of six randomized controlled trials. Diabetes Obes Metab 17:533–540

Kautzky-Willer A, Harreiter J, Pacini G (2016) Sex and gender differences in risk, pathophysiology and complications of type 2 diabetes mellitus. Endocr Rev 37:278–316

Kim B, Kim YY, Nguyen PT-T, Nam H, Suh JG (2020) Sex differences in glucose metabolism of streptozotocin-induced diabetes inbred mice (C57bl/6j). Appl Biol Chem 63:59

Lansey MN, Walker NN, Hargett SR, Stevens JR, Keller SR (2012) Deletion of Rab gap As160 modifies glucose uptake and Glut4 translocation in primary skeletal muscles and adipocytes and impairs glucose homeostasis. Am J Physiol Endocrinol Metab 303:E1273–E1286

Li Q, Liu F, Zheng TS, Tang JL, Lu HJ, Jia WP (2010) Slc22a2 gene 808 G/T variant is related to plasma lactate concentration in Chinese type 2 diabetics treated with metformin. Acta Pharmacol Sin 31:184–190

Macotela Y, Boucher J, Tran TT, Kahn CR (2009) Sex and depot differences in adipocyte insulin sensitivity and glucose metabolism. Diabetes 58:803–812

Manrique C, Lastra G, Habibi J, Mugerfeld I, Garro M, Sowers JR (2012) Loss of estrogen receptor a signaling leads to insulin resistance and obesity in young and adult female mice. Cardiorenal Med 2:200–210

Markle JG, Frank DN, Mortin-Toth S, Robertson CE, Feazel LM, Rolle-Kampczyk U, Von Bergen M, Mccoy KD, Macpherson AJ, Danska JS (2013) Sex differences in the gut microbiome drive hormone-dependent regulation of autoimmunity. Science 339:1084–1088

Mauvais-Jarvis F (2016) Role of sex steroids in B cell function, growth, and survival. Trends Endocrinol Metab 27:844–855

Mauvais-Jarvis F (2017) Epidemiology of gender differences in diabetes and obesity. Adv Exp Med Biol 1043:3–8

Mauvais-Jarvis F (2018) Gender differences in glucose homeostasis and diabetes. Physiol Behav 187:20–23

Mauvais-Jarvis F, Clegg DJ, Hevener AL (2013) The role of estrogens in control of energy balance and glucose homeostasis. Endocr Rev 34:309–338

Mauvais-Jarvis F, Arnold AP, Reue K (2017a) A guide for the design of pre-clinical studies on sex differences in metabolism. Cell Metab 25:1216–1230

Mauvais-Jarvis F, Manson JE, Stevenson JC, Fonseca VA (2017b) Menopausal hormone therapy and type 2 diabetes prevention: evidence, mechanisms, and clinical implications. Endocr Rev 38:173–188

Mcewan S, Kwon H, Tahiri A, Shanmugarajah N, Cai W, Ke J, Huang T, Belton A, Singh B, Wang L, Pang ZP, Dirice E, Engel EA, El Ouaamari A (2021) Deconstructing the origins of sexual dimorphism in sensory modulation of pancreatic B cells. Mol Metab 53:101260

Menke A, Casagrande S, Geiss L, Cowie CC (2015) Prevalence of and trends in diabetes among adults in the United States, 1988-2012. JAMA 314:1021–1029

Morino K, Petersen KF, Dufour S, Befroy D, Frattini J, Shatzkes N, Neschen S, White MF, Bilz S, Sono S, Pypaert M, Shulman GI (2005) Reduced mitochondrial density and increased Irs-1 serine phosphorylation in muscle of insulin-resistant offspring of type 2 diabetic parents. J Clin Invest 115:3587–3593

Mousavy Gharavy SN, Owen BM, Millership SJ, Chabosseau P, Pizza G, Martinez-Sanchez A, Tasoez E, Georgiadou E, Hu M, Fine NHF, Jacobson DA, Dickerson MT, Idevall-Hagren O, Montoya A, Kramer H, Mehta Z, Withers DJ, Ninov N, Gadue PJ, Cardenas-Diaz FL, Cruciani-Guglielmacci C, Magnan C, Ibberson M, Leclerc I, Voz M, Rutter GA (2021) Sexually dimorphic roles for the type 2 diabetes-associated C2cd4b gene in murine glucose homeostasis. Diabetologia 64:850–864

Movérare-Skrtic S, Venken K, Andersson N, Lindberg MK, Svensson J, Swanson C, Vanderschueren D, Oscarsson J, Gustafsson JA, Ohlsson C (2006) Dihydrotestosterone treatment results in obesity and altered lipid metabolism in orchidectomized mice. Obesity (Silver Spring) 14:662–672

Muthusamy T, Murugesan P, Balasubramanian K (2009) Sex steroids deficiency impairs glucose transporter 4 expression and its translocation through defective Akt phosphorylation in target tissues of adult male rat. Metabolism 58:1581–1592

Newsholme EA, Dimitriadis G (2001) Integration of biochemical and physiologic effects of insulin on glucose metabolism. Exp Clin Endocrinol Diabetes 109(Suppl 2):S122–S134

Niswender KD (2011) Basal insulin: physiology, pharmacology, and clinical implications. Postgrad Med 123:17–26

Noda K, Melhorn MI, Zandi S, Frimmel S, Tayyari F, Hisatomi T, Almulki L, Pronczuk A, Hayes KC, Hafezi-Moghadam A (2010) An animal model of spontaneous metabolic syndrome: Nile grass rat. FASEB J 24:2443–2453

Nookaew I, Svensson P-A, Jacobson P, Jernås M, Taube M, Larsson I, Andersson-Assarsson JC, Sjöström L, Froguel P, Walley A, Nielsen J, Carlsson LMS (2013) Adipose tissue resting energy expenditure and expression of genes involved in mitochondrial function are higher in women than in men. J Clin Endocrinol Metabol 98:E370–E378

Norheim F, Hasin-Brumshtein Y, Vergnes L, Chella Krishnan K, Pan C, Seldin MM, Hui ST, Mehrabian M, Zhou Z, Gupta S, Parks BW, Walch A, Reue K, Hofmann SM, Arnold AP, Lusis AJ (2019) Gene-by-sex interactions in mitochondrial functions and cardio-metabolic traits. Cell Metab 29:932–949.E4

Nyström L, Dahlquist G, Ostman J, Wall S, Arnqvist H, Blohmé G, Lithner F, Littorin B, Scherstén B, Wibell L (1992) Risk of developing insulin-dependent diabetes mellitus (Iddm) before 35 years of age: indications of climatological determinants for age at onset. Int J Epidemiol 21:352–358

Olivotto I, Oreziak A, Barriales-Villa R, Abraham TP, Masri A, Garcia-Pavia P, Saberi S, Lakdawala NK, Wheeler MT, Owens A, Kubanek M, Wojakowski W, Jensen MK, Gimeno-Blanes J, Afshar K, Myers J, Hegde SM, Solomon SD, Sehnert AJ, Zhang D, Li W, Bhattacharya M, Edelberg JM, Waldman CB, Lester SJ, Wang A, Ho CY, Jacoby D (2020) Mavacamten for treatment of symptomatic obstructive hypertrophic cardiomyopathy (explorer-Hcm): a randomised, double-blind, placebo-controlled, phase 3 trial. Lancet 396:759–769

Olofsson CS, Göpel SO, Barg S, Galvanovskis J, Ma X, Salehi A, Rorsman P, Eliasson L (2002) Fast insulin secretion reflects exocytosis of docked granules in mouse pancreatic B-cells. Pflugers Arch 444:43–51

Ostman J, Lönnberg G, Arnqvist HJ, Blohmé G, Bolinder J, Ekbom Schnell A, Eriksson JW, Gudbjörnsdottir S, Sundkvist G, Nyström L (2008) Gender differences and temporal variation in the incidence of type 1 diabetes: results of 8012 cases in the nationwide diabetes incidence study in Sweden 1983-2002. J Intern Med 263:386–394
Paloma Álvarez-Rendón J, Manuel Murillo-Maldonado J, Rafael Riesgo-Escovar J (2023) The insulin signaling pathway A century after its discovery: sexual dimorphism in insulin signaling. Gen Comp Endocrinol 330:114146
Pang H, Li J, Wang Y, Su X, Gao Y, Li SJ (2021) Mice lacking the proton channel Hv1 exhibit sex-specific differences in glucose homeostasis. J Biol Chem 297:101212
Paula FJ, Pimenta WP, Saad MJ, Paccola GM, Piccinato CE, Foss MC (1990) Sex-related differences in peripheral glucose metabolism in normal subjects. Diabete Metab 16:234–239
Penniman CM, Suarez Beltran PA, Bhardwaj G, Junck TL, Jena J, Poro K, Hirshman MF, Goodyear LJ, O'neill, B. T. (2019) Loss of Foxos in muscle reveals sex-based differences in insulin sensitivity but mitigates diet-induced obesity. Mol Metab 30:203–220
Petersen KF, Befroy D, Dufour S, Dziura J, Ariyan C, Rothman DL, Dipietro L, Cline GW, Shulman GI (2003) Mitochondrial dysfunction in the elderly: possible role in insulin resistance. Science 300:1140–1142
Petersen KF, Dufour S, Befroy D, Garcia R, Shulman GI (2004) Impaired mitochondrial activity in the insulin-resistant offspring of patients with type 2 diabetes. N Engl J Med 350:664–671
Pilkis SJ, Granner DK (1992) Molecular physiology of the regulation of hepatic gluconeogenesis and glycolysis. Annu Rev Physiol 54:885–909
Porte D Jr (1991) Banting lecture 1990. Beta-cells in type ii diabetes mellitus. Diabetes 40:166–180
Ramamani A, Aruldhas MM, Govindarajulu P (1999) Differential response of rat skeletal muscle glycogen metabolism to testosterone and estradiol. Can J Physiol Pharmacol 77:300–304
Rebolledo-Solleiro D, Fernandez-Guasti A (2018) Influence of sex and estrous cycle on blood glucose levels, body weight gain, and depressive-like behavior in streptozotocin-induced diabetic rats. Physiol Behav 194:560–567
Regitz-Zagrosek V, Lehmkuhl E, Weickert MO (2006) Gender differences in the metabolic syndrome and their role for cardiovascular disease. Clin Res Cardiol 95:136–147
Regitz-Zagrosek V, Lehmkuhl E, Mahmoodzadeh S (2007) Gender aspects of the role of the metabolic syndrome as a risk factor for cardiovascular disease. Gend Med 4 Suppl B:S162–S177
Rossi MC, Cristofaro MR, Gentile S, Lucisano G, Manicardi V, Mulas MF, Napoli A, Nicolucci A, Pellegrini F, Suraci C, Giorda C (2013) Sex disparities in the quality of diabetes care: biological and cultural factors may play a different role For different outcomes: a cross-sectional observational study from the Amd annals initiative. Diabetes Care 36:3162–3168
Santos RS, Frank AP, Fátima LA, Palmer BF, Öz OK, Clegg DJ (2018) Activation of estrogen receptor alpha induces Beiging of adipocytes. Mol Metab 18:51–59
Schneider J, Han WH, Matthew R, Sauvé Y, Lemieux H (2020) Age and sex as confounding factors in the relationship between cardiac mitochondrial function and type 2 diabetes in the Nile grass rat. PloS One 15:E0228710
Seidell JC, Björntorp P, Sjöström L, Kvist H, Sannerstedt R (1990) Visceral fat accumulation in men is positively associated with insulin, glucose, and C-peptide levels, but negatively with testosterone levels. Metabolism 39:897–901
Seino S (2012) Cell signalling in insulin secretion: the molecular targets of Atp, camp and sulfonylurea. Diabetologia 55:2096–2108
Shi H, Strader AD, Sorrell JE, Chambers JB, Woods SC, Seeley RJ (2008) Sexually different actions of leptin in proopiomelanocortin neurons to regulate glucose homeostasis. Am J Physiol Endocrinol Metab 294:E630–E639
Shi H, Seeley RJ, Clegg DJ (2009) Sexual differences in the control of energy homeostasis. Front Neuroendocrinol 30:396–404
Shi H, Sorrell JE, Clegg DJ, Woods SC, Seeley RJ (2010) The roles of leptin receptors on Pomc neurons in the regulation of sex-specific energy homeostasis. Physiol Behav 100:165–172

Sicree RA, Zimmet PZ, Dunstan DW, Cameron AJ, Welborn TA, Shaw JE (2008) Differences in height explain gender differences in the response to the oral glucose tolerance test- the Ausdiab study. Diabet Med 25:296–302

Susan B-W (2004) Endocrine pancreas. In: Johnson LR (ed) Encyclopedia of gastroenterology. Elsevier, New York

Szalat A, Raz I (2008) Gender-specific care of diabetes mellitus: particular considerations in the management of diabetic women. Diabetes Obes Metab 10:1135–1156

Szendroedi J, Schmid AI, Chmelik M, Toth C, Brehm A, Krssak M, Nowotny P, Wolzt M, Waldhausl W, Roden M (2007) Muscle mitochondrial Atp synthesis and glucose transport/phosphorylation in type 2 diabetes. PLoS Med 4:E154

Szendroedi J, Phielix E, Roden M (2011) The role of mitochondria in insulin resistance and type 2 diabetes mellitus. Nat Rev Endocrinol 8:92–103

Tibblin G, Adlerberth A, Lindstedt G, Björntorp P (1996) The pituitary-gonadal axis and health in elderly men: a study of men born in 1913. Diabetes 45:1605–1609

Tonolo G (2021) Sex-gender awareness in diabetes. Diabetology 2:117–122

Tramunt B, Smati S, Grandgeorge N, Lenfant F, Arnal JF, Montagner A, Gourdy P (2020) Sex differences in metabolic regulation and diabetes susceptibility. Diabetologia 63:453–461

Tsai SY, Rodriguez AA, Dastidar SG, Del Greco E, Carr KL, Sitzmann JM, Academia EC, Viray CM, Martinez LL, Kaplowitz BS, Ashe TD, La Spada AR, Kennedy BK (2016) Increased 4e-Bp1 expression protects against diet-induced obesity and insulin resistance in male mice. Cell Rep 16:1903–1914

Tschritter O, Fritsche A, Shirkavand F, Machicao F, Häring H, Stumvoll M (2003) Assessing the shape of the glucose curve during an oral glucose tolerance test. Diabetes Care 26:1026–1033

Tsou PL, Jiang YD, Chang CC, Wei JN, Sung FC, Lin CC, Chiang CC, Tai TY, Chuang LM (2004) Sex-related differences between adiponectin and insulin resistance in schoolchildren. Diabetes Care 27:308–313

Tura A, Pacini G, Moro E, Vrbíková J, Bendlová B, Kautzky-Willer A (2018) Sex- and age-related differences of metabolic parameters in impaired glucose metabolism and type 2 diabetes compared to normal glucose tolerance. Diabetes Res Clin Pract 146:67–75

Utzschneider KM, Younes N, Rasouli N, Barzilay JI, Banerji MA, Cohen RM, Gonzalez EV, Ismail-Beigi F, Mather KJ, Raskin P, Wexler DJ, Lachin JM, Kahn SE (2021) Shape of the Ogtt glucose response curve: relationship with B-cell function and differences by sex, race, and Bmi in adults with early type 2 diabetes treated with metformin. BMJ Open Diabetes Res Care:9

Virtanen KA, Lidell ME, Orava J, Heglind M, Westergren R, Niemi T, Taittonen M, Laine J, Savisto N-J, Enerbäck S, Nuutila P (2009) Functional Brown adipose tissue in healthy adults. N Engl J Med 360:1518–1525

Vital P, Larrieta E, Hiriart M (2006) Sexual dimorphism in insulin sensitivity and susceptibility to develop diabetes in rats. J Endocrinol 190:425–432

Wang Y, Zhou Y, Graves DT (2014) Foxo transcription factors: their clinical significance and regulation. Biomed Res Int 2014:925350

Wild S, Roglic G, Green A, Sicree R, King H (2004) Global prevalence of diabetes: estimates for the year 2000 and projections for 2030. Diabetes Care 27:1047–1053

Xu Y, Nedungadi TP, Zhu L, Sobhani N, Irani BG, Davis KE, Zhang X, Zou F, Gent LM, Hahner LD, Khan SA, Elias CF, Elmquist JK, Clegg DJ (2011) Distinct hypothalamic neurons mediate estrogenic effects on energy homeostasis and reproduction. Cell Metab 14:453–465

Xu YXZ, Ande SR, Mishra S (2018) Gonadectomy in mito-Ob mice revealed a sex-dimorphic relationship between prohibitin and sex steroids in adipose tissue biology and glucose homeostasis. Biol Sex Differ 9:37

Yassin A, Haider A, Haider KS, Caliber M, Doros G, Saad F, Garvey WT (2019) Testosterone therapy in men with hypogonadism prevents progression from prediabetes to type 2 diabetes: eight-year data from a registry study. Diabetes Care 42:1104–1111

Yu M, Bean JC, Liu H, He Y, Yang Y, Cai X, Yu K, Pei Z, Liu H, Tu L, Conde KM, Wang M, Li Y, Yin N, Zhang N, Han J, Scarcelli NA, Xu P, He Y, Xu Y, Wang C (2022) Sk3 in Pomc neurons plays A sexually dimorphic role in energy and glucose homeostasis. Cell Biosci 12:170
Yurkovetskiy L, Burrows M, Khan AA, Graham L, Volchkov P, Becker L, Antonopoulos D, Umesaki Y, Chervonsky AV (2013) Gender bias in autoimmunity is influenced by microbiota. Immunity 39:400–412

Sex-Gender-Based Differences in Metabolic Diseases

Ilaria Campesi, Margherita Ruoppolo, Flavia Franconi,
Marianna Caterino, and Michele Costanzo

Contents

Abstract

Sexual dimorphism creates different biological and cellular activities and selective regulation mechanisms in males and females, thus generating differential responses in health and disease. In this scenario, the sex itself is a source of physiologic metabolic disparities that depend on constitutive genetic and epigenetic features that characterize in a specific manner one sex or the other. This has

I. Campesi
Department of Biomedical Sciences, University of Sassari, Sassari, Italy

Laboratory of Sex-Gender Medicine, National Institute of Biostructures and Biosystems, Sassari, Italy

M. Ruoppolo · M. Caterino · M. Costanzo (✉)
Department of Molecular Medicine and Medical Biotechnology, University of Naples Federico II, Naples, Italy

CEINGE – Biotecnologie Avanzate Franco Salvatore s.c.ar.l., Naples, Italy
e-mail: michele.costanzo@unina.it

F. Franconi
Laboratory of Sex-Gender Medicine, National Institute of Biostructures and Biosystems, Sassari, Italy

S. E. Tsirka, M. Acosta-Martinez (eds.), *Sex and Gender Effects in Pharmacology*,
Handbook of Experimental Pharmacology 282,
https://doi.org/10.1007/164_2023_683

as a direct consequence a huge impact on the metabolic routes that drive the phenotype of an individual. The impact of sex is being clearly recognized also in disease, whereas male and females are more prone to the development of some disorders, or have selective responses to drugs and therapeutic treatments. Actually, very less is known regarding the probable differences guided by sex in the context of inherited metabolic disorders, owing to the scarce consideration of sex in such restricted field, accompanied by an intrinsic bias connected with the rarity of such diseases. Metabolomics technologies have been ultimately developed and adopted for being excellent tools for the investigation of metabolic mechanisms, for marker discovery or monitoring, and for supporting diagnostic procedures of metabolic disorders. Hence, metabolomic approaches can excellently embrace the discovery of sex differences, especially when associated to the outcome or the management of certain inborn errors of the metabolism.

Keywords

Metabolomics · Precision medicine · Sex metabolites · Gender metabolomics · Sex in metabolism · Mass spectrometry

1 Introduction

In the last decades, the aim of discovering sex-gender differences is driving the medical research on several aspects, most of which include metabolic diseases (Rich-Edwards et al. 2018).

Before delving into the specific aspects, it is essential to clarify adequately the concepts of sex and gender. Sex (genetic, epigenetic, hormonal, and other biological factors) and gender (socially constructed characteristics of women and men, the rules, roles and relationships between groups of men and women) are two distinct concepts that interact and intersect each other forming Gordians nodes. Therefore, numerous international authors use the term "sex-gender-based differences" and we too adhere to this choice, because it gives equal dignity to the two terms (Mauvais-Jarvis et al. 2021; Campesi et al. 2021b).

Biochemical disparities in males and females are partly due to sexual hormones and chromosomes but they also include sex-based differences in fetal or neonatal programming, and epigenetic modifications (Tramunt et al. 2020; Campesi et al. 2021a; Braun et al. 2022). The existence of such sex and gender differences provides, as a direct consequence, that the metabolic homeostasis has a differential regulation in males and females (Wang and Xu 2019), thus differentially influencing both the development of a metabolic disorder, the diagnosis, the outcomes, and the response to pharmacological treatments.

The discovery of sex-gender-based differences able to find solutions to predict the onset or prevent the damages induced by some metabolic conditions is blinded by the over-reliance of research on male animals (Stotland 2001; Campesi et al. 2021b). In fact, including female subjects in basic science designs or pre-clinical studies is pivotal to generate data with relevant application to individuals of both the sexes (Kwiatkowski et al. 2013; Prakash et al. 2018). On the verge of development of precision and/or personalized medicine approaches, this aspect overshadows the added complexity of research plans that include female animals, with the worthy cause to improve health and medicine for both males and females (Franconi et al. 2015; Mauvais-Jarvis et al. 2017). Expanding such considerations to a social level, focusing on both the sexes in the early phases of scientific research relies on the economic advantages to reduce the medical interventions, hospitalizations, and the costs for pharmaceutical production and testing (Clegg and Mauvais-Jarvis 2018).

Sex and gender matter also in relationship with genetic metabolic disorders, which occur owing to mutated genes that cause an enzyme deficiency or organ dysfunction as for the liver or pancreas (Kautzky-Willer and Handisurya 2009). Conventionally, they are comprised in the group of inborn errors of metabolism (IEMs) and are usually inherited and rare diseases, strongly influenced by sexual hormones (Ruoppolo et al. 2014), nutritional habits and lifestyles (Campesi et al. 2020, 2021c, 2022).

From a biochemical point of view, IEMs show alterations in the anabolic or catabolic processes related to proteins, lipids, and sugars synthesis or degradation. Therefore, approximately all the aspects of metabolism involving energy balance as well as glucose and lipid metabolism are controlled in a sexually dimorphic manner, thus influencing differently the pathogenesis of several disorders, including obesity and diabetes (Link et al. 2013; Clegg and Mauvais-Jarvis 2018; Seghieri et al. 2022).

Metabolomics methodologies are in these contexts the gold-standard approaches used to unravel mechanisms connected with perturbations of metabolism. The most modern, mass spectrometry-based metabolomics platforms allow the screening of hundreds of molecules that can be quantitatively monitored to assess metabolic differences between diverse conditions. Eventually, metabolomics could be useful in metabolic disorders to highlight existing differences driven by the influence of sex.

In this chapter, we focus our attention onto the use of metabolomics methodology with a special attention to IEMs research and on the possible influence of sex-gender on specific IEMs. In addition, we provide evidence of using metabolomics as a tool to discover possible connections between altered metabolism and sex.

2 Metabolomics in the Study of Metabolic Diseases

In the last two decades, scientific interest has turned onto the study of the phenomena and molecular mechanisms that orchestrate the biology of an organism. These holistic and large-scale approaches define the modern Systems Biology, dominating the scientific scenarios with respect to the classic and reductionist approaches (Nicholson and Lindon 2008; Tavassoly et al. 2018). In this context, "omics" sciences are systemic approaches capable of capturing the entirety of complex biological phenomena through sophisticated analyses and computational methodologies that allow the definition of precise functional activities and

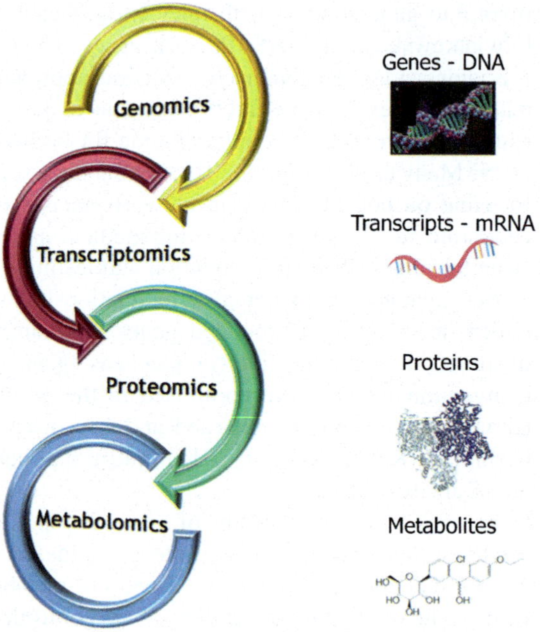

Fig. 1 Genome, transcriptome, proteome, and metabolome are concatenated as the biological information is transferred through different molecules, from DNA to proteins and metabolites. Appropriate omics technologies have been developed for the large-scale description of a biological system from diverse perspectives

interaction networks (Tavassoly et al. 2018; Costanzo et al. 2021; Santorelli et al. 2022). A scheme representing the flow of the biologic information at different levels and the corresponding omics associated is shown in Fig. 1.

Among the omics sciences, metabolomics aims at studying all the small molecules called "metabolites" that reflect the metabolic state of a cell, a tissue, or an individual (Joyce and Palsson 2006). Metabolites are small molecules (i.e., sugars, lipids, vitamins, hormones, pigments, etc.) naturally produced by an organism as a product of biochemical reactions and metabolism intermediates (i.e., from the conversion of food nutrients, drugs metabolism, etc.).

Accordingly, the metabolome is closer to describing the phenotype of an organism, covering the endpoint of genomic, transcriptomic, and proteomic processes. Taking part in numerous reactions in the organism, metabolites are subjected to extreme spatial and temporal variability especially in response to exogenous and environmental stimuli. Thus, while the proteome allows the definition of perturbed pathways upon environmental changes or endogenous stimuli (Costanzo et al. 2020a, b, 2022b; Manganelli et al. 2021), the metabolomic signature of an organism mirrors its metabolic profile as a function of the genome. In the field of human biomedical science, metabolomics can be employed to perform diagnosis, discover new disease biomarkers, study the effects of drugs or the mechanisms altered in pathological conditions in order to retrieve novel therapeutic targets. Usually, metabolomics analyses can be carried out employing different analytical platforms such as mass spectrometry (MS) and nuclear magnetic resonance (NMR) spectroscopy (Roviello et al. 2014; Costanzo et al. 2022a). As further advance in MS, lipidomics platforms allow the identification of several hundreds of lipid molecules, thus covering a quota of the metabolome that comprises the lipidome (Costanzo and Caterino 2023). Whatever the technique used, the ideal analytical metabolomic platform should provide a combination of high sensitivity, high specificity, high resolution, and high throughput.

NMR spectroscopy allows to both identify and quantify metabolites in a sample. Its great advantage lies in the non-destructive nature of the technique. It can be employed in the analysis of larger (>500 Da) molecules, such as sugars, amines, or volatile liquids (Wishart 2011). However, the high cost of the instrumentation, lower sensitivity, and difficulty in the analysis of complex mixtures limit the use of NMR to only few laboratories. On the other hand, MS offers the possibility of conducting quantitative analyses with high specificity and sensitivity in a picomolar and nanomolar dynamic range. In addition, the coupling of MS with separation techniques such as gas chromatography (GC), liquid chromatography (LC), or capillary electrophoresis (CE) allows to reduce the complexity of the mixture of metabolites, making easier the interpretation of the data. The disadvantages of MS techniques are related to their destructive nature and the fact that different compounds have different ionization capacities with a consequent bias in the quantitative analysis. A comparison between NMR, LC-MS, and GC-MS, including advantages and disadvantages, and the molecular classes that are able to detect, is reported in Fig. 2.

Instrumentation costs ↑ … ↓ *Sample preparation and analysis costs*

Analytical platform	Advantages	Disadvantages	Molecules detected
NMR	Non-destructive Quantitative Simple sample preparation Very reproducible	Low sensitivity (1-10 μmol/L) Requires large volumes	Sugars Amines Volatile liquids Large metabolites
LC-MS	Short separation time High resolution and mass accuracy Simple sample preparation High sensitivity (< 1 μmol/L)	Destructive Low reproducibility of retention times between different LC systems Ion suppression with co-eluting compounds Volatile coumpounds can not be measured	Medium-to-high non-polar metabolites: Nucleosides and nucleotides Lysophosphatidylcholines Acylacarnitines Acylglycines Polar metabolites: Amino and organic acids ↕ Non-polar metabolites:
GC-MS	High reproducibility of retention times No ion suppression with co-eluting compounds Comprehensive database for the identification High sensitivity (< 1 μmol/L)	Elaborate sample preparation Samples must be volatile Non-volatile samples require derivatization Manual sample preparation can introduce variability	Fatty acids Steroids Eicosanoids Carbohydrates Esters Cholesterol Volatile metabolites

Fig. 2 Comparison between the analytical platforms used in metabolomics. Advantages and disadvantages, including the type of molecules preferentially detected, are summarized

Currently, MS-based metabolomics is being widely used and MS-studies largely exceed the number of studies conducted using NMR. MS is a powerful analytical technique that allows to measure the mass of compounds. In particular, a mass spectrometer is able to separate and detect different molecular species present in a mixture according to their mass-to-charge ratio (m/z). The molecules in a sample are first ionized and then their mass is measured. The output of a MS analysis is a mass spectrum, a plot that shows the distribution of ions (along a m/z range) in relation to their intensity (recorded as relative abundance or total ion current). As representing the pattern of distribution of ions within one sample, each mass spectrum generated from a mass spectrometer is unique.

The high sensitivity and specificity of MS instrumentations allow the selective, accurate, and rapid identification and quantification of many metabolites, despite the high heterogeneity and the different chemical structures. As mentioned, coupling MS analysis with upstream separation techniques (formally known as hyphenated techniques, GC-MS, LC-MS, CE-MS) is a winning choice in the way that extremely reduces the complexity of the analyzed matrices, increasing the coverage of identified metabolites (Nicholson and Lindon 2008; Johnson and Gonzalez 2012; Schrimpe-Rutledge et al. 2016; Beale et al. 2018). The choice of which platform to use for metabolomics investigations depends on the experimental design, the expected outcome of the experiment, and the finances of the laboratory.

Currently, MS-based techniques are routinely used for the screening of IEMs in newborns (Ruoppolo et al. 2022). In fact, since metabolic disorders are due to defects in enzymes or transport proteins, which often result in the accumulation or the lack of certain metabolites, the metabolic profiling of biological fluids can mirror systemic alterations in patients providing precious information on their metabolic status. Therefore, the screening of the levels of certain metabolites allows the identification of more than 40 distinct metabolic defects than can be grouped into four main categories: aminoacidemias, organic acidemias, urea cycle defects, and fatty acid oxidation disorders. As an example, by targeted metabolomics is possible the diagnosis of aminoacidemias and urea cycle defects through the detection of increased levels of amino acids, such as phenylalanine (Phe) in case of phenylketonuria (PKU) or hyperphenylalaninemia (HPA), tyrosine (Tyr) for the tyrosinemias, valine, leucine, and isoleucine for the maple syrup urine disease (MSUD), citrulline for citrullinemias, etc. Instead, other molecules targeted by mass spectrometry belong to the class of acylcarnitines, which are used the most for detection of organic acidemias and fatty acid oxidation disorders. Among these, the propionylcarnitine (C3) is detected in case of propionic acidemia (PA) or methylmalonic acidemia (MMA), the valerylcarnitine (C5) in case of isovaleric acidemia (IVA) or 2-methylbutyryl-CoA dehydrogenase deficiency (2-MBG), the glutarylcarnitine (C5DC) for the glutaric acidemia type I (GAI) (Gonzalez Melo et al. 2021a, b; Ruoppolo et al. 2022).

3 Metabolomics as Technology to Discover Sex-Gender Differences

The biology of the two sexes is extremely different (Stotland 2001), thus having a great impact also on the metabolome. Although sex is not still adequately considered in metabolomics studies, the omics approach results are extremely helpful to discover sex differences in healthy or pathological conditions through the analysis of small molecules present in many biological fluids or tissues, in humans as well as animal models (Ruoppolo et al. 2018; Costanzo et al. 2022c). Hence, metabolic profiles can be significantly different in males and females and this is often driven by specific genetic variants in metabolism-related genes that enhance the sexual dimorphism (Mittelstrass et al. 2011). These considerations strongly suggest that sex-related and sex-specific effects should be punctually considered in the design and interpretation of studies. In fact, the specific and accurate characterization of the differences induced by sex at the metabolome and lipidome level would allow to define and deliver personalized healthcare services, incorporating the concept of personalized medicine (Brennan and Gibbons 2020; Campesi et al. 2021b).

Notwithstanding, sex can highly affect the metabolome in an age-dependent manner, as also reported for some serum or plasma and urine biomarkers (Campesi et al. 2016; Caterino et al. 2020). As reported by several sex-gender-based studies, male and female newborns display distinct metabolomic patterns (Ruoppolo et al. 2015). In particular, amino acid levels have been detected as significantly higher in females than in males, while males showed significantly higher free carnitine, total esterified carnitine, and saturated acylcarnitines (Ruoppolo et al. 2015).

In addition, the characterization of the urinary metabolome in healthy children between 1 and 36 months of age, showed that sex differences predominate in the first 6 months of life, where the majority of urinary organic acids were higher in males, indicating and confirming that sexual dimorphism starts in very early life (Caterino et al. 2020).

Furthermore, another metabolomics investigation conducted in premature neonates showed the presence of a sex-dependent metabolome that is further influenced by sex in conditions of diverse gestational age and pharmacological treatments, such as caffeine, which is often used to treat premature infants showing respiratory symptoms (e.g., apnea, intermittent hypoxemia, etc.). Precisely, the sex is responsible for the qualitative and quantitative variations in several amino acids and acylcarnitines, making male and female infants at different stages of prematurity metabolically distinct (Caterino et al. 2021).

Thus, in the light of these considerations, it appears increasingly relevant to integrate sex-gender-based differences and age variables into metabolomics. Studying the sex differences in healthy individuals' metabolome offers the possibility to define concentrations ranges within the population and discover differences at the baseline, without implications on health. On the other hand, as already mentioned, the evidence that sex influences the metabolome also in various pathological situations is relevant because it offers the opportunity to characterize sex-specific disease biomarkers and direct the person-disease management toward personalized medicine approaches (Di Minno et al. 2022). To date, only few investigations consider the variations of the metabolome as directly commanded by sex and gender, so the majority of the findings regard anthropometrics measurements and clinical features. However, as the common interest lies in describing sex and gender differences connected within pathological status, below will be shown the main known sex differences observed on a classical inborn error of metabolism, the PKU.

4 One Example: The PKU

PKU is a rare inborn error of metabolism characterized by defects in the enzymatic activity of phenylalanine hydroxylase (PAH), which guides the conversion of the essential amino acid Phenylalanine (Phe) into Tyrosine (Tyr). The PAH reaction, which predominantly occurs in the liver and kidney, requires reduced tetrahydrobiopterin (BH4) as cofactor (Fig. 3). BH4 is oxidized to quinonoid dihydrobiopterin (qBH2) in the course of the hydroxylation reaction, and qBH2 is enzymatically converted into BH4 to sustain other Phe hydroxylation reactions (Fig. 3) (van Spronsen et al. 2021).

98% of PKU patients show mutations in the *PAH* gene, with clinical phenotypes that range in severity from classic PKU to more moderate HPA conditions (de Baulny et al. 2007). Other cases of PKU may be caused by defects in the metabolism of BH4, accounting for 1–2% of all HPA cases (Vela-Amieva et al. 2022). Since BH4 is needed as cofactor for the transformation of tyrosine and tryptophan into catecholamine and serotonin, disorders caused by defects in BH4 metabolism may be considered as neurotransmitter-related diseases (de Baulny et al. 2007).

The clinical presentation of PKU patients comprises severe and irreversible neurological alterations. Major manifestations include progressive encephalopathy, seizures, abnormal behavior/hyperactivity, autistic or schizophrenic signs, eczema and lightly pigmented skin, and a musty odor. Instead, as already mentioned, non-classical PKU may clinically manifest as a wide range of forms that show mild alterations and classified as mild HPA (Hanley 2011).

The high levels of Phe that accumulate in the brain are responsible for the neurological impairment and, currently, dietary guidelines are targeted to maintaining blood Phe concentrations at low levels (Firman et al. 2022). In fact,

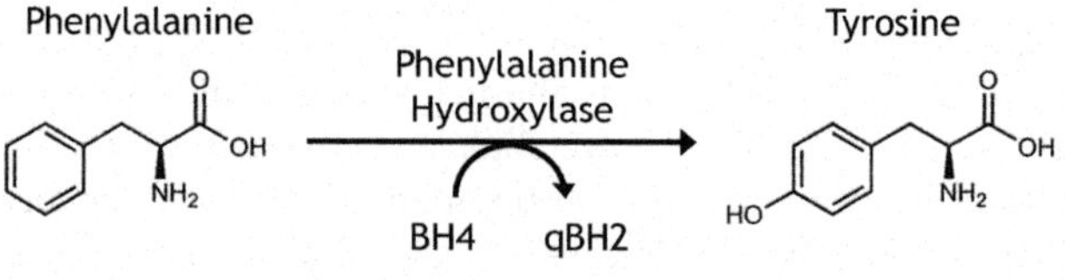

Fig. 3 Schematic representation of the reaction catalyzed by phenylalanine hydroxylase enzyme in the conversion of phenylalanine into tyrosine. The reactions for the biopterin regeneration were not reported

neurological damage can be partially avoided if patients are treated with a Phe-restricted diet shortly after birth. For this reason, the early diagnosis of PKU/HPA in the neonatal period through the national newborn screening programs and subsequent treatments are essential to reduce the metabolic disregulation in these patients, who are globally identified with a prevalence of 1:10,000 (van Spronsen et al. 2021). Actually, many therapeutic options to treat PKU are under investigation, such as gene therapy, which is becoming an increasingly valuable tool for several monogenic metabolic disorders (Bell et al. 2017; Maestro et al. 2021).

Whilst current knowledge is fairly comprehensive regarding the biochemical and genetic characterization of PKU, less is known about the impact of sex-gender on PKU and HPA-associated conditions (Lichter-Konecki and Vockley 2019; Elhawary et al. 2022).

In this regard, one main remarkable factor directly causative of this lack of information is the rarity of the disease, which penalizes the possibility of in-depth investigations of sex-gender-based effects, as the representative population under study is too small to provide sufficient statistical power for drawing definitive conclusions. In addition, in those cases where the sample size is small, statistical p-values are particularly vulnerable to small deviations in the observed number of outcomes (Mitani and Haneuse 2020). However, despite such limitations, some conclusions that explain sex-gender-based differences in PKU-associated conditions have been drawn, especially in children.

First, the major differences are observed in children when anthropometric measurements are compared between PKU patients and healthy controls. One recent study from Sailer et al. (2020) focused on the determination of several body composition measurements that include weight, height, BMI, lean body mass (LBM), and fat mass (FM), and explored the potential relationship between body composition and dietary intake in PKU. The results of this study revealed significant differences in male PKU children compared to healthy ones. In detail, the normalized height was significantly lower in the male PKU group, as well as the percentage of LBM. On the other hand, PKU males showed significantly higher FM than controls (Sailer et al. 2020). The majority of the studies cited in the literature do not report big differences in the percentage of FM between males and females affected by PKU when compared to controls, with only few evidences indicating an increasing trend for FM in PKU patients with more differences within the female group (Allen et al. 1995; Dobbelaere et al. 2003; Huemer et al. 2007; Albersen et al. 2010; Rocha et al. 2013).

Earlier, Allen et al. (1995, 1996) had discovered that female children had lower total body fat-free mass (FFM) and total body nitrogen (TBN) in comparison with control subjects (Allen et al. 1995, 1996). In contrast, no sex differences in the body composition were described in another study, which instead showed some differences when comparing pubertal to prepubertal subjects from a mild HPA group, identifying increased LBM in pubertal participants (Doulgeraki et al. 2014).

Notwithstanding, among the factors that modulate the nutritional outcomes of protein status in PKU, the sex was identified during some investigations (Firman et al. 2022). Sailer et al. initially did not find significant differences in total energy,

energy per kg of body weight, and total grams of protein per kg of body weight comparing the PKU patients and controls. Additionally, no differences were detected between males and females with PKU (Sailer et al. 2020). On the other hand, when analyzing the differences within the sexes (intra-sex analysis), some sex-specific features were documented. In particular, the protein-to-energy ratio was significantly lower in male PKU children compared to their respective sex-matched controls. In fact, the percentage of total energy obtained from protein was lower in male PKU patients than male controls, as well as the percentage of energy deriving from fat. By contrast, the percentage of energy deriving from carbohydrate source was found statistically increased in male PKU subjects compared with the male control group (Sailer et al. 2020). The above-mentioned disparities regarding the influence of sex on the protein status in PKU were not observed in the female cohort. Unfortunately other studies did not report sex comparisons of dietary protein intake (Allen et al. 1995, 1996). However, increased Phe levels in PKU patients have been associated with augmented weight in girls more than boys (McBurnie et al. 1991).

PKU has been for long associated with defects in the physical growth of patients. In many cases, bone and skeleton fragilities caused by a diminished bone mineral density (BMD) have emerged as a long-term complication increasing the risk of fractures. Male PKU individuals were characterized by lower total body BMD Z-scores and tended to have lower L1–L4 spine and total femur BMD Z-scores in comparison with female PKU patients (Stroup et al. 2018). The hypothesis supporting this is based on the fact that male PKU subjects tended to have higher intakes of protein equivalents from low-Phe amino acid medical foods (AA-MF). Given that AA-MF provide a high dietary acid load and increase the urinary excretion of calcium and magnesium, it was suggested that the amino acid intake by medical foods could negatively impact on bone mineral density in PKU males with respect to female patients (Stroup et al. 2017). For these reasons, male individuals with PKU showing lower total body BMD Z-scores may be at higher risk for osteoporosis than female PKU patients (Stroup et al. 2018).

Physiological and nutritional habits as well as the quality of physical activity can strongly impact on carbohydrate and glucose metabolism in both sexes (Tarnopolsky and Ruby 2001), especially in individuals carrying defects in primary metabolic routes. Thus, since the treatment of PKU is based on the restriction in the intake of natural proteins, patients can show severe growth impairment when remain untreated. Actually, a longitudinal retrospective study over the course of 31 years showed no significant growth changes between treated PKU and mild HPA individuals when compared to a healthy population (Couce et al. 2015). Only for PKU individuals, there was a tendency for height to be slightly lower and for weight to be slightly higher than the control group. Nevertheless, an acceleration of growth was observed for PKU girls up to 8 years old, leading to a slightly lower final height. Nowadays, in fact, long-term normal growth standards are achievable for PKU patients that undergo an appropriate dietary treatment (Couce et al. 2015).

5 Sex-Gender-Biased Treatment of Metabolic Disorders: The Case of Propionic Acidemia

Attempts to treat many IEMs through gene therapy have been made in humans or in disease animal models with some interesting results (Guenzel et al. 2014; Jiang et al. 2020; Maestro et al. 2021). The case of propionic acidemia (PA) revealed a sex-specific bias while testing a therapeutic intervention for this rare inherited metabolic disease using gene therapy, which was tested in a PA mouse model. In this example, while strong and durable efficacy was obtained in male mice, female animals showed a tissue-specific loss for the adeno-associated virus (AAV) gene therapy-mediated gene expression, thereby reducing the durability and efficacy of the therapy. Whether similar sex-biased outcomes may be determined with the AAV vectors employed for the gene therapy in humans is still under investigation (Guenzel et al. 2015).

PA is an inborn error of propionate metabolism that results from mutations in the alpha or beta subunits of propionyl-CoA carboxylase (PCC). PCC is a 750 kDa heterododecamer constituted by 6 alpha (*PCCA*) and 6 beta (*PCCB*) propionyl-CoA carboxylase subunits that uses biotin as cofactor. Although sharing a common structure with other acyl-CoA carboxylases, which includes a biotin carboxylase domain, a carboxytransferase domain, and biotin-carboxyl carrier protein domain, PCC has a unique biotin transfer domain in the alpha subunit that is essential for the interactions with the beta subunit (Huang et al. 2010; Wongkittichote et al. 2017). PCC is involved in the carboxylation of propionyl-CoA produced from the catabolism of odd-chain fatty acids, cholesterol, valine, methionine, isoleucine, and threonine to form methylmalonyl-CoA. The latter is then converted by the methylmalonyl-CoA mutase (and its cofactor adenosylcobalamin) into succinyl-CoA for energy production in the Krebs cycle (Costanzo et al. 2020a, b) (Fig. 4).

Mutations in the *PCCA* or *PCCB* genes are directly causative of PA, which can present as early- and late-onset forms characterized by metabolic acidosis, hyperammonemia, lethargy, vomiting, coma and, finally, death when not properly treated. Despite the exact mechanisms that lead to PA complications are still uncertain, as common trait with other organic acidemias PA pathogenesis depends on the accumulation of toxic metabolites (like propionic acid and ammonia), and on secondary unbalances in energy production and mitochondrial functions (Knerr et al. 2012).

Considering that no effective pharmacological therapy is disposable for PA, the liver transplant has been presented as a therapeutic solution to partially reduce the metabolic decompensation in patients. However, such intervention enables the correction of PCC deficiency solely in the liver with the patients possibly showing other PA-related complications (Critelli et al. 2018).

With these concerns, gene therapy approaches have been explored to provide transgene expression in multiple tissues in organic acidemias (Chandler and Venditti 2019). In particular, the ability of AAV vectors to correct systemic PA symptoms has been tested by Guenzel and collaborators in a *PCCA null* mouse model of PA (Guenzel et al. 2015). Results from this study showed that AAV therapy allowed

Fig. 4 Schematic representation of the propionyl-CoA metabolism

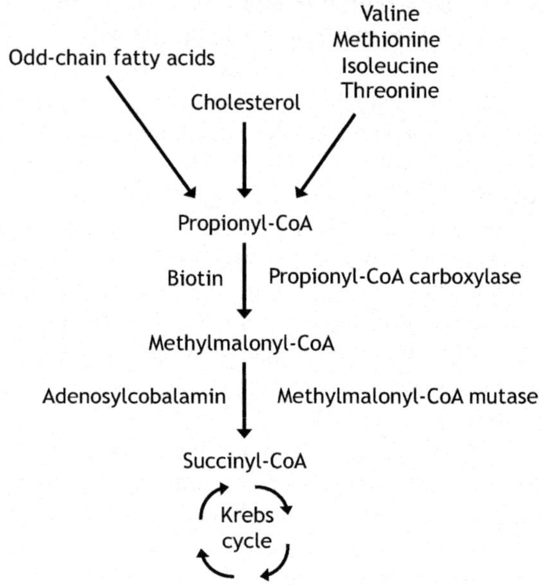

persistent long-term expression of the PCCA protein over 1.5 years after single injection in mice, with rescued activity of PCC. However, the authors found significant sex differences in the transgene expression between females and males.

Previous research revealed that AAV therapy delivers a significantly different short-term expression of transgenes in liver when comparing male and female mice, and that the increased amount of proteins produced in males is mediated by the higher content of androgens in male animals (Davidoff et al. 2003; Pañeda et al. 2009; Dane et al. 2009).

Basing on such considerations, Guenzel et al. speculated that the female mice also showed diminished vector-mediated expression due to a scarcity of androgens, whereas higher therapeutic PCCA protein expression was observed in the livers of male mice. These results at 4 weeks after the AAV therapy were confirmed only in the liver; therapeutic levels of PCCA in muscle tissue were comparable between males and females showing no effect of sex. Extending these observations for a longer period of time, 1.5 years after the treatment, the authors revealed a remarkable effect of sex, with female mice showing low PCAA levels in either the liver or skeletal muscle, while having similar levels compared with males in the cardiac tissue or in other tissues. Even though the liver PCCA levels were lower in females than in males after AAV therapy, female mice exhibited a therapeutic advantage from 1 to 45 weeks after treatment (Guenzel et al. 2015). The reason behind this sex-biased effects in response to the therapy is still unknown, and could be due to the AAV vectors themselves, or to still undiscovered mechanisms diverse among the sexes.

6 Conclusions

Mass-spectrometry based metabolomics has become an essential component of "omics" studies, with its main intrinsic features that allow building a bridge between the genetic, epigenetic, and the phenotypical endpoint of biological systems.

It is clear that several aspects of the metabolism are differently controlled in men and women of different ages starting from prenatal life, thus influencing their behavior in health and disease in terms of metabolic regulation, diagnosis, and therapeutic intervention. Unfortunately, much less is known regarding the probable differences guided by sex and gender in the context of inherited metabolic disorders, and this is mostly due to the rarity of such conditions that do not allow to perform powerful statistical sex-analyses and -correlations.

On the path toward precision, personalized and holistic health and medicine, deciphering sex-gender-specific traits in metabolic control is certainly a pivotal issue to improve individual approaches for the management and treatment of metabolic disorders. Therefore, the elucidation of sex-gender specific biological variations would be considered extremely relevant from several perspectives and should be advised as a necessary requisite by the whole scientific community.

References

Albersen M, Bonthuis M, de Roos NM et al (2010) Whole body composition analysis by the BodPod air-displacement plethysmography method in children with phenylketonuria shows a higher body fat percentage. J Inherit Metab Dis 33:283–288. https://doi.org/10.1007/s10545-010-9149-8

Allen J, McCauley J, Waters D et al (1995) Resting energy expenditure in children with phenylketonuria. Am J Clin Nutr 62:797–801. https://doi.org/10.1093/ajcn/62.4.797

Allen JR, Baur LA, Waters DL et al (1996) Body protein in prepubertal children with phenylketonuria. Eur J Clin Nutr 50:178–186

Beale DJ, Pinu FR, Kouremenos KA et al (2018) Review of recent developments in GC–MS approaches to metabolomics-based research. Metabolomics

Bell SM, Wendt DJ, Zhang Y et al (2017) Formulation and PEGylation optimization of the therapeutic PEGylated phenylalanine ammonia lyase for the treatment of phenylketonuria. PLoS One 12:e0173269. https://doi.org/10.1371/journal.pone.0173269

Braun AE, Mitchel OR, Gonzalez TL et al (2022) Sex at the interface: the origin and impact of sex differences in the developing human placenta. Biol Sex Differ 13:50. https://doi.org/10.1186/s13293-022-00459-7

Brennan L, Gibbons H (2020) Sex matters: a focus on the impact of biological sex on metabolomic profiles and dietary interventions. Proc Nutr Soc 79:205–209. https://doi.org/10.1017/S002966511900106X

Campesi I, Occhioni S, Tonolo G et al (2016) Ageing/menopausal status in healthy women and ageing in healthy men differently affect cardiometabolic parameters. Int J Med Sci 13:124–132. https://doi.org/10.7150/ijms.14163

Campesi I, Milella L, Palermo M et al (2020) Cigarette smoking affects the differences between male and female phenotypes. Am J Transl Res 12:2998–3010

Campesi I, Franconi F, Montella A et al (2021a) Human umbilical cord: information mine in sex-specific medicine. Life 11:52. https://doi.org/10.3390/life11010052

Campesi I, Montella A, Seghieri G, Franconi F (2021b) The person's care requires a sex and gender approach. J Clin Med 10:4770. https://doi.org/10.3390/jcm10204770
Campesi I, Montella A, Sotgiu G et al (2021c) Combined oral contraceptives modify the effect of smoking on inflammatory cellular indexes and endothelial function in healthy subjects. Eur J Pharmacol 891:173762. https://doi.org/10.1016/j.ejphar.2020.173762
Campesi I, Montella A, Sotgiu G et al (2022) Smoking and combined oral contraceptives should be considered as an independent variable in sex and gender-oriented studies. Toxicol Appl Pharmacol 457:116321. https://doi.org/10.1016/j.taap.2022.116321
Caterino M, Ruoppolo M, Villani GRD et al (2020) Influence of sex on urinary organic acids: a cross-sectional study in children. Int J Mol Sci 21:582. https://doi.org/10.3390/ijms21020582
Caterino M, Ruoppolo M, Costanzo M et al (2021) Sex affects human premature neonates' blood metabolome according to gestational age, parenteral nutrition, and caffeine treatment. Metabolites 11:158. https://doi.org/10.3390/metabo11030158
Chandler RJ, Venditti CP (2019) Gene therapy for methylmalonic acidemia: past, present, and future. Hum Gene Ther 30:1236–1244. https://doi.org/10.1089/hum.2019.113
Clegg DJ, Mauvais-Jarvis F (2018) An integrated view of sex differences in metabolic physiology and disease. Mol Metab 15:1–2. https://doi.org/10.1016/j.molmet.2018.06.011
Costanzo M, Caterino M (2023) Targeted lipidomics data of COVID-19 patients. Data Br 48: 109089. https://doi.org/10.1016/j.dib.2023.109089
Costanzo M, Caterino M, Cevenini A et al (2020a) Data independent acquisition mass spectrometry for proteomic advances into isolated methylmalonic acidemia. In: NATO science for peace and security series A: chemistry and biology. Springer Science and Business Media B.V, pp 221–223
Costanzo M, Caterino M, Cevenini A et al (2020b) Dataset of a comparative proteomics experiment in a methylmalonyl-CoA mutase knockout HEK 293 cell model. Data Br 33:106453. https://doi.org/10.1016/j.dib.2020.106453
Costanzo M, Fiocchetti M, Ascenzi P et al (2021) Proteomic and bioinformatic investigation of altered pathways in neuroglobin-deficient breast cancer cells. Molecules 26:2397. https://doi.org/10.3390/molecules26082397
Costanzo M, Caterino M, Ruoppolo M (2022a) Targeted metabolomics. In: Metabolomics perspectives. Elsevier, pp 219–236
Costanzo M, Caterino M, Salvatori I et al (2022b) Proteome data of neuroblastoma cells overexpressing neuroglobin. Data Br 41:107843. https://doi.org/10.1016/j.dib.2022.107843
Costanzo M, Caterino M, Sotgiu G et al (2022c) Sex differences in the human metabolome. Biol Sex Differ 13:30. https://doi.org/10.1186/s13293-022-00440-4
Couce ML, Guler I, Anca-Couce A et al (2015) New insights in growth of phenylketonuric patients. Eur J Pediatr 174:651–659. https://doi.org/10.1007/s00431-014-2446-8
Critelli K, McKiernan P, Vockley J et al (2018) Liver transplantation for propionic acidemia and methylmalonic acidemia: perioperative management and clinical outcomes. Liver Transpl 24: 1260–1270. https://doi.org/10.1002/lt.25304
Dane AP, Cunningham SC, Graf NS, Alexander IE (2009) Sexually dimorphic patterns of episomal rAAV genome persistence in the adult mouse liver and correlation with hepatocellular proliferation. Mol Ther 17:1548–1554. https://doi.org/10.1038/mt.2009.139
Davidoff AM, Ng CYC, Zhou J et al (2003) Sex significantly influences transduction of murine liver by recombinant adeno-associated viral vectors through an androgen-dependent pathway. Blood 102:480–488. https://doi.org/10.1182/blood-2002-09-2889
de Baulny HO, Abadie V, Feillet F, de Parscau L (2007) Management of phenylketonuria and hyperphenylalaninemia. J Nutr 137:1561S–1563S. https://doi.org/10.1093/jn/137.6.1561S
Di Minno A, Gelzo M, Caterino M et al (2022) Challenges in metabolomics-based tests, biomarkers revealed by metabolomic analysis, and the promise of the application of metabolomics in precision medicine. Int J Mol Sci 23:5213. https://doi.org/10.3390/ijms23095213

Dobbelaere D, Michaud L, Debrabander A et al (2003) Evaluation of nutritional status and pathophysiology of growth retardation in patients with phenylketonuria. J Inherit Metab Dis 26:1–11. https://doi.org/10.1023/A:1024063726046

Doulgeraki A, Skarpalezou A, Theodosiadou A et al (2014) Body composition profile of young patients with phenylketonuria and mild hyperphenylalaninemia. Int J Endocrinol Metab 12. https://doi.org/10.5812/ijem.16061

Elhawary NA, AlJahdali IA, Abumansour IS et al (2022) Genetic etiology and clinical challenges of phenylketonuria. Hum Genomics 16:22. https://doi.org/10.1186/s40246-022-00398-9

Firman SJ, Ramachandran R, Whelan K et al (2022) Protein status in phenylketonuria: a scoping review. Clin Nutr 41:894–922. https://doi.org/10.1016/j.clnu.2022.02.010

Franconi F, Rosano G, Campesi I (2015) Need for gender-specific pre-analytical testing: the dark side of the moon in laboratory testing. Int J Cardiol 179:514–535. https://doi.org/10.1016/j.ijcard.2014.11.019

Gonzalez Melo M, Fontana A, Viertl D et al (2021a) A knock-in rat model unravels acute and chronic renal toxicity in glutaric aciduria type I. Mol Genet Metab. https://doi.org/10.1016/j.ymgme.2021.10.003

Gonzalez Melo M, Remacle N, Cudré-Cung H-P et al (2021b) The first knock-in rat model for glutaric aciduria type I allows further insights into pathophysiology in brain and periphery. Mol Genet Metab 133:157–181. https://doi.org/10.1016/j.ymgme.2021.03.017

Guenzel AJ, Hillestad ML, Matern D, Barry MA (2014) Effects of adeno-associated virus serotype and tissue-specific expression on circulating biomarkers of propionic acidemia. Hum Gene Ther 25:837–843. https://doi.org/10.1089/hum.2014.012

Guenzel AJ, Collard R, Kraus JP et al (2015) Long-term sex-biased correction of circulating propionic acidemia disease markers by adeno-associated virus vectors. Hum Gene Ther 26: 153–160. https://doi.org/10.1089/hum.2014.126

Hanley WB (2011) Non-PKU mild hyperphenylalaninemia (MHP) – the dilemma. Mol Genet Metab 104:23–26. https://doi.org/10.1016/j.ymgme.2011.05.007

Huang CS, Sadre-Bazzaz K, Shen Y et al (2010) Crystal structure of the α6β6 holoenzyme of propionyl-coenzyme A carboxylase. Nature 466:1001–1005. https://doi.org/10.1038/nature09302

Huemer M, Huemer C, Möslinger D et al (2007) Growth and body composition in children with classical phenylketonuria: results in 34 patients and review of the literature. J Inherit Metab Dis 30:694–699. https://doi.org/10.1007/s10545-007-0549-3

Jiang L, Park J-S, Yin L et al (2020) Dual mRNA therapy restores metabolic function in long-term studies in mice with propionic acidemia. Nat Commun 11:5339. https://doi.org/10.1038/s41467-020-19156-3

Johnson CH, Gonzalez FJ (2012) Challenges and opportunities of metabolomics. J Cell Physiol

Joyce AR, Palsson B (2006) The model organism as a system: integrating "omics" data sets. Nat Rev Mol Cell Biol

Kautzky-Willer A, Handisurya A (2009) Metabolic diseases and associated complications: sex and gender matter! Eur J Clin Investig 39:631–648. https://doi.org/10.1111/j.1365-2362.2009.02161.x

Knerr I, Weinhold N, Vockley J, Gibson KM (2012) Advances and challenges in the treatment of branched-chain amino/keto acid metabolic defects. J Inherit Metab Dis 35:29–40. https://doi.org/10.1007/s10545-010-9269-1

Kwiatkowski K, Coe K, Bailar JC, Swanson GM (2013) Inclusion of minorities and women in cancer clinical trials, a decade later: have we improved? Cancer 119:2956–2963. https://doi.org/10.1002/cncr.28168

Lichter-Konecki U, Vockley J (2019) Phenylketonuria: current treatments and future developments. Drugs 79:495–500. https://doi.org/10.1007/s40265-019-01079-z

Link JC, Chen X, Arnold AP, Reue K (2013) Metabolic impact of sex chromosomes. Adipocytes 2: 74–79. https://doi.org/10.4161/adip.23320

Maestro S, Weber ND, Zabaleta N et al (2021) Novel vectors and approaches for gene therapy in liver diseases. JHEP Rep 3:100300. https://doi.org/10.1016/j.jhepr.2021.100300

Manganelli V, Salvatori I, Costanzo M et al (2021) Overexpression of neuroglobin promotes energy metabolism and autophagy induction in human neuroblastoma SH-SY5Y cells. Cell 10:3394. https://doi.org/10.3390/cells10123394

Mauvais-Jarvis F, Arnold AP, Reue K (2017) A guide for the design of pre-clinical studies on sex differences in metabolism. Cell Metab 25:1216–1230. https://doi.org/10.1016/j.cmet.2017.04.033

Mauvais-Jarvis F, Berthold HK, Campesi I et al (2021) Sex- and gender-based pharmacological response to drugs. Pharmacol Rev 73:730–762. https://doi.org/10.1124/pharmrev.120.000206

McBurnie MA, Kronmal RA, Schuett VE et al (1991) Physical growth of children treated for phenylketonuria. Ann Hum Biol 18:357–368. https://doi.org/10.1080/03014469100001662

Mitani AA, Haneuse S (2020) Small data challenges of studying rare diseases. JAMA Netw Open 3: e201965. https://doi.org/10.1001/jamanetworkopen.2020.1965

Mittelstrass K, Ried JS, Yu Z et al (2011) Discovery of sexual dimorphisms in metabolic and genetic biomarkers. PLoS Genet. https://doi.org/10.1371/journal.pgen.1002215

Nicholson JK, Lindon JC (2008) Systems biology: metabonomics. Nature

Pañeda A, Vanrell L, Mauleon I et al (2009) Effect of adeno-associated virus serotype and genomic structure on liver transduction and biodistribution in mice of both genders. Hum Gene Ther 20: 908–917. https://doi.org/10.1089/hum.2009.031

Prakash VS, Mansukhani NA, Helenowski IB et al (2018) Sex bias in interventional clinical trials. J Women's Health 27:1342–1348. https://doi.org/10.1089/jwh.2017.6873

Rich-Edwards JW, Kaiser UB, Chen GL et al (2018) Sex and gender differences research design for basic, clinical, and population studies: essentials for investigators. Endocr Rev 39:424–439. https://doi.org/10.1210/er.2017-00246

Rocha JC, van Spronsen FJ, Almeida MF et al (2013) Early dietary treated patients with phenylketonuria can achieve normal growth and body composition. Mol Genet Metab 110:S40–S43. https://doi.org/10.1016/j.ymgme.2013.10.009

Roviello GN, Roviello G, Musumeci D et al (2014) Synthesis and supramolecular assembly of 1,3-bis(1′-uracilyl)-2- propanone. RSC Adv 4:28691–28698. https://doi.org/10.1039/c4ra03713h

Ruoppolo M, Campesi I, Scolamiero E et al (2014) Serum metabolomic profiles suggest influence of sex and oral contraceptive use. Am J Transl Res

Ruoppolo M, Scolamiero E, Caterino M et al (2015) Female and male human babies have distinct blood metabolomic patterns. Mol BioSyst. https://doi.org/10.1039/c5mb00297d

Ruoppolo M, Caterino M, Albano L et al (2018) Targeted metabolomic profiling in rat tissues reveals sex differences. Sci Rep 8:4663. https://doi.org/10.1038/s41598-018-22869-7

Ruoppolo M, Malvagia S, Boenzi S et al (2022) Expanded newborn screening in Italy using tandem mass spectrometry: two years of national experience. Int J Neonatal Screen 8:47. https://doi.org/10.3390/ijns8030047

Sailer M, Elizondo G, Martin J et al (2020) Nutrient intake, body composition, and blood phenylalanine control in children with phenylketonuria compared to healthy controls. Mol Genet Metab Rep 23:100599. https://doi.org/10.1016/j.ymgmr.2020.100599

Santorelli L, Caterino M, Costanzo M (2022) Dynamic interactomics by cross-linking mass spectrometry: mapping the daily cell life in postgenomic era. Omi A J Integr Biol 26:633–649. https://doi.org/10.1089/omi.2022.0137

Schrimpe-Rutledge AC, Codreanu SG, Sherrod SD, McLean JA (2016) Untargeted metabolomics strategies – challenges and emerging directions. J Am Soc Mass Spectrom. https://doi.org/10.1007/s13361-016-1469-y

Seghieri G, Franconi F, Campesi I (2022) Why we need sex-gender medicine: the striking example of type 2 diabetes. Diabetology 3:460–469. https://doi.org/10.3390/diabetology3030034

Stotland NL (2001) Gender-based biology. Am J Psychiatry 158:161–162. https://doi.org/10.1176/appi.ajp.158.2.161

Stroup BM, Sawin EA, Murali SG et al (2017) Amino acid medical foods provide a high dietary acid load and increase urinary excretion of renal net acid, calcium, and magnesium compared with glycomacropeptide medical foods in phenylketonuria. J Nutr Metab 2017:1–12. https://doi.org/10.1155/2017/1909101
Stroup BM, Hansen KE, Krueger D et al (2018) Sex differences in body composition and bone mineral density in phenylketonuria: a cross-sectional study. Mol Genet Metab Rep 15:30–35. https://doi.org/10.1016/j.ymgmr.2018.01.004
Tarnopolsky MA, Ruby BC (2001) Sex differences in carbohydrate metabolism. Curr Opin Clin Nutr Metab Care 4:521–526. https://doi.org/10.1097/00075197-200111000-00010
Tavassoly I, Goldfarb J, Iyengar R (2018) Systems biology primer: the basic methods and approaches. Essays Biochem 62:487–500. https://doi.org/10.1042/EBC20180003
Tramunt B, Smati S, Grandgeorge N et al (2020) Sex differences in metabolic regulation and diabetes susceptibility. Diabetologia 63:453–461. https://doi.org/10.1007/s00125-019-05040-3
van Spronsen FJ, Blau N, Harding C et al (2021) Phenylketonuria. Nat Rev Dis Primers 7:36. https://doi.org/10.1038/s41572-021-00267-0
Vela-Amieva M, Alcántara-Ortigoza MA, Ibarra-González I et al (2022) Genotypic spectrum underlying tetrahydrobiopterin metabolism defects: experience in a single Mexican reference center. Front Genet 13. https://doi.org/10.3389/fgene.2022.993612
Wang C, Xu Y (2019) Mechanisms for sex differences in energy homeostasis. J Mol Endocrinol 62: R129–R143. https://doi.org/10.1530/JME-18-0165
Wishart DS (2011) Advances in metabolite identification. Bioanalysis
Wongkittichote P, Ah Mew N, Chapman KA (2017) Propionyl-CoA carboxylase – a review. Mol Genet Metab 122:145–152. https://doi.org/10.1016/j.ymgme.2017.10.002

Hypothalamic-Pituitary-Gonadal Axis Disorders Impacting Fertility in Both Sexes and the Potential of Kisspeptin-Based Therapies to Treat Them

Maricedes Acosta-Martínez

Contents

M. Acosta-Martínez (✉)
Department of Physiology and Biophysics, Renaissance School of Medicine at Stony Brook, Stony Brook, NY, USA
e-mail: maricedes.acosta@stonybrook.edu

S. E. Tsirka, M. Acosta-Martinez (eds.), *Sex and Gender Effects in Pharmacology*, Handbook of Experimental Pharmacology 282,
https://doi.org/10.1007/164_2023_666

Abstract

Impaired function of the hypothalamic-pituitary-gonadal (HPG) axis can lead to a vast array of reproductive disorders some of which are inherited or acquired, but many are of unknown etiology. Among the clinical consequences of HPG impairment, infertility is quite common. According to the latest report from the World Health Organization, the global prevalence of infertility during a person's lifetime is a staggering 17.5% which translate into 1 out of every 6 people experiencing it. In both sexes, infertility is associated with adverse health events, and if unresolved, infertility can cause substantial psychological stress, social stigmatization, and economic strain. Even though significant advances have been made in the management and treatment of infertility, low or variable efficacy of treatments and medication adverse effects still pose a significant problem. However, the discovery that in humans inactivating mutations in the gene encoding the kisspeptin receptor (Kiss1R) results in pubertal failure and infertility has expanded our understanding of the mechanisms underlying the neuroendocrine control of reproduction, opening up potential new therapies for the treatment of infertility disorders. In this chapter we provide an overview of common infertility disorders affecting men and women, their recommended treatments, and the potential of kisspeptin-based pharmacotherapies to treat them.

Keywords

Fertility · Gonadotropins · Hypothalamus · In vitro fertilization · Kisspeptin · Male hypogonadism · Ovulatory disorders · Sex steroids

Abbreviations

AMH	Anti-mullerian hormone
ART	Assisted reproductive technology
BMI	Body mass index
BMSCs	Bone marrow derived mesenchymal stem cells
BPA	Bisphenol A
CBAVD	Congenital absence of vas deferens
CC	Clomiphene citrate
CHH	Congenital hypogonadotropic hypogonadism
COS	Controlled ovarian stimulation
DA	Dopamine
E_2	Estradiol
EDCs	Endocrine disrupting chemicals

EMT	Empirical medical therapy
ERα	Estrogen receptor alpha
FHA	Functional hypothalamic amenorrhea
FSH	Follicle stimulating hormone
GABA	γ-Amino butyric acid
GnRH	Gonadotropin releasing hormone
hCG	Human chorionic gonadotropin
hMG	Human menopausal gonadotropin
HPG	Hypothalamic pituitary gonadal
ICSI	Intracytoplasmic sperm injection
IUI	Intrauterine insemination
IVF	In vitro fertilization
Kiss1R	Kisspeptin receptor
KP10	Kisspeptin 10
KP54	Kisspeptin 54
LH	Luteinizing hormone
LTZ	Letrozole
MKRN3	Makorin RING-finger protein 3
NK3R	Neurokinin B receptor
NKB	Neurokinin B
NPY	Neuropeptide Y
OHSS,	Ovarian hyperstimulation syndrome
OS	Oxidative stress
PCOS	Polycystic ovarian syndrome
POA	Preoptic area
POI	Premature ovarian insufficiency
PVC	Polyvinyl chloride
ROS	Reactive oxygen species
RP3V	Rostral periventricular region of the third ventricle
T	Testosterone
T2D	Type 2 diabetes

1 Introduction

Impaired function of the hypothalamic-pituitary-gonadal (HPG) axis can lead to a vast array of reproductive disorders some of which are inherited or acquired but many are of unknown etiology. These can occur early on, disrupting the onset and/or tempo of reproductive maturation (puberty), or they can manifest in the adult individual. Among the clinical consequences of HPG impairment, infertility is quite common. In fact, the global disease burden of infertility is growing, with the age-standardized prevalence rate increasing by 0.37% per year for females and 0.29% per year for males from 1990 to 2017 (Sun et al. 2019). Infertility represents an important public health issue because if not resolved, it can cause considerable psychological stress, social stigmatization, and economic strain (Boivin et al. 2022). Moreover, in both sexes, infertility is associated with a higher incidence of non-communicable diseases such as diabetes, cardiovascular disease, and certain cancers (Choy and Eisenberg 2018; Senapati 2018). Alarmingly, the inability to conceive has been associated with premature mortality in women (Wang et al. 2022b). While awareness about infertility as an important medical condition has increased in recent years, low or variable efficacy of treatments and medication side effects still beset its clinical management.

Underlying the control of reproduction is a tightly coordinated communication between specialized gonadotropin releasing hormone (GnRH)-containing neurons in the hypothalamus, the gonadotropin cells of the pituitary, and the germ cells and supportive tissue of the gonads (ovaries and testes). The intermittent discharge of GnRH into the pituitary portal vasculature is essential for the pulsatile secretion of the gonadotropins, luteinizing hormone (LH), and follicle stimulating hormone (FSH), by the pituitary (Christian and Moenter 2010). These in turn act on target cells in the testes and ovaries to direct gametogenesis, as well as the secretion of gonadal steroid hormones. Impaired GnRH secretion might lead to abnormally high or abnormally low gonadotropin levels affecting the secretion of gonadal hormones, which in turn negatively impacts follicular development in females and spermatogenesis in males. However, malfunction can occur at any level of the HPG axis and progress in the clinical diagnosis and treatment of infertility has relied on our understanding of the cellular hierarchy and the molecular mechanisms governing its physiology. In this regard, the discovery almost two decades ago that inactivating mutations in the gene encoding the kisspeptin receptor (*KISS1R*) were associated with hypogonadotropic hypogonadism and absence of puberty in humans has expanded the field of reproductive biology (de Roux et al. 2003; Seminara et al. 2003). Beyond its fundamental role governing mammalian puberty, this sexually dimorphic neural network is now recognized as part of the "GnRH pulse generator," responsible for pulsatile gonadotropin secretion.

In this chapter we will focus on HPG axis disorders that impact fertility in both sexes and discuss the recommended medical interventions. We will also review the findings supporting the future utilization of kisspeptin-based therapies for some of these reproductive disorders.

2 Development and Function of the HPG Axis: An Overview

Fertility critically depends on what is termed as the "GnRH pulse generator," a neural network located in the infundibular nucleus (equivalent to the arcuate nucleus in rodents), that co-expresses the neuropeptides kisspeptin, neurokinin B and dynorphin A, the *KNDy* (*K*iss/*N*KB/*D*yn) neurons (Fig. 1; (Moore et al. 2018). Through paracrine and autocrine signaling, neurokinin B stimulates, whereas dynorphin A inhibits kisspeptin output and hence GnRH secretion from the median eminence, and subsequent pulsatile LH release from the anterior pituitary. GnRH

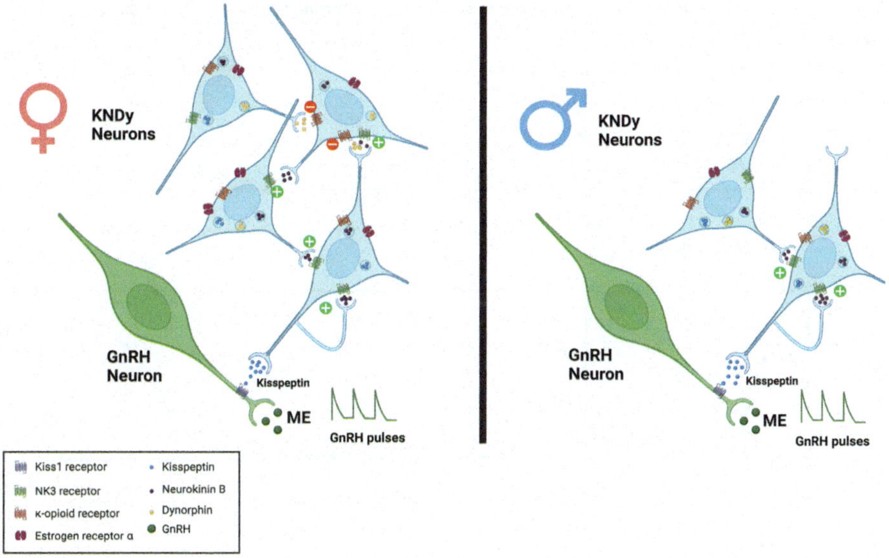

Fig. 1 Model of the GnRH pulse generator. Pulsatile GnRH release is controlled by the activity of hypothalamic neurons that co-express the neuropeptides kisspeptin, neurokinin B and dynorphin A, the KnDy neurons. NKB secreted from KnDy neurons bind to NK3R stimulating kisspeptin release which in turn binds to Kiss1Rs on GnRH neurons to stimulate GnRH release. In contrast, Dyn released from KnDy neurons binds to κ-ORs thereby inhibiting KNDy neuronal activity and kisspeptin release. It has been proposed that alternate episodes of facilitation and inhibition of kisspeptin release by NKB and Dyn induce pulsatile secretion of GnRH at the ME. Negative feedback actions of sex-steroid hormones like estradiol act on estrogen receptors expressed in KnDy neurons to maintain pulsatile GnRH release. Made using Biorender.com *Dyn* Dynorphin, *GnRH* gonadotropin releasing hormone, *Kiss1R* kisspeptin receptor, *κ-OR* kappa opioid receptor, *ME* median eminence, *NKB* Neurokinin B, *NK3R* Neurokinin B receptor

neurons express kisspeptin receptors, hence they are direct targets of kisspeptin actions. Furthermore, KNDy neurons express receptors for neuromodulators known to control GnRH function, hence, they can serve as a bridge system, relying information about changes in the internal and external environment, including the positive and negative feedback control by gonadal steroid hormones.

The activity of the GnRH pulse generator and hence of the HPG axis varies throughout the lifespan (Fig. 2; (Howard 2021). Pulsatile production of GnRH starts in utero, at around 10–12 weeks of gestation, shortly after GnRH neurons have completed their embryonic migration from the olfactory placode to the hypothalamus (Casoni et al. 2016). Independent of GnRH release however, there is a sharp rise in fetal LH and FSH during mid-pregnancy, which coincides with the beginnings of follicular or seminiferous tubule development. Due to the suppressive actions of fetal testosterone (T), higher levels of LH and FSH are observed in female compared to male fetuses (O'Shaughnessy and Fowler 2011). Then, increasing production of estrogen and progesterone by the placenta blocks fetal gonadotropin levels for the remaining of pregnancy. After birth, the absence of negative feedback by placental

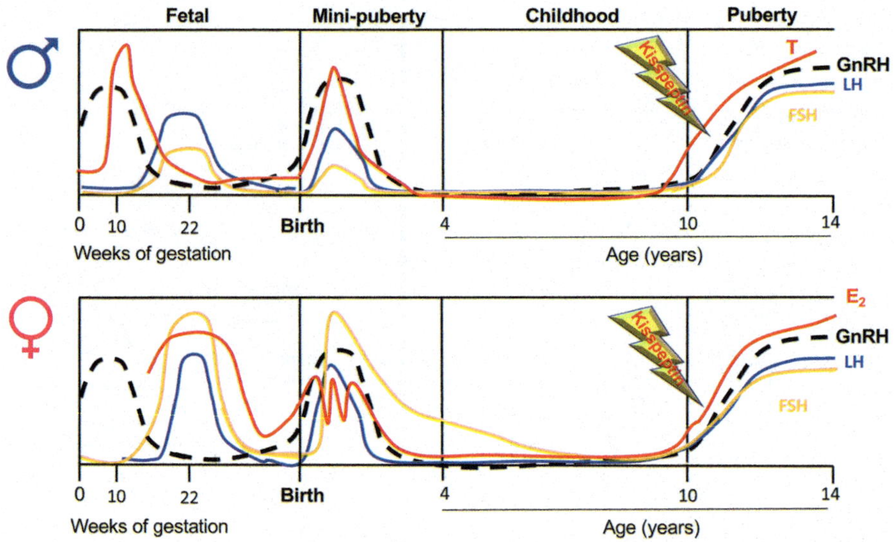

Fig. 2 Schematic representation of the changes in reproductive hormone levels during the fetal, postnatal, childhood, and pubertal periods in boys (top panel) and girls (lower panel). GnRH secretion starts early in gestation, followed by an increase in fetal LH and FSH levels during mid-gestation. In boys, fetal production of T also starts early and accompanies the production of LH and FSH at mid-gestation. In girls, however, gonadotropin and E_2 levels increase during mid-gestation. Then, negative feedback exerted by placenta hormones suppresses fetal reproductive hormone secretion for the remaining of pregnancy. After birth, a strong adult-like activity of the HPG axis occurs, a period termed minipuberty. Gonadotropin levels peak 1–2 months after birth in both sexes, however, while in boys both LH and FSH levels slowly decline afterwards, in girls, FSH levels remain high for up to 4 years after birth. Minipuberty is followed by a period of quiescent HPG axis activity until puberty, when reactivation of a strong GnRH pulse generator, which includes the release of the neuropeptide kisspeptin, occurs. Adapted from Howard (2021). *GnRH* Gonadotropin releasing hormone, *HPG* hypothalamic pituitary gonadal, *LH* luteinizing hormone, *FSH* follicle stimulating hormone, *T* testosterone, E_2 estradiol

hormones gives rise to a second phase of HPG activation called minipuberty (Renault et al. 2020). The gonadotropins and sex hormones produced during this period are important for the maturation of the sexual organs, laying the ground for future fertility. For instance, in boys, for about 1–6 months after birth, HPG axis activity produces FSH, LH, and T at adult levels, the latter contributing to penile and testicular growth. Girls also experience minipuberty but in contrast to boys, FSH levels remain elevated for up to 3–4 years. Fluctuating levels of estradiol (E_2) are also observed in females during this period; however, its physiological significance is less understood (Renault et al. 2020).

Minipuberty is followed by a period of quiescent HPG axis activity until puberty, when reactivation of a strong GnRH pulse generator occurs. Loss of function mutations in *KISS1 (*encoding kisspeptin*), KISS1R, TAC3* (encoding Neurokinin B) or its receptor *TACR3* (NK3R), results in congenital gonadotropin deficiency and pubertal failure in humans, supporting a key role of KNDy neurons in triggering pulsatile GnRH release at puberty (Uenoyama et al. 2019; Witchel and Plant 2021). However, the mechanisms driving the prepubertal suppression of kisspeptin in mammals vary by species. For example, the prepubertal inhibition of kisspeptin synthesis in rodents is driven primarily by estrogen through the activation of estrogen receptor alpha (ERα) (Mayer et al. 2010). In contrast, estrogen-independent mechanisms are at play in primates, which might include the regulation of kisspeptin by γ-amino butyric acid (GABA), neuropeptide Y (NPY), and more recently, by the intracellular protein Makorin RING-finger Protein 3 (MKRN3) (Uenoyama et al. 2019). Loss of function mutations in *MKRN3* were identified in patients exhibiting premature activation of the HPG axis known as central precocious puberty (Schreiner et al. 2014; Simon et al. 2016). MKRN3 represses *KISS1* and *TAK3* promoter activity, thereby acting as a prepubertal repressor of the upstream control of GnRH neurons (Abreu et al. 2020). Accordingly, hypothalamic MKRN3 expression is high in rodents and in nonhuman primates early in life but decreases as puberty approaches. Similarly, circulating MKRN3 levels decline prior to pubertal onset and throughout puberty in girls (Hagen et al. 2015) and boys (Busch et al. 2016).

In the adult, the regulation of KNDy neurons by gonadal sex steroids, particularly E_2, produces two modes of GnRH/LH release: pulsatile and as a surge, the latter occurring only in females. During the follicular phase of the menstrual cycle, pulsatile gonadotropin secretion stimulates the maturation of ovarian follicles and the production of ovarian sex hormones. This tonic GnRH/LH release is maintained by the negative feedback action of E_2 on hypothalamic kisspeptin neurons (Skorupskaite et al. 2014). At the end of the follicular phase, ovarian E_2 exerts positive feedback to induce the LH surge required for ovulation. Studies in rodents suggest that arcuate kisspeptin neurons mediate E_2 negative feedback on GnRH/LH release (Yeo and Herbison 2014), whereas E_2 acting on ERα in kisspeptin neurons located in the rostral periventricular region of the third ventricle (RP3V) mediates positive feedback (Dubois et al. 2015). Even though in humans a rostral preoptic area (POA) kisspeptin population has been identified (Hrabovszky et al. 2010) the consensus is that KNDy neurons in the infundibular nucleus "relay" both E_2 negative and positive feedback, with the role of the POA kisspeptin population still unclear (Skorupskaite et al. 2014).

Similar mechanisms control pulsatile GnRH/LH release in males. For example, androgens, which are converted to estrogen, act on hypothalamic kisspeptin neurons to exert negative feedback regulation of GnRH/LH release, which is necessary to maintain spermatogenesis and steroidogenesis (O'Shaughnessy and Fowler 2011). At the gonad level, LH acts on Leydig cells to stimulate T release, whereas FSH and T act on Sertoli cells to support the initiation and maintenance of spermatogenesis. FSH also stimulates Sertoli cells to produce inhibin B which aids T in regulating pituitary FSH secretion.

It is important to point out that strong sexual dimorphism characterizes hypothalamic kisspeptin expression. Few kisspeptin-expressing cells and fibers are present in the male infundibular nucleus and none in the rostral POA. In contrast in the female there is abundance of kisspeptin cells and fibers in both regions (Hrabovszky et al. 2010). These sex differences are thought to be established perinatally, through the actions of sex steroids (Taziaux et al. 2016). While pulsatile release of GnRH is crucial for the maintenance of anterior pituitary cell (gonadotrophs) responsiveness to GnRH stimulation in both sexes, the sex differences in kisspeptin expression might contribute to sex differences in the neuroendocrine control and hence pattern of GnRH/LH release.

The pharmacotherapy utilized to treat infertility disorders in men and women involves targeting different levels of the HPG axis to stimulate or inhibit reproductive hormone secretion. Recent clinical studies have shown that the administration of kisspeptin, kisspeptin receptor agonists, and even Neurokinin B receptor antagonists can efficiently stimulate or inhibit endogenous gonadotropin and gonadal hormone levels. Hence, in Sect. 5 we will provide a detailed description of kisspeptin pharmacology as well as the reproductive disorders in which the use of kisspeptin pharmacotherapy is being explored.

3 Female Infertility

The causes of infertility in women can be attributed to structural problems such as damage to the fallopian tubes, uterine disorders like endometriosis and fibroids, and to ovulatory disorders (Carson and Kallen 2021). However, ovulatory disorders, which are linked to the episodic or chronic dysfunction of the HPG axis, are the most common factor of female infertility, accounting for approximately 25% of infertility cases (Carson and Kallen 2021).

Until recently, ovulatory disorders were classified based on the WHO system, which primarily relies on circulating levels of gonadotropin and gonadal sex hormones. As such, ovulatory disorders were grouped into three categories: *group I* (hypogonadotropic hypogonadism), *Group II* (normo-gonadotropic, normo-estrogenic anovulation), and *Group III* (hypergonadotropic hypoestrogenic anovulation); (reviewed in Koysombat et al. (2023)). In 2022, however, the International Federation of Gynecology and Obstetrics (FIGO) developed a new classification system meant to be applied after identifying the presence of an ovulatory disorder (Munro et al. 2022). The new system, summarized by its acronym HyPO-P, employs three anatomical categories, *hy*pothalamic (Type I), *p*ituitary (Type II), and *o*varian (Type III) and a fourth separate category for polycystic ovarian syndrome (*P*COS, Type IV). Then, a second level of classification frames each of the anatomic categories (I-III) into presumed etiologies summarized by the GAIN-FIT-PIE acronym; GAIN stands for Genetic, Autoimmune, Iatrogenic, or Neoplasm etiologies, FIT stands for Functional, Infectious/inflammatory, or Trauma and vascular etiologies, and PIE stands for Physiological, Idiopathic, and Endocrine etiologies. A third level of classification consists of specific diagnosis. The goal of the updated classification is to have a standardized language that can be universally used by researchers, clinicians, educators, and patients, and in this way advance research, facilitate diagnosis and, importantly, improve the communication between doctors and their patients. Supporters of the new classification system argue that in contrast to the previous WHO system, HyPO-P explicitly recognizes that many causes of ovulatory disorders are not related to ovarian function and that many occur on a spectrum.

3.1 Examples of Ovulatory Disorders

3.1.1 Functional Hypothalamic Amenorrhea (FHA)

A common cause of secondary amenorrhea, which occurs when a woman who already menstruates does not get her period for 3 months or more, is functional hypothalamic amenorrhea (FHA), accounting for approximately 1–2% of cases (Phylactou et al. 2021). Impaired GnRH release resulting in gonadotropin levels that are too low to stimulate follicular development and E_2 production characterize patients with FHA. FHA is caused by stress, negative energy balance due to poor nutrition or decreased caloric intake, or by excessive exercise, but often a combination of these is responsible (Morrison et al. 2021). Not surprisingly, the prevalence of FHA is higher in women athletes, with one study reporting that half of women who exercise regularly experience subtle menstrual disorders and approximately 30% have amenorrhea (De Souza et al. 2010). In fact, the term female athlete triad refers to the co-occurrence of menstrual dysfunction, low energy availability, and decreased bone mineral density and was first coined in 1992 by the American College of Sports Medicine after experts in the field noticed this pattern among young female athletes (Nazem and Ackerman 2012). Importantly, in addition to impaired reproduction, the chronic absence of E_2, if untreated, will negatively impact cardiac, skeletal, and brain functions.

FHA is a reversible condition, and the elimination of causative factors is often times enough to reverse it. For example, lifestyle changes such as reducing exercise and increasing caloric intake will reverse amenorrhea (Roberts et al. 2020). In the case of FHA due to emotional or psychological stress, cognitive behavioral therapy and/or pharmacotherapy for anxiety or depression might help reverse amenorrhea. In other cases, such as those due to eating disorders, a multidisciplinary approach is needed. However, when lifestyle changes are unsuccessful in reversing amenorrhea and infertility, pharmacotherapy is recommended to induce ovulation. In such cases, clinicians are advised to induce ovulation only after attempts to normalize energy balance, and when a body mass index (BMI) of at least 18.5 kg/m^2 has been reached, otherwise the risk for pregnancy complications such as small-for-gestational-age babies, preterm labor, and even miscarriage is high (Gordon et al. 2017).

3.1.2 Congenital Hypogonadotropic Hypogonadism (CHH)

The term congenital hypogonadotropic hypogonadism (CHH) is used to describe a heterogeneous group of genetic disorders in which genes that control GnRH neuronal migration and function are mutated (Young et al. 2019). These rare genetic disorders are associated with deficient GnRH secretion and/or action, resulting in pubertal failure and infertility. In approximately 50% of cases, CHH patients also suffer from a reduced or deficient sense of smell, which is termed Kallmann syndrome. Over 30 genes have been associated with CHH which can act either alone or in combination resulting in a spectrum of clinical presentations, including non-reproductive phenotypes (Stamou et al. 2015). However, 50% of CHH cases remain without an identified genetic cause. The genetic complexity of CHH is also reflected in its different modes of inheritance, which can be X-linked, autosomal dominant, or autosomal recessive (Young et al. 2019).

Diagnosis of CHH in early adolescence can be challenging because the clinical presentation is very similar to that of constitutional delay of growth and puberty. Timely diagnosis and treatment will induce puberty, leading to improved sexual, bone, metabolic, and psychological health. While infertility in adult women with CHH is treatable (Sect. 3.2), some studies suggest that these patients are diagnosed late (after the age of 18) and experience a lower quality of life when compared to women with other forms of infertility (Dzemaili et al. 2017).

3.1.3 Hyperprolactinemia

In women, a major consequence of hyperprolactinemia is hypogonadotropic anovulation which results in amenorrhea, hypogonadism, and infertility (Melmed et al. 2011). Suppression of the hypothalamic pulsatile GnRH release by prolactin underlies this hypogonadotropic hypogonadal state. In addition, if untreated, hyperprolactinemia increases the risk for osteoporosis, a consequence of the estrogen deficiency. Possible causes of hyperprolactinemia include physiological (pregnancy and breast feeding), iatrogenic (drug-induced), a neoplasm, and endocrine. However, the most common cause of hyperprolactinemia are prolactin-secreting adenomas (prolactinomas), with microadenomas (<10 mm) being the most frequent type observed in women (Kaiser 2012).

3.1.4 Premature Ovarian Insufficiency (POI)

POI (premature ovarian failure) occurs when a woman's ovaries fail to function before the age of 40. It is associated with low estrogen production and the depletion of ovarian follicles, leading to menstrual abnormalities and infertility (Rudnicka et al. 2018). The prevalence of POI in the general population is estimated to be around 1% and while most cases of POI are idiopathic, genetic abnormalities, metabolic disorders, iatrogenic interventions, and other causes can also contribute to this disorder. The most common treatment for POI is hormone replacement therapy, which is effective at inducing regular menstrual cycles, prevents menopausal symptoms, and maintains bone health (Chon et al. 2021).

While there is no proven fertility treatment for women with POI, transplantation of stem cells might be a future clinical option to recover ovarian function in these patients (Wang et al. 2022a). Stem cells are thought to promote tissue repair through paracrine actions, inducing the release of bioactive factors that promote angiogenesis, block apoptosis and fibrosis, and exert anti-inflammatory and immunoregulatory effects (He et al. 2018). In rodent models of POI, such as chemically-induced ovarian damage, stem cell therapy improved ovarian function and stimulated reproductive hormone secretion (Wang et al. 2022a). Studies about the therapeutic effects of stem cell transplantation in patients with POI are few but encouraging. One study evaluated the therapeutic effects of autologous bone marrow derived mesenchymal stem cells (BMSCs) injected via laparoscopy into the ovaries of 10 women suffering from POI and reported that two patients resumed menstruation 3 months after transplantation and one became pregnant and delivered a healthy full-term baby (Edessy et al. 2016). Another study showed that the levels of estrogen and of anti-mullerian hormone (AMH), an indicator or ovarian reserve, rose significantly 1 month after autologous BMSCs transplantation in 26 out of 30 patients, and this change was maintained throughout the 48-week follow-up period (Gabr et al. 2016). Moreover, 60% of patients showed ovulation with ovum sizes ranging from 12 to 20 mm. Future studies are needed to address challenges pertaining to cell dose as well as determining the best route of injection so that a higher therapeutic success can be achieved.

3.1.5 Polycystic Ovarian Syndrome (PCOS)

PCOS affects approximately 4–20% of women worldwide, often leading to anovulatory infertility (Deswal et al. 2020). In fact, PCOS is considered to be the most common single cause of ovulatory dysfunction, responsible for 2–13% of secondary oligo/amenorrhea cases (Phylactou et al. 2021). To diagnose PCOS, the new FIGO system utilizes the "Rotterdam criteria" in which oligo-ovulation/anovulation with either hyperandrogenism, diagnosed either clinically (excessive hair growth, hirsutism) or biochemically (raised T serum levels), or polycystic ovaries on ultrasonogram, define the syndrome (Fauser et al. 2004). Increased GnRH pulsatility is a hallmark of PCOS; the increase in GnRH pulse frequency (from every 90 min to hourly) results in elevated LH secretion which in turn increases ovarian androgen production (Phylactou et al. 2021). Also contributing to high LH and androgen secretion is a reduced sensitivity to negative feedback by sex-steroid hormones (Abbara and Dhillo 2021). However, only a reported 40–60% of PCOS patients have elevated LH levels which leaves a significant proportion of PCOS patients with gonadotropin levels in the normal range.

PCOS is a complex and heterogenous disease whose manifestations are not limited to ovarian dysfunction. Women with PCOS have intrinsic insulin resistance and are at increased risk of type 2 diabetes (T2D), irrespective of age and BMI (Kakoly et al. 2019). In fact, it is estimated that the metabolic syndrome, a conglomerate of conditions including hypertension, hyperglycemia, obesity, and abnormal cholesterol or triglyceride levels, affects 33% of women with PCOS (Chandrasekaran and Sagili 2018). Although lifestyle changes, such as increased exercise and dietary modifications, have demonstrated substantial improvements in clinical symptoms, effects on ovulation or on pregnancy rates have not been examined.

3.2 Pharmacotherapy for Ovulatory Disorder-Related Infertility

3.2.1 Pulsatile GnRH Therapy

Pulsatile GnRH is considered the best treatment to induce ovulation and fertility in women with FHA or with CHH without pituitary dysfunction. Intravenous (iv.) or subcutaneous (sc.) pulsatile delivery is achieved by a portable pump, which contains gonadorelin, a synthetic peptide that is chemically and biologically identical to GnRH (Scheiber and Liu 2011). In this way, the pump mimics the physiological delivery of GnRH to the pituitary which increases the release LH and FSH, inducing ovulation in a way that closely resembles a normal menstrual cycle.

The GnRH pump has been shown to be safe and efficient, results in ovulation in more than 90% of cycles. In hypogonadotropic patients, pregnancy rates per GnRH-induced cycle ranged from 18% to 32% (Scheiber and Liu 2011). Moreover, compared to spontaneous pregnancies in the normal population, the GnRH pump is associated with only a slight increase in the rate of multiple pregnancies (1–2% vs. 5%) (Tranoulis et al. 2018). Cases of ovarian hyperstimulation syndrome (OHSS), a rare but potentially life-threatening complication in which the ovaries swell and leak fluid into the body, have not been reported using the GnRH pump (Christou et al. 2017). Surprisingly however, this FDA approved method for inducing ovulation is not widely utilized. In fact, in the USA, pulsatile treatment with GnRH (sc. or iv.) is only available in a research setting, whereas in Europe the sc. pump is available for clinical use.

3.2.2 Gonadotropin Injections

In anovulatory women with LH and FSH deficiency, such as women with CHH or FHA, an alternative therapeutic option to the GnRH pump is daily injections of gonadotropin preparations. Because FSH and LH work in synergy to stimulate an adequate follicular response, steroidogenesis, and ovulation, gonadotropin preparations containing LH are preferred to those containing FSH only. For example, human menopausal gonadotropin (hMG), which contains FSH and LH at a physiological 1:1 ratio, can effectively induce ovulation in women with FHA (Shoham et al. 1991). Highly purified recombinant gonadotropins are also available.

Regardless of the gonadotropin preparation utilized, the goal is to obtain a single ovulation and minimize the risks for OHSS and multiple pregnancies. The ovary has a threshold level for FSH below which follicular development does not occur (O'Dea et al. 2008). Therefore, a low-dose step-up protocol is utilized to reach the FSH threshold gradually and minimize risks (Matsuzaki et al. 2018). For instance, the starting dose of FSH can be increased or decreased depending on the ovarian response, as determined by repeated serum E_2 measurements or by counting maturing follicles using ultrasonography. Then, FSH treatment is followed by human chorionic gonadotropin (hCG) or LH to trigger ovulation and progesterone secretion.

Gonadotropin therapy can also be used to induce ovulation and restore fertility in women with PCOS but only in patients that show resistance to first-line treatments. This is because women with PCOS are at high risk of developing multiple follicles inducing multiple pregnancies and of OHSS (Sun et al. 2020). In general, women with PCOS have enough endogenous LH levels, hence ovulation can be induced with low-dose FSH. However, due to the difficulty in predicting when the follicles will respond to FSH and when follicular growth will start, long-term daily FSH injections are often required in PCOS patients, which can lead to significant economic burden (Homburg 2003).

3.2.3 Dopamine Receptor Agonists

Pharmacological intervention with dopamine (DA) receptor agonists such as cabergoline and bromocriptine is the first line of medical therapy for women with prolactinomas and for those with ovulatory disorders secondary to hyperprolactinemia (Majumdar and Mangal 2013; Nunes et al. 2011). A systematic review of the literature suggested that DA agonists are effective in resolving amenorrhea (median 78%; range 40–100%) and in restoring fertility (53%; 10–100%), (Melmed et al. 2011). However, the use of these drugs is associated with gastrointestinal (nausea, vomiting, constipation) and neurological (hypotension, dizziness, headache, fatigue) side effects which can be severe (Nunes et al. 2011), resulting in discontinuation of treatment in a significant number of patients. Moreover, resistance to DA agonist is observed in some patients (Maiter 2019), with a prevalence of 20–30% for bromocriptine and around 10% for cabergoline. Interestingly, the two principal predictive factors of resistance to DA agonists are being male, and in the case of hyperprolactinemia due to prolactinomas, tumor invasiveness.

3.2.4 Clomiphene Citrate

Clomiphene citrate (CC) is an oral medication of relatively low cost when compared to injectable gonadotropins. Clomiphene blocks estrogen negative feedback by binding to hypothalamic ERs, thereby increasing GnRH pulse frequency and the production of LH and FSH by the pituitary, which stimulates the growth of the ovarian follicle. However, in patients with FHA, which are hypoestrogenic, CC can't antagonize estrogen's actions, hence this population shows poor response to ovulation induction by CC (Gordon 2010). Clinicians are advised to perform a trial with CC for ovulation induction if a woman has sufficient endogenous E_2 levels (Gordon et al. 2017).

CC has been the first-line method for ovulation induction in patients with PCOS-associated infertility (Brown and Farquhar 2016). However, around 20–25% of patients are resistant to CC treatment (Homburg 2003). In such cases, intermittent CC treatment in which high serum FSH levels are maintained by repeating the administration of CC was recently shown to induce follicular growth in 80% of CC-resistant PCOS women (Takasaki et al. 2018). Other well-known disadvantages of CC treatment in PCOS women include a significant discrepancy between ovulation and pregnancy rates (70–90%; 40–70%) and a high rate of miscarriages compared to the general population (Franks et al. 1985). In addition, the peripheral anti-estrogenic effects of CC result in the chronic depletion of ERs, adversely affecting endometrial growth and development as well as quantity and quality of cervical mucus, contributing to decrease in pregnancy success (Randall and Templeton 1991).

3.2.5 Aromatase Inhibitors

The aromatase inhibitor letrozole (LTZ) is rapidly replacing CC as the first line of treatment to induce ovulation in women with PCOS. This is because, compared with CC, LTZ is associated with higher live birth and ovulation rates among infertile women with PCOS (Legro et al. 2014; Sakar and Oglak 2020). Moreover, LTZ treatment induces ovulation and pregnancy rates similar to hMGs, but with lower incidence of OHSS, making LTZ a good alternative in patients resistant to CC (Shi et al. 2020).

LTZ reduces E_2 levels and might act centrally to prevent E_2 negative feedback on FSH, inducing ovulation (Yang et al. 2021). Letrozole is not an FDA approved treatment of infertility and ovulation. However, comprehensive meta-analysis, in which the effectiveness and safety of various ovulation induction treatments in women with PCOS were evaluated, concluded that LTZ is more effective than CC in improving live birth and pregnancy rates when used to cause ovulation followed by timed intercourse or intrauterine insemination (IUI) (Franik et al. 2018; Wang et al. 2017). As with CC, LTZ is administered orally, however, due to its short half-life elimination time of 48 h there are fewer adverse effects on estrogen target tissues such as the endometrium and cervix (Yang et al. 2021).

3.2.6 Metformin

Metformin is the most studied insulin lowering agent in PCOS as it is able to ameliorate many of the endocrine, metabolic, and reproductive abnormalities associated with this complex syndrome (Moghetti et al. 2000). Compared to placebo, metformin monotherapy is effective in achieving ovulation in women with PCOS. However, many women treated with metformin experience gastrointestinal side effects such as nausea and vomiting (Tso et al. 2009). A study that compared the effectiveness of CC, metformin or the combination of both drugs in Asian Indian women with PCOS found that the combination of CC and metformin was superior to CC alone in improving ovulation and pregnancy rates (Kar and Sanchita 2015). In addition, while metformin was as good as CC inducing ovulation, a lower risk of multiple pregnancy was associated with metformin monotherapy (Kar and Sanchita 2015; Tso et al. 2009). On the other hand, metformin effectiveness as a monotherapy or in combination with CC may be influenced by obesity, as lower rates of pregnancy and ovulation have been reported in obese women compared to non-obese women with PCOS (Tziomalos and Dinas 2018). Hence, the use of metformin and other insulin sensitizing agents as adjuncts is limited and might be favorable only in women who are resistant to CC alone (Legro et al. 2007).

4 Male Infertility

A myriad of factors can result in male infertility including: (1) Obstruction of the reproductive tract, causing dysfunction in semen ejaculation, (2) Endocrine disorders associated with altered productions of hypothalamic and/or pituitary hormones, which in turn negatively affect T and sperm production, (3) Testicular failure to produce sperm, and (4) Abnormal sperm function and quality, (e.g. abnormal sperm shape and/or movement) (Agarwal et al. 2021a).

4.1 Risk Factors Linked to Male Infertility

Several studies support the notion that men today produce fewer and less healthy sperm than in the past. For example, a series of meta-analysis have shown a trend of continuing decline in sperm counts globally, with the most recent analysis suggesting that this decline is restricted to Western countries (North America, Europe, Australia, and New Zealand (Levine et al. 2017). A retrospective study that evaluated the semen analysis from almost 120,000 men examined for infertility concerns at two fertility clinics found that over a span of 16 years (2002–2017) the proportion of men with a normal total motile sperm count had declined by about 10% (Tiegs et al. 2019). Moreover, below-normal serum T levels are being encountered more often in men seeking fertility. The question then is what are the factors causing the decline in sperm counts and motility which in turn can negatively impact male fertility?

One possibility is that this decline in sperm quality occurs secondary to lifestyle changes. For example, the modern trend of delaying conception until later in life might bias for males already at risk for low T levels (Liu et al. 2021). The impact of obesity and related comorbidities, which are associated with subfertility in both sexes, cannot be discounted (Pivonello et al. 2019). Additionally, unhealthy lifestyles such as excessive alcohol consumption and smoking are strongly associated with poor sperm quality (Agarwal et al. 2021a). However, deeper analysis suggests that the trend in global decline of sperm quality is still observed after controlling for these risk factors. Therefore, environmental factors such as exposure to *endocrine disruptors* might play a significant role. Endocrine disrupting chemicals (EDCs) mimic the body endogenous hormones interfering with endocrine functions including the HPG axis. These chemicals are present in hundreds of commonly used compounds like plastics, pesticides, herbicides, and others. Examples of EDCs include phthalate metabolites used in plastic to soften polyvinyl chloride (PVC) polymers, the plasticizer Bisphenol A (BPA), and dioxins. A significant number of animal studies support a direct association between EDCs and impaired reproductive function in males and females (Rattan et al. 2017; Rehman et al. 2018). Moreover, human exposure to EDCs has been correlated to decrease semen quality (Rehman et al. 2018). However, controversies and a lack of consensus exist about the management of this environmental problem (Bergman et al. 2015).

4.2 Male Hypogonadism

Male hypogonadism is a decrease in testicular function manifested by low T levels and/or impaired sperm production, and it accounts for over 10% of male-factor infertility (Fallara et al. 2021). Male hypogonadism can be classified into primary or secondary, the former is caused by testicular failure, and the latter occurs as a result of a hypothalamic and/or pituitary dysfunction (Agarwal et al. 2021a; Fraietta et al. 2013). Both can be due to congenital or acquired factors that ultimately impair spermatogenesis. However, the most common form of hypogonadisms is primary, which is characterized by low T levels accompanied by high LH and FSH levels (hypergonadotropic).

4.2.1 Primary Hypogonadism

Varicocele is an acquired form of hypogonadisms and the most common and correctable cause of infertility in men, with a prevalence of 15% of healthy men and of 25% of men with abnormal semen analysis (Agarwal et al. 2021a). Varicocele is a condition where the veins in the testicles are dilated increasing testicular temperature which promotes the production of reactive oxygen species (ROS). Men with severe varicocele produce abnormally shaped sperm and low sperm counts. Surgical varicocele repair (varicocelectomy) improves serum T level in men with hypogonadism and infertility and also improves erectile dysfunction (Srini and Veerachari 2011).

Other acquired forms of primary hypogonadism include aging and exposure to gonadotoxic agents like chemotherapy and radiotherapy since they negatively impact Leydig cell and Sertoli cell function.

Cytogenetic or chromosomal abnormalities are important causes of male infertility. For instance, karyotype anomalies have a prevalence of 12–15% in azoospermia, 5% in severe oligospermia, and less than 1% in normal semen (Agarwal et al. 2021a). Klinefelter syndrome (also known as 47, XXY) is the most common congenital manifestation of primary hypogonadisms, affecting about 1 in every 500 men. Patients with Klinefelter syndrome or its mosaic variants present with impaired spermatogenesis with severe oligospermia or azoospermia (Martin 2008). Assisted reproductive technology (ART), in which sperm retrieval is followed by intracytoplasmic sperm injection (ICSI) during the in vitro fertilization (IVF) process, is recommended for patients with Klinefelter syndrome seeking to father their own biological children (Corona et al. 2017); for more on ART, refer to Sect. 6.

4.2.2 Secondary Hypogonadism

Secondary or central male hypogonadism is characterized by low T and low gonadotropin levels (hypogonadotropic hypogonadism). As with primary testicular failure, central hypogonadism can be the result of congenital or acquired diseases (Fraietta et al. 2013).

Secondary hypogonadism that is of acquired origin can be caused by drugs (sex steroids, GnRH analogues), pituitary lesions, hyperprolactinemia, previous anabolic steroids abuse, encephalic trauma, pituitary/brain radiation, excessive exercise, alcohol abuse, or illicit drug intake (Agarwal et al. 2021a; Fraietta et al. 2013).

As discussed in Sect. 3.1, CHH is linked to mutations of genes affecting GnRH neuron or pituitary function. Kallmann syndrome is a common cause of CHH in men, with an estimated prevalence of 1 in 30,000 males vs. 1 in 120,000 females. Kallmann syndrome is often X-linked, which might explain its higher prevalence in men (Laitinen et al. 2011). However, it is possible that this genetic disease is underestimated in females, as affected women tend to have milder symptoms.

Central hypogonadism is one of the few medically treatable causes of male infertility. Human CG and hMG are commonly used in clinical practice to substitute for LH and FSH, respectively, and induce fertility in patients with central hypogonadism (Rajkanna et al. 2016). For example, successful pregnancies were reported for female partners of 16–57% of men with CHH after treatment (Young et al. 2019).

4.3 Post-Testicular Defects

Male-factor infertility may not be associated with abnormal pituitary or gonadal hormones levels. These post-testicular factors affect the ability of the sperm to travel from the testicle to leave the body in the ejaculate. For example, congenital absence of vas deferens (CBAVD) accounts for 1–2% of all cases of infertility and up to 5% of men with azoospermia (Cai and Li 2022). Patients with CBAVD have no palpable vas deferens (one or both sides) on physical examination. CBAVD may be accompanied by congenital abnormalities in the urogenital system and cystic fibrosis related clinical manifestations. Other examples include ejaculatory duct abnormalities, retrograde ejaculation, and erectile dysfunction.

4.4 Idiopathic Infertility in Men

Up to 50% of male infertility cases are idiopathic, however, no evidence-based treatment guidelines are currently available for idiopathic male infertility. It has been reported that most clinicians in the USA use what is termed empirical medical therapy (EMT) which includes the utilization of SERMs, aromatase inhibitors, and gonadotropins to treat idiopathic male-factor infertility (Ko et al. 2012). However, their use can be costly and often associated with side effects. Moreover, very few placebo-controlled trials have been done to investigate whether EMTs do in fact improve live birth outcomes. Therefore, the concept of male oxidative stress infertility (MOSI) has been proposed to describe infertile men with abnormal semen characteristics and oxidative stress (OS), and in this way include patients who were previously classified as having idiopathic male infertility (Agarwal et al. 2019).

Oxidative stress is caused by an imbalance between production and accumulation of ROS in cells and tissues and the ability of a biological system to detoxify these reactive products. While small quantities of ROS are required to ensure normal cellular physiological functions, including spermatogenesis, excessive ROS production results in OS, which can negatively impact fertility (Sanocka and Kurpisz 2004). For example, OS interferes with capacitation and may cause sperm membrane and DNA damage, thereby affecting the sperm's potential to fertilize an egg. In fact, about 30% to 80% of infertile men have elevated seminal ROS levels (Agarwal et al. 2019). Therefore, antioxidants may offer a relatively safe and inexpensive way to treat male infertility, with various studies supporting their effectiveness at improving semen parameters and live birth rates (Agarwal et al. 2021b).

5 Kisspeptin-Based Therapies for Infertility

Clinical manipulation of gonadotropin levels with kisspeptin treatment results in physiological responses that lack the side effects associated with many first-line infertility medications. Therefore, development and testing of kisspeptin-based therapies for certain HPG disorders impacting fertility is an area of great interest.

5.1 Kisspeptin Pharmacology

The kisspeptins are derived from the proteolytic processing of a 145 amino acid long precursor, giving rise to kisspeptin-54 (KP54) which can be further cleaved into shorter, biologically active amidated peptides, including kisspeptin-10 (KP10) (Mills and Dhillo 2022). All kisspeptin isoforms share a common C-terminal decapeptide sequence, corresponding to KP10, which confers biological activity at the Kiss1R. KP54 and KP10 have been the most extensively studied, both having similar receptor binding affinities and efficacies. However, in humans, KP54 is presumed to be the most abundant subtype of the two. In addition, compared to KP10, KP54 is more resistant to proteolytic degradation and in male mice, KP54 but not KP10, was shown to cross the blood brain barrier (de Tassigny et al. 2017; Dhillo et al. 2005). These characteristics might explain why in several studies compared to KP54, KP10 is less effective at eliciting an LH response when administered peripherally as a single injection (de Tassigny et al. 2017).

KP10 and KP54 potently stimulate LH release and the number of LH pulses in healthy individuals of both sexes. However, in women, the internal gonadal hormone environment greatly influences the HPG response to kisspeptin administration. For example, Dhillo examined the effect of a single sc. bolus injection of KP54 on LH in healthy females and found that the stimulatory effect of KP54 on LH was greatest in the preovulatory phase and least in the follicular phase of the menstrual cycle (Dhillo et al. 2007). KP10 also stimulates gonadotropin levels at the preovulatory (Jayasena et al. 2011) and early follicular phase (George et al. 2012). Furthermore, when the gonadotropin response to KP10 administration was investigated in women taking sex-steroid contraceptives in the form of combined estrogen and progesterone pill and in women with progesterone contraceptive implants, KP10 failed to elevate LH levels in women taking the combination pill, suggesting that the form of sex-steroid feedback influences the gonadotropin response to KP10 (George et al. 2012).

In healthy men, administration of KP54 or KP10 has consistently been reported to potently stimulate gonadotropin release and T levels. For example, serum LH and FSH levels were elevated after a single iv. bolus injection of KP10 (Jayasena et al. 2011), and continuous KP10 infusion potently stimulated T, LH pulse frequency and pulse size (George et al. 2011). Similarly, iv. infusion of KP54 stimulates LH, FSH, and T release in men (Dhillo et al. 2005; Jayasena et al. 2015). On the other hand, the stimulatory effects of kisspeptin on T levels seem to be age-dependent; while increased plasma LH levels were observed in healthy adult, middle-aged, and advanced age men, plasma T concentrations were elevated only in the youngest cohort of adult men (Ullah et al. 2019). Hence, while the central hypothalamic-pituitary axis remains responsive to kisspeptin stimulation throughout adult life, the ability of kisspeptin-induced LH to stimulate T secretion by Leydig cell decreases with age.

5.2 Kisspeptin Treatment in Women with FHA

Overall, kisspeptin treatment in women with FHA can stimulate reproductive hormone secretion and increase LH pulsatility. However, mode and frequency of treatment is key to avoid rapid desensitization (tachyphylaxis). For example, while twice daily sc. administration of KP54 to women with FHA resulted in desensitization by the second week of treatment, women with FHA who were treated with twice-weekly KP54 injections had significantly elevated levels of reproductive hormones after 8 weeks (Jayasena et al. 2009, 2010). Also important is the fact that when the same KP54 dose was administered sc. twice daily to healthy women, it did not induce desensitization, suggesting that sensitivity to kisspeptin can modulate the susceptibility to tachyphylaxis (Jayasena et al. 2013). Subsequent studies showed that constant iv. infusion of KP54 temporarily increased both basal and pulsatile LH secretion in women with FHA, with desensitization occurring only at the highest dose (Jayasena et al. 2014b). Hence, similar to the GnRH pump, constant administration of KP54 might be a viable option to treat infertility due to FHA and in other ovulatory disorders.

Kiss1R agonists such as MVT-602 offer an alternative to endogenous kisspeptin peptides to treat women with FHA. A study comparing the effects of MVT-602 to those of KP54 in healthy women found that although the peak amplitude of LH response was similar after administration of either compound, the timing of the LH peak occurred much later after administration of MVT-602, which translated into a fourfold increase in the area under the curve of LH rise (Abbara et al. 2020). Moreover, when the effects of MVT-602 were tested in women with FHA or PCOS, the rise in gonadotropin levels after MVT-602 occurred much sooner and more potently in women with FHA, compared to the PCOS or control groups. The prolonged and potent gonadotropin response observed after a single MVT-606 is encouraging, as it might imply that less frequent injections will be needed, which would limit the risk of desensitization. However, additional studies are needed to investigate if chronic administration of MVT-602 is effective in stimulating follicular development and fertility in women with FHA.

5.3 Kisspeptin Treatment in Women with Hyperprolactinemia

The observation that in hyperprolactinemic mice hypothalamic kisspeptin expression is reduced and that KP administration restored hypothalamic GnRH release, gonadotropin secretion, and ovarian cyclicity led to the hypothesis that reduced hypothalamic kisspeptin secretion plays a role in hyperprolactinemia-induced hypogonadotropic amenorrhea (Sonigo et al. 2012). In support of this hypothesis, iv. infusion of KP10 in hyperprolactinemic women with chronic amenorrhea was found to increase gonadotropin levels and LH pulses, and these effects were accompanied by elevation of serum E_2, T, and inhibin B levels (Millar et al. 2017). Although the study was exploratory with only 2 subjects, their findings support a future utilization of kisspeptin or analogues to restore ovarian function and fertility in women with hyperprolactinemia that are intolerant or resistant DA agonists and in whom surgery to remove the adenoma is not a viable option.

5.4 Neurokinin 3 Receptor Antagonists in PCOS

Neurokinin B via its receptor NK3R stimulates hypothalamic kisspeptin release which in turn increases GnRH neurosecretory activity (Moore et al. 2018). Therefore, antagonizing NK3Rs has been proposed to dampen the GnRH hypersecretion observed in PCOS patients, leading to decreased LH and androgen production. Two NK3R antagonists, MLE4901 and fezolinetant, have been investigated for their effects on T and LH levels in women with PCOS. MLE4901 was tested in women that presented all PCOS clinical criteria, namely hyperandrogenism, oligomenorrhea/amenorrhea, and polycystic ovarian morphology on ultrasound (George et al. 2016). MLE4901 treatment dose-dependently reduced LH pulse frequency, basal LH and total T. However, the study was of short duration (28 days) and did not focus on other clinical outcomes such as ovulation. On the other hand, fezolinetant which has a shorter half-life than MLE4901 was found to dose-dependently suppress T levels and to reduce the LH-to-FSH ratio in PCOS women with hyperandrogenemia (Fraser et al. 2021). The fezolinetant-induced reductions were maintained for the duration of the 12-week intervention. However, not all women receiving fezolinetant were anovulatory and compared to placebo, circulating levels of progesterone and E_2 did not change significantly. Hence, while the effects of these NK3R antagonists in PCOS, particularly the strong suppression of hyperandrogenemia are promising, larger and longer-term studies are needed in order to determine their potential to treat anovulation in PCOS.

5.5 Kisspeptin Treatment in T2D-Associated Male Hypogonadism

At least 25% of men with T2D have low T and low gonadotropin levels, with an additional 4% with low T levels and elevated LH and FSH concentrations (Dandona and Dhindsa 2011). The relationship between low T and T2D is bidirectional, as low T levels predisposes to T2D. While low sperm counts, erectile dysfunction, and a decrease in sex drive are all associated with hypogonadism, hyperglycemia per se can negatively impact sperm quality, resulting in a reduction of fertility (Maresch et al. 2019). The hypothalamic kisspeptin system plays a central role in the integration of energy status and reproduction (Acosta-Martinez 2011). Hence, suppression of kisspeptin release might contribute to the T deficiency observed in men with T2D and obesity. This hypothesis was investigated in a study testing the effects of KP10 administration on reproductive hormone secretion in a cohort of men with obesity (BMI >40 kg/m^2) and low T levels (George et al. 2013). Both a single iv. bolus injection and a continuous iv. infusion of KP10 significantly increased LH secretion in healthy men and in men with T2DM. Moreover, continuous iv. KP10 also augmented LH pulse frequency and serum T levels in T2D men. Since kisspeptin administration has been shown to enhance glucose-stimulated insulin secretion in healthy men (Izzi-Engbeaya et al. 2018), kisspeptin agonists could be utilized to stimulate endogenous T secretion and insulin release in men with T2DM.

Kisspeptin may be also served as a marker of male reproductive health. For example, serum kisspeptin levels were found to be lower in infertile males with abnormal sperm parameters compared to fertile men with normal sperm parameters (Rehman et al. 2019). Furthermore, levels of kisspeptin protein in seminal plasma have been positively associated with semen quality, i.e., higher sperm concentration, total sperm number, and total motile sperm count (Zou et al. 2019). Hence, future studies should examine whether treatment with kisspeptin or kisspeptin agonists also benefits men affected by central hypogonadism and/or infertility not related to T2D.

6 Assisted Reproductive Technology (ART)

Close to 2% of all US infants are born using ART, the most common type being IVF. IVF is recommended when ovulation induction with timed intercourse or IUI has not resulted in a successful pregnancy. IVF involves the collection of oocytes from the ovary, followed by fertilization in vitro, ending with the transfer of the resulting embryo into the uterus. If infertility is due to very poor sperm quality, ICSI can be part of IVF. Fertilization and pregnancy rates in IVFs that utilize ICSI were reported to be comparable to those observed with normal sperm (Wu et al. 2023).

A critical component of IVF is controlled ovarian stimulation (COS), which is aimed at producing the synchronous growth of multiple follicles and at preventing premature spontaneous ovulation (Melo et al. 2022). The following 5 steps are utilized in most COS protocols: (1) Use of birth control pills to achieve synchronization of ovarian follicles, (2) Treatment with a GnRH antagonist to suppress the secretion of pituitary gonadotropins and in this way prevent premature ovulation, (3) Stimulation of the ovaries by daily injections of gonadotropins (FSH alone or in combination with LH), (4) Final oocyte maturation or timed trigger with hCG injection, and (5) Egg retrieval 36 h later.

Due to its similarity to LH, hCG has been the trigger of choice for oocyte maturation. However, its much longer half-life (about 2 days) contributes to the occurrence of OHSS in high responders. In fact, an estimated 3% to 6% of women, who go through IVF, experience some form of OHSS (Schirmer et al. 2020). In susceptible patient groups such as PCOS, the risk for OHSS is increased fivefold after IVF (Sun et al. 2020). Alternatively, GnRH agonist can be used to trigger ovulation since they are associated with less incidence of OHSS in high responders and are able to induce endogenous FSH and LH release (Gonen et al. 1990). However, GnRH agonists might produce a sub-optimal LH surge, with several studies reporting increased early pregnancy loss and decreased rates of ongoing pregnancies associated with their utilization (Kolibianakis et al. 2005).

On the other hand, as part of the GnRH pulse generator, kisspeptin signaling is necessary for the occurrence of the preovulatory gonadotropin surge. As such, a "kisspeptin trigger" could be utilized instead of hCG or GnRH agonist to induce oocyte maturation. For example, a single sc. bolus administration of KP54 induces an LH rise that safely matures oocytes in women undergoing IVF therapy (Jayasena et al. 2014a). Successful stimulation of oocyte maturation and pregnancies without the development of OHSS were observed when KP54 was tested in high-risk populations undergoing IVF (Abbara et al. 2015). Moreover, extending the duration of the LH response with a second dose of KP54 further improved oocyte maturation without increasing the occurrence of OHSS (Abbara et al. 2017). Additional studies are needed to directly compare KP54 use as ovulation trigger with hCG or GnRH.

7 Conclusion

Regardless of whether infertility is attributed to a male-, a female-factor, or both, its clinical diagnosis and management can be challenging. Cost, side effects and resistance to medications are prevailing obstacles encountered by many patients seeking to conceive. In a substantial number of cases the underlying cause of infertility is unknown, leaving doctors with limited guidelines and tools to treat them. Moreover, more individuals are choosing to delay conception until later years, posing additional challenges regarding treatment options and effectiveness. Advancement in ART continues to offer hope to these individuals. Furthermore, kisspeptin treatment might be a more physiological and cost-effective option for oocyte maturation preceding IVF and for the treatment of infertility disorders related to the dysfunction of the GnRH pulse generator. However, larger randomized control trials are needed to compare the efficacy of kisspeptin to that of other first-line interventions.

References

Abbara A, Dhillo WS (2021) Targeting elevated GnRH pulsatility to treat polycystic ovary syndrome. J Clin Endocrinol Metab 106:e4275–e4277

Abbara A, Jayasena CN, Christopoulos G, Narayanaswamy S, Izzi-Engbeaya C, Nijher GMK, Comninos AN, Peters D, Buckley A, Ratnasabapathy R, Prague JK, Salim R, Lavery SA, Bloom SR, Szigeti M, Ashby DA, Trew GH, Dhillo WS (2015) Efficacy of Kisspeptin-54 to trigger oocyte maturation in women at high risk of ovarian hyperstimulation syndrome (OHSS) during in vitro fertilization (IVF) therapy. J Clin Endocrinol Metab 100:3322–3331

Abbara A, Clarke S, Islam R, Prague JK, Comninos AN, Narayanaswamy S, Papadopoulou D, Roberts R, Izzi-Engbeaya C, Ratnasabapathy R, Nesbitt A, Vimalesvaran S, Salim R, Lavery SA, Bloom SR, Huson L, Trew GH, Dhillo WS (2017) A second dose of kisspeptin-54 improves oocyte maturation in women at high risk of ovarian hyperstimulation syndrome: a phase 2 randomized controlled trial. Hum Reprod 32:1915–1924

Abbara A, Eng PC, Phylactou M, Clarke SA, Richardson R, Sykes CM, Phumsatitpong C, Mills E, Modi M, Izzi-Engbeaya C, Papadopoulou D, Purugganan K, Jayasena CN, Webber L, Salim R, Owen B, Bech P, Comninos AN, McArdle CA, Voliotis M, Tsaneva-Atanasova K, Moenter S, Hanyaloglu A, Dhillo WS (2020) Kisspeptin receptor agonist has therapeutic potential for female reproductive disorders. J Clin Invest 130:6739–6753

Abreu AP, Toro CA, Song YB, Navarro VM, Bosch MA, Eren A, Liang JN, Carroll RS, Latronico AC, Ronnekleiv OK, Aylwin CF, Lomniczi A, Ojeda S, Kaiser UB (2020) MKRN3 inhibits the reproductive axis through actions in kisspeptin-expressing neurons. J Clin Invest 130:4486–4500

Acosta-Martinez M (2011) PI3K: an attractive candidate for the central integration of metabolism and reproduction. Front Endocrinol (Lausanne) 2:110

Agarwal A, Parekh N, Selvam MKP, Henkel R, Shah R, Homa ST, Ramasamy R, Ko E, Tremellen K, Esteves S, Majzoub A, Alvarez JG, Gardner DK, Jayasena CN, Ramsay JW, Cho CL, Saleh R, Sakkas D, Hotaling JM, Lundy SD, Vij S, Marmar J, Gosalvez J, Sabanegh E, Park HJ, Zini A, Kavoussi P, Micic S, Smith R, Busetto GM, Bakircioglu ME, Haidl G, Balercia G, Puchalt NG, Ben-Khalifa M, Tadros N, Kirkman-Browne J, Moskovtsev S, Huang XF, Borges E, Franken D, Bar-Chama N, Morimoto Y, Tomita K, Srini VS, Ombelet W, Baldi E, Muratori M, Yumura Y, La Vignera S, Kosgi R, Martinez MP, Evenson DP, Zylbersztejn DS, Roque M, Cocuzza M, Vieira M, Ben-Meir A, Orvieto R, Levitas E, Wiser A, Arafa M, Malhotra V, Parekattil SJ, Elbardisi H, Carvalho L, Dada R, Sifer C, Talwar P, Gudeloglu A, Mahmoud AMA, Terras K, Yazbeck C, Nebojsa B, Durairajanayagam D, Mounir A, Kahn LG, Baskaran S, Pai RD, Paoli D, Leisegang K, Moein MR, Malik S, Yaman O, Samanta L, Bayane F, Jindal SK, Kendirci M, Altay B, Perovic D, Harlev A (2019) Male oxidative stress infertility (MOSI): proposed terminology and clinical practice guidelines for management of idiopathic male infertility. World J Mens Health 37:296–312

Agarwal A, Baskaran S, Parekh N, Cho CL, Henkel R, Vij S, Arafa M, Selvam MKP, Shah R (2021a) Male infertility. Lancet 397:319–333

Agarwal A, Leisegang K, Majzoub A, Henkel R, Finelli R, Selvam MKP, Tadros N, Parekh N, Ko EY, Cho CL, Arafa M, Alves MG, Oliveira PF, Alvarez JG, Shah R (2021b) Utility of antioxidants in the treatment of male infertility: clinical guidelines based on a systematic review and analysis of evidence. World J Mens Health 39:233–290

Bergman A, Becher G, Blumberg B, Bjerregaard P, Bornman R, Brandt I, Casey SC, Frouin H, Giudice LC, Heindel JJ, Iguchi T, Jobling S, Kidd KA, Kortenkamp A, Lind PM, Muir D, Ochieng R, Ropstad E, Ross PS, Skakkebaek NE, Toppari J, Vandenberg LN, Woodruff TJ, Zoeller RT (2015) Manufacturing doubt about endocrine disrupter science – a rebuttal of industry-sponsored critical comments on the UNEP/WHO report "State of the Science of Endocrine Disrupting Chemicals 2012". Regul Toxicol Pharmacol 73:1007–1017

Boivin J, Vassena R, Costa M, Vegni E, Dixon M, Collura B, Markert M, Samuelsen C, Guiglotto J, Roitmann E, Domar A (2022) Tailored support may reduce mental and relational impact of infertility on infertile patients and partners. Reprod Biomed Online 44:1045–1054

Brown J, Farquhar C (2016) Clomiphene and other antioestrogens for ovulation induction in polycystic ovarian syndrome. Cochrane Database Syst Rev 12(12):CD002249

Busch AS, Hagen CP, Almstrup K, Juul A (2016) Circulating MKRN3 levels decline during puberty in healthy boys. J Clin Endocrinol Metab 101:2588–2593

Cai Z, Li H (2022) Congenital bilateral absence of the vas deferens. Front Genet 13:775123

Carson SA, Kallen AN (2021) Diagnosis and management of infertility a review. JAMA 326:65–76

Casoni F, Malone SA, Belle M, Luzzati F, Collier F, Allet C, Hrabovszky E, Rasika S, Prevot V, Chedotal A, Giacobini P (2016) Development of the neurons controlling fertility in humans: new insights from 3D imaging and transparent fetal brains. Development 143:3969–3981

Chandrasekaran S, Sagili H (2018) Metabolic syndrome in women with polycystic ovary syndrome. Obstet Gynaecol 20:245–252
Chon SJ, Umair Z, Yoon MS (2021) Premature ovarian insufficiency: past, present, and future. Front Cell Dev Biol 9:672890
Choy JT, Eisenberg ML (2018) Male infertility as a window to health. Fertil Steril 110:810–814
Christian CA, Moenter SM (2010) The neurobiology of preovulatory and estradiol-induced gonadotropin-releasing hormone surges. Endocr Rev 31:544–577
Christou F, Pitteloud N, Gomez F (2017) The induction of ovulation by pulsatile administration of GnRH: an appropriate method in hypothalamic amenorrhea. Gynecol Endocrinol 33:598–601
Corona G, Pizzocaro A, Lanfranco F, Garolla A, Pelliccione F, Vignozzi L, Ferlin A, Foresta C, Jannini EA, Maggi M, Lenzi A, Pasquali D, Francavilla S, King KIG (2017) Sperm recovery and ICSI outcomes in Klinefelter syndrome: a systematic review and meta-analysis. Hum Reprod Update 23:265–275
Dandona P, Dhindsa S (2011) Update: hypogonadotropic hypogonadism in type 2 diabetes and obesity. J Clin Endocrinol Metab 96:2643–2651
de Roux N, Genin E, Carel JC, Matsuda F, Chaussain JL, Milgrom E (2003) Hypogonadotropic hypogonadism due to loss of function of the KiSS1-derived peptide receptor GPR54. Proc Natl Acad Sci U S A 100:10972–10976
De Souza MJ, Toombs RJ, Scheid JL, O'Donnell E, West SL, Williams NI (2010) High prevalence of subtle and severe menstrual disturbances in exercising women: confirmation using daily hormone measures. Hum Reprod 25:491–503
de Tassigny XD, Jayasena C, Murphy KG, Dhillo WS, Colledge WH (2017) Mechanistic insights into the more potent effect of KP-54 compared to KP-10 in vivo. PloS One 12
Deswal R, Narwal V, Dang A, Pundir CS (2020) The prevalence of polycystic ovary syndrome: a brief systematic review. J Hum Reprod Sci 13:261–271
Dhillo WS, Chaudhri OB, Patterson M, Thompson EL, Murphy KG, Badman MK, McGowan BM, Amber V, Patel S, Ghatei MA, Bloom SR (2005) Kisspeptin-54 stimulates the hypothalamic-pituitary gonadal axis in human males. J Clin Endocrinol Metab 90:6609–6615
Dhillo WS, Chaudhri OB, Thompson EL, Murphy KG, Patterson M, Ramachandran R, Nijher GK, Amber V, Kokkinos A, Donaldson M, Ghatei MA, Bloom SR (2007) Kisspeptin-54 stimulates gonadotropin release most potently during the Preovulatory phase of the menstrual cycle in women. J Clin Endocrinol Metab 92:3958–3966
Dubois SL, Acosta-Martinez M, DeJoseph MR, Wolfe A, Radovick S, Boehm U, Urban JH, Levine JE (2015) Positive, but not negative feedback actions of estradiol in adult female mice require estrogen receptor alpha in kisspeptin neurons. Endocrinology 156:1111–1120
Dzemaili S, Tiemensma J, Quinton R, Pitteloud N, Morin D, Dwyer AA (2017) Beyond hormone replacement: quality of life in women with congenital hypogonadotropic hypogonadism. Endocr Connect 6:404–412
Edessy M, Hosni NH, Shady Y, Waf Y, Bakry S, Kamel M (2016) Autologous stem cells therapy, the first baby of idiopathic premature ovarian failure. Acta Med Int 3:19–23
Fallara G, Cazzaniga W, Boeri L, Capogrosso P, Candela L, Pozzi E, Belladelli F, Schifano N, Ventimiglia E, Abbate C, Papaleo E, Vigano P, Montorsi F, Salonia A (2021) Male factor infertility trends throughout the last 10 years: report from a tertiary-referral academic andrology centre. Andrology 9:610–617
Fauser BCJM, Chang J, Azziz R, Legro R, Dewailly D, Franks S, Tarlatzis BC, Fauser B, Balen A, Bouchard P, Dahlgren E, Devoto L, Diamanti E, Dunaif A, Filicori M, Homburg R, Ibanez L, Laven J, Magoffin D, Nestler J, Norman RJ, Pasquali R, Pugeat M, Strauss J, Tan S, Taylor A, Wild R, Wild S, Ehrmann D, Lobo R, ESHRE-ASRM-sponsored, R. (2004) Revised 2003 consensus on diagnostic criteria and long-term health risks related to polycystic ovary syndrome (PCOS). Hum Reprod 19:41–47
Fraietta R, Zylberstejn DS, Esteves SC (2013) Hypogonadotropic hypogonadism revisited. Clinics (Sao Paulo) 68(Suppl 1):81–88

Franik S, Eltrop S, Kremer J, Kiesel L, Farquhar C (2018) Aromatase inhibitors (letrozole) for subfertile women with polycystic ovary syndrome – a cochrane systematic review. Hum Reprod 33:131–132

Franks S, Adams J, Mason H, Polson D (1985) Ovulatory disorders in women with polycystic ovary syndrome. Clin Obstet Gynaecol 12:605–632

Fraser GL, Obermayer-Pietsch B, Laven J, Griesinger G, Pintiaux A, Timmerman D, Fauser BCJM, Lademacher C, Combalbert J, Hoveyda HR, Ramael S (2021) Randomized controlled trial of neurokinin 3 receptor antagonist Fezolinetant for treatment of polycystic ovary syndrome. J Clin Endocrinol Metab 106:E3519–E3532

Gabr H, Elkheir WA, El-Gazzar A (2016) Autologous stem cell transplantation in patients with idiopathic premature ovarian failure. J Tissue Sci Eng 7:3(Suppl)

George JT, Anderson RA, Millar RP (2012) Kisspeptin-10 stimulation of gonadotrophin secretion in women is modulated by sex steroid feedback. Hum Reprod 27:3552–3559

George JT, Veldhuis JD, Roseweir AK, Newton CL, Faccenda E, Millar RP, Anderson RA (2011) Kisspeptin-10 is a potent stimulator of LH and increases pulse frequency in men. J Clin Endocrinol Metab 96(8):E1228–E1236. https://doi.org/10.1210/jc.2011-0089. Epub 2011 Jun 1. PMID: 21632807; PMCID: PMC3380939.

George JT, Veldhuis JD, Tena-Sempere M, Millar RP, Anderson RA (2013) Exploring the pathophysiology of hypogonadism in men with type 2 diabetes: Kisspeptin-10 stimulates serum testosterone and LH secretion in men with type 2 diabetes and mild biochemical hypogonadism. Clin Endocrinol (Oxf) 79:100–104

George JT, Kakkar R, Marshall J, Scott ML, Finkelman RD, Ho TW, Veldhuis J, Skorupskaite K, Anderson RA, McIntosh S, Webber L (2016) Neurokinin B receptor antagonism in women with polycystic ovary syndrome: a randomized, placebo-controlled trial. J Clin Endocrinol Metab 101:4313–4321

Gonen Y, Balakier H, Powell W, Casper RF (1990) Use of gonadotropin-releasing hormone agonist to trigger follicular maturation for in vitro fertilization. J Clin Endocrinol Metab 71:918–922

Gordon CM (2010) Functional hypothalamic amenorrhea. New Engl J Med 363:365–371

Gordon CM, Ackerman KE, Berga SL, Kaplan JR, Mastorakos G, Misra M, Murad MH, Santoro NF, Warren MP (2017) Functional hypothalamic amenorrhea: an endocrine society clinical practice guideline. J Clin Endocrinol Metab 102:1413–1439

Hagen CP, Sorensen K, Mieritz MG, Johannsen TH, Almstrup K, Juul A (2015) Circulating MKRN3 levels decline prior to pubertal onset and through puberty: a longitudinal study of healthy girls. J Clin Endocrinol Metab 100:1920–1926

He Y, Chen D, Yang L, Hou Q, Ma H, Xu X (2018) The therapeutic potential of bone marrow mesenchymal stem cells in premature ovarian failure. Stem Cell Res Ther 9:263

Homburg R (2003) The management of infertility associated with polycystic ovary syndrome. Reprod Biol Endocrinol 1:109

Howard SR (2021) Interpretation of reproductive hormones before, during and after the pubertal transition-identifying health and disordered puberty. Clin Endocrinol (Oxf) 95:702–715

Hrabovszky E, Ciofi P, Vida B, Horvath MC, Keller E, Caraty A, Bloom SR, Ghatei MA, Dhillo WS, Liposits Z, Kallo I (2010) The kisspeptin system of the human hypothalamus: sexual dimorphism and relationship with gonadotropin-releasing hormone and neurokinin B neurons. Eur J Neurosci 31:1984–1998

Izzi-Engbeaya C, Comninos AN, Clarke SA, Jomard A, Yang L, Jones S, Abbara A, Narayanaswamy S, Eng PC, Papadopoulou D, Prague JK, Bech P, Godsland IF, Bassett P, Sands C, Camuzeaux S, Gomez-Romero M, Pearce JTM, Lewis MR, Holmes E, Nicholson JK, Tan T, Ratnasabapathy R, Hu M, Carrat G, Piemonti L, Bugliani M, Marchetti P, Johnson PR, Hughes SJ, James Shapiro AM, Rutter GA, Dhillo WS (2018) The effects of kisspeptin on beta-cell function, serum metabolites and appetite in humans. Diabetes Obes Metab 20:2800–2810

Jayasena CN, Nijher GM, Chaudhri OB, Murphy KG, Ranger A, Lim A, Patel D, Mehta A, Todd C, Ramachandran R, Salem V, Stamp GW, Donaldson M, Ghatei MA, Bloom SR, Dhillo WS (2009) Subcutaneous injection of kisspeptin-54 acutely stimulates gonadotropin secretion in

women with hypothalamic amenorrhea, but chronic administration causes tachyphylaxis. J Clin Endocrinol Metab 94:4315–4323
Jayasena CN, Nijher GM, Abbara A, Murphy KG, Lim A, Patel D, Mehta A, Todd C, Donaldson M, Trew GH, Ghatei MA, Bloom SR, Dhillo WS (2010) Twice-weekly administration of kisspeptin-54 for 8 weeks stimulates release of reproductive hormones in women with hypothalamic amenorrhea. Clin Pharmacol Ther 88:840–847
Jayasena CN, Nijher GMK, Comninos AN, Abbara A, Januszewki A, Vaal ML, Sriskandarajah L, Murphy KG, Farzad Z, Ghatei MA, Bloom SR, Dhillo WS (2011) The effects of Kisspeptin-10 on reproductive hormone release show sexual dimorphism in humans. J Clin Endocrinol Metab 96:E1963–E1972
Jayasena CN, Comninos AN, Nijher GM, Abbara A, De Silva A, Veldhuis JD, Ratnasabapathy R, Izzi-Engbeaya C, Lim A, Patel DA, Ghatei MA, Bloom SR, Dhillo WS (2013) Twice-daily subcutaneous injection of kisspeptin-54 does not abolish menstrual cyclicity in healthy female volunteers. J Clin Endocrinol Metab 98:4464–4474
Jayasena CN, Abbara A, Comninos AN, Nijher GMK, Christopoulos G, Narayanaswamy S, Izzi-Engbeaya C, Sridharan M, Mason AJ, Warwick J, Ashby D, Ghatei MA, Bloom SR, Carby A, Trew GH, Dhillo WS (2014a) Kisspeptin-54 triggers egg maturation in women undergoing in vitro fertilization. J Clin Invest 124:3667–3677
Jayasena CN, Abbara A, Veldhuis JD, Comninos AN, Ratnasabapathy R, De Silva A, Nijher GM, Ganiyu-Dada Z, Mehta A, Todd C, Ghatei MA, Bloom SR, Dhillo WS (2014b) Increasing LH pulsatility in women with hypothalamic amenorrhoea using intravenous infusion of Kisspeptin-54. J Clin Endocrinol Metab 99:E953–E961
Jayasena CN, Abbara A, Narayanaswamy S, Comninos AN, Ratnasabapathy R, Bassett P, Mogford JT, Malik Z, Calley J, Ghatei MA, Bloom SR, Dhillo WS (2015) Direct comparison of the effects of intravenous kisspeptin-10, kisspeptin-54 and GnRH on gonadotrophin secretion in healthy men. Hum Reprod 30:1934–1941
Kaiser UB (2012) Hyperprolactinemia and infertility: new insights. J Clin Invest 122:3467–3468
Kakoly NS, Earnest A, Teede HJ, Moran LJ, Joham AE (2019) The impact of obesity on the incidence of type 2 diabetes among women with polycystic ovary syndrome. Diabetes Care 42: 560–567
Kar S, Sanchita S (2015) Clomiphene citrate, metformin or a combination of both as the first line ovulation induction drug for Asian Indian women with polycystic ovarian syndrome: a randomized controlled trial. J Hum Reprod Sci 8:197–201
Ko EY, Siddiqi K, Brannigan RE, Sabanegh ES Jr (2012) Empirical medical therapy for idiopathic male infertility: a survey of the American Urological Association. J Urol 187:973–978
Kolibianakis EM, Schultze-Mosgau A, Schroer A, van Steirteghem A, Devroey P, Diedrich K, Griesinger G (2005) A lower ongoing pregnancy rate can be expected when GnRH agonist is used for triggering final oocyte maturation instead of HCG in patients undergoing IVF with GnRH antagonists. Hum Reprod 20:2887–2892
Koysombat K, Abbara A, Dhillo WS (2023) Current pharmacotherapy and future directions for neuroendocrine causes of female infertility. Expert Opin Pharmacother 24:37–47
Laitinen EM, Vaaralahti K, Tommiska J, Eklund E, Tervaniemi M, Valanne L, Raivio T (2011) Incidence, phenotypic features and molecular genetics of kallmann syndrome in Finland. Orphanet J Rare Dis:6
Legro RS, Barnhart HX, Schlaff WD, Carr BR, Diamond MP, Carson SA, Steinkampf MP, Coutifaris C, McGovern PG, Cataldo NA, Gosman GG, Nestler JE, Giudice LC, Leppert PC, Myers ER, Med CMR (2007) Clomiphene, metformin, or both for infertility in the polycystic ovary syndrome. New Engl J Med 356:551–566
Legro RS, Brzyski RG, Diamond MP, Coutifaris C, Schlaff WD, Casson P, Christman GM, Huang H, Yan QS, Alvero R, Haisenleder DJ, Barnhart KT, Bates GW, Usadi R, Lucidi S, Baker V, Trussell JC, Krawetz SA, Snyder P, Ohl D, Santoro N, Eisenberg E, Zhang H, Network NRM (2014) Letrozole versus clomiphene for infertility in the polycystic ovary syndrome. New Engl J Med 371:119–129

Levine H, Jorgensen N, Martino-Andrade A, Mendiola J, Weksler-Derri D, Mindlis I, Pinotti R, Swan SH (2017) Temporal trends in sperm count: a systematic review and meta-regression analysis. Hum Reprod Update 23:646–659

Liu YJ, Shen XB, Yu N, Shang XJ, Gu YQ, Zuo LD, Xiong CL, Ye Z, Zhou YZ (2021) Prevalence of late-onset hypogonadism among middle-aged and elderly males in China: results from a national survey. Asian J Androl 23

Maiter D (2019) Management of Dopamine Agonist-Resistant Prolactinoma. Neuroendocrinology 109:42–50

Majumdar A, Mangal NS (2013) Hyperprolactinemia. J Hum Reprod Sci 6:168–175

Maresch CC, Stute DC, Fleming T, Lin J, Hammes HP, Linn T (2019) Hyperglycemia induces spermatogenic disruption via major pathways of diabetes pathogenesis. Sci Rep 9:13074

Martin RH (2008) Cytogenetic determinants of male fertility. Hum Reprod Update 14:379–390

Matsuzaki T, Iwasa T, Yanagihara R, Komasaka M, Yano K, Mayila Y, Tachibana A, Yamamoto Y, Kato T, Kuwahara A, Irahara M (2018) Pilot study of the optimal protocol of low dose step-up follicle stimulating hormone therapy for infertile women. Reprod Med Biol 17: 315–324

Mayer C, Acosta-Martinez M, Dubois SL, Wolfe A, Radovick S, Boehm U, Levine JE (2010) Timing and completion of puberty in female mice depend on estrogen receptor alpha-signaling in kisspeptin neurons. Proc Natl Acad Sci U S A 107:22693–22698

Melmed S, Casanueva FF, Hoffman AR, Kleinberg DL, Montori VM, Schlechte JA, Wass JAH (2011) Diagnosis and treatment of hyperprolactinemia: an endocrine society clinical practice guideline. J Clin Endocrinol Metab 96:273–288

Melo P, Eapen A, Chung Y, Jeve Y, Price MJ, Sunkara SK, Macklon NS, Bhattacharya S, Khalaf Y, Tobias A, Broekmans F, Khairy M, Gallos I, Coomarasamy A (2022) Controlled ovarian stimulation (COS) protocols for assisted reproduction: a Cochrane systematic review and network meta-analysis. Hum Reprod 37

Millar RP, Sonigo C, Anderson RA, George J, Maione L, Brailly-Tabard S, Chanson P, Binart N, Young J (2017) Hypothalamic-pituitary-ovarian axis reactivation by Kisspeptin-10 in hyperprolactinemic women with chronic amenorrhea. J Endocr Soc 1:1362–1371

Mills EG, Dhillo WS (2022) Invited review: translating kisspeptin and neurokinin B biology into new therapies for reproductive health. J Neuroendocrinol 34:e13201

Moghetti P, Castello R, Negri C, Tosi F, Perrone F, Caputo M, Zanolin E, Muggeo M (2000) Metformin effects on clinical features, endocrine and metabolic profiles, and insulin sensitivity in polycystic ovary syndrome: a randomized, double-blind, placebo-controlled 6-month trial, followed by open, long-term clinical evaluation. J Clin Endocrinol Metab 85:139–146

Moore AM, Coolen LM, Porter DT, Goodman RL, Lehman MN (2018) KNDy cells revisited. Endocrinology 159:3219–3234

Morrison AE, Fleming S, Levy MJ (2021) A review of the pathophysiology of functional hypothalamic amenorrhoea in women subject to psychological stress, disordered eating, excessive exercise or a combination of these factors. Clin Endocrinol (Oxf) 95:229–238

Munro MG, Balen AH, Cho S, Critchley HOD, Diaz I, Ferriani R, Henry L, Mocanu E, van der Spuy ZM, Rela FCMD, Endocrinology FCRM (2022) The FIGO ovulatory disorders classification system. Fertil Steril 118:768–786

Nazem TG, Ackerman KE (2012) The female athlete triad. Sports Health 4:302–311

Nunes VD, El Dib R, Boguszewski CL, Nogueira CR (2011) Cabergoline versus bromocriptine in the treatment of hyperprolactinemia: a systematic review of randomized controlled trials and meta-analysis. Pituitary 14:259–265

O'Dea L, O'Brien F, Currie K, Hemsey G (2008) Follicular development induced by recombinant luteinizing hormone (LH) and follicle-stimulating hormone (FSH) in anovulatory women with LH and FSH deficiency: evidence of a threshold effect. Curr Med Res Opin 24:2785–2793

O'Shaughnessy PJ, Fowler PA (2011) Endocrinology of the mammalian fetal testis. Reproduction 141:37–46

Phylactou M, Clarke SA, Patel B, Baggaley C, Jayasena CN, Kelsey TW, Comninos AN, Dhillo WS, Abbara A (2021) Clinical and biochemical discriminants between functional hypothalamic amenorrhoea (FHA) and polycystic ovary syndrome (PCOS). Clin Endocrinol (Oxf) 95:239–252

Pivonello R, Menafra D, Riccio E, Garifalos F, Mazzella M, de Angelis C, Colao A (2019) Metabolic disorders and male hypogonadotropic hypogonadism. Front Endocrinol (Lausanne) 10:345

Rajkanna J, Tariq S, Oyibo SO (2016) Successful fertility treatment with gonadotrophin therapy for male hypogonadotrophic hypogonadism. Endocrinol Diabetes Metab Case Rep 2016:150124

Randall JM, Templeton A (1991) Cervical mucus score and in vitro sperm mucus interaction in spontaneous and clomiphene citrate cycles. Fertil Steril 56:465–468

Rattan S, Zhou C, Chiang C, Mahalingam S, Brehm E, Flaws JA (2017) Exposure to endocrine disruptors during adulthood: consequences for female fertility. J Endocrinol 233:R109–R129

Rehman S, Usman Z, Rehman S, AlDraihem M, Rehman N, Rehman I, Ahmad G (2018) Endocrine disrupting chemicals and impact on male reproductive health. Transl Androl Urol 7:490–503

Rehman R, Fatima SS, Alam F, Ashraf M, Zafar S (2019) Kisspeptin and attributes of infertile males and females: a cross-sectional study in a subset of Pakistani population. Andrologia 51: e13370

Renault CH, Aksglaede L, Wojdemann D, Hansen AB, Jensen RB, Juul A (2020) Minipuberty of human infancy – a window of opportunity to evaluate hypogonadism and differences of sex development? Ann Pediatr Endocrin 25:84–91

Roberts RE, Farahani L, Webber L, Jayasena C (2020) Current understanding of hypothalamic amenorrhoea. Ther Adv Endocrinol 11

Rudnicka E, Kruszewska J, Klicka K, Kowalczyk J, Grymowicz M, Skorska J, Pieta W, Smolarczyk R (2018) Premature ovarian insufficiency – aetiopathology, epidemiology, and diagnostic evaluation. Menopause Rev 17:105–108

Sakar MN, Oglak SC (2020) Letrozole is superior to clomiphene citrate in ovulation induction in patients with polycystic ovary syndrome. Pak J Med Sci 36:1460–1465

Sanocka D, Kurpisz M (2004) Reactive oxygen species and sperm cells. Reprod Biol Endocrinol 2: 12

Scheiber M, Liu J (2011) The use of gonadotropin-releasing hormone to induce ovulation. Glob Libr Women's Med

Schirmer DA 3rd, Kulkarni AD, Zhang Y, Kawwass JF, Boulet SL, Kissin DM (2020) Ovarian hyperstimulation syndrome after assisted reproductive technologies: trends, predictors, and pregnancy outcomes. Fertil Steril 114:567–578

Schreiner F, Gohlke B, Hamm M, Korsch E, Woelfle J (2014) MKRN3 mutations in familial central precocious puberty. Horm Res Paediatr 82:122–126

Seminara SB, Messager S, Chatzidaki EE, Thresher RR, Acierno JS, Shagoury JK, Bo-Abbas Y, Kuohung W, Schwinof KM, Hendrick AG, Zahn D, Dixon J, Kaiser UB, Slaugenhaupt SA, Gusella JF, O'Rahilly S, Carlton MBL, Crowley WF, Aparicio SAJR, Colledge WH (2003) The GPR54 gene as a regulator of puberty. New Engl J Med 349:1614–U1618

Senapati S (2018) Infertility: a marker of future health risk in women? Fertil Steril 110:783–789

Shi SQ, Hong T, Jiang FF, Zhuang Y, Chen L, Huang XL (2020) Letrozole and human menopausal gonadotropin for ovulation induction in clomiphene resistance polycystic ovary syndrome patients a randomized controlled study. Medicine 99

Shoham Z, Balen A, Patel A, Jacobs HS (1991) Results of ovulation induction using human menopausal gonadotropin or purified follicle-stimulating-hormone in hypogonadotropic hypogonadism patients. Fertil Steril 56:1048–1053

Simon D, Ba I, Mekhail N, Ecosse E, Paulsen A, Zenaty D, Houang M, Jesuran Perelroizen M, de Filippo GP, Salerno M, Simonin G, Reynaud R, Carel JC, Leger J, de Roux N (2016) Mutations in the maternally imprinted gene MKRN3 are common in familial central precocious puberty. Eur J Endocrinol 174:1–8

Skorupskaite K, George JT, Anderson RA (2014) The kisspeptin-GnRH pathway in human reproductive health and disease. Hum Reprod Update 20:485–500

Sonigo C, Bouilly J, Carre N, Tolle V, Caraty A, Tello J, Simony-Conesa FJ, Millar R, Young J, Binart N (2012) Hyperprolactinemia-induced ovarian acyclicity is reversed by kisspeptin administration. J Clin Invest 122:3791–3795

Srini VS, Veerachari SB (2011) Does varicocelectomy improve gonadal function in men with hypogonadism and infertility? Analysis of a prospective study. Int J Endocrinol 2011:916380

Stamou MI, Cox KH, Crowley WF (2015) Discovering genes essential to the hypothalamic regulation of human reproduction using a human disease model: adjusting to life in the "-Omics" era. Endocr Rev 36:603–621

Sun H, Gong TT, Jiang YT, Zhang S, Zhao YH, Wu QJ (2019) Global, regional, and national prevalence and disability-adjusted life-years for infertility in 195 countries and territories, 1990-2017: results from a global burden of disease study, 2017. Aging (Albany NY) 11:10952–10991

Sun B, Ma Y, Li L, Hu L, Wang F, Zhang Y, Dai S, Sun Y (2020) Factors associated with ovarian hyperstimulation syndrome (OHSS) severity in women with polycystic ovary syndrome undergoing IVF/ICSI. Front Endocrinol (Lausanne) 11:615957

Takasaki A, Tamura I, Okada-Hayashi M, Orita T, Tanabe M, Maruyama S, Shimamura K, Morioka H (2018) Usefulness of intermittent clomiphene citrate treatment for women with polycystic ovarian syndrome that is resistant to standard clomiphene citrate treatment. Reprod Med Biol 17:454–458

Taziaux M, Staphorsius AS, Ghatei MA, Bloom SR, Swaab DF, Bakker J (2016) Kisspeptin expression in the human infundibular nucleus in relation to sex, gender identity, and sexual orientation. J Clin Endocrinol Metab 101:2380–2389

Tiegs AW, Landis J, Garrido N, Scott RT, Hotaling JM (2019) Total motile sperm count trend over time: evaluation of semen analyses from 119,972 men from subfertile couples. Urology 132:109–116

Tranoulis A, Laios A, Pampanos A, Yannoukakos D, Loutradis D, Michala L (2018) Efficacy and safety of pulsatile gonadotropin-releasing hormone therapy among patients with idiopathic and functional hypothalamic amenorrhea: a systematic review of the literature and a meta-analysis. Fertil Steril 109:708

Tso LO, Costello MF, Albuquerque LE, Andriolo RB, Freitas V (2009) Metformin treatment before and during IVF or ICSI in women with polycystic ovary syndrome. Cochrane Database Syst Rev

Tziomalos K, Dinas K (2018) Obesity and outcome of assisted reproduction in patients with polycystic ovary syndrome. Front Endocrinol 9

Uenoyama Y, Inoue N, Nakamura S, Tsukamura H (2019) Central mechanism controlling pubertal onset in mammals: a triggering role of Kisspeptin. Front Endocrinol 10

Ullah H, Nabi G, Zubair H, Ullah R, Shahab M (2019) Age-dependent changes in the reproductive axis responsiveness to kisspeptin-10 administration in healthy men. Andrologia 51

Wang R, Kim BV, van Wely M, Johnson NP, Costello MF, Zhang HW, Ng EHY, Legro RS, Bhattacharya S, Norman RJ, Mol BJ (2017) Treatment strategies for women with WHO group II anovulation: systematic review and network meta-analysis. Br Med J 356

Wang MY, Wang YX, Li-Ling J, Xie HQ (2022a) Adult stem cell therapy for premature ovarian failure: from bench to bedside. Tissue Eng Part B Rev 28:63–78

Wang YX, Farland LV, Wang SW, Gaskins AJ, Wang L, Rich-Edwards JW, Tamimi R, Missmer SA, Chavarro JE (2022b) Association of infertility with premature mortality among US women: prospective cohort study. Lancet Reg Health Am 7

Witchel SF, Plant TM (2021) Neurobiology of puberty and its disorders. Handb Clin Neurol 181: 463–496

Wu CY, Huang TJ, Hwu YM, Lee RKK, Lin MH (2023) Comparison of clinical outcomes between conventional in vitro fertilization and intracytoplasmic sperm injection in poor responders with only single oocyte retrieved. Taiwan J Obstet Gynecol 62:55–58

Yang AM, Cui N, Sun YF, Hao GM (2021) Letrozole for female infertility. Front Endocrinol 12

Yeo SH, Herbison AE (2014) Estrogen-negative feedback and estrous cyclicity are critically dependent upon estrogen receptor-alpha expression in the arcuate nucleus of adult female mice. Endocrinology 155:2986–2995

Young J, Xu C, Papadakis GE, Acierno JS, Maione L, Hietamaki J, Raivio T, Pitteloud N (2019) Clinical management of congenital hypogonadotropic hypogonadism. Endocr Rev 40:669–710

Zou P, Wang XG, Chen Q, Yang H, Zhou NY, Sun L, Chen HQ, Liu JY, Ao L, Cui ZH, Cao J (2019) Kisspeptin protein in seminal plasma is positively associated with semen quality: results from the MARHCS study in Chongqing, China. Biomed Res Int 2019:5129263

The manufacturer's authorised representative in the EU is Springer Nature Customer Service Centre GmbH, Europaplatz 3, 69115 Heidelberg, Germany. If you have any concerns regarding our products, please contact ProductSafety@springernature.com

Printed and bound by CPI Group (UK) Ltd, Croydon, CR0 4YY
01/10/2026
02225866-0005